Physiological Basis of Rehabilitation Medicine

edited by

JOHN A. DOWNEY, M.D., D. Phil. (*Oxon.*)
Professor of Rehabilitation Medicine,
College of Physicians and Surgeons,
Columbia University

and

ROBERT C. DARLING, M.D.
Simon Baruch Professor and Chairman of the
Department of Rehabilitation Medicine, College of
Physicians and Surgeons, Columbia University

W. B. Saunders Company • Philadelphia • London • Toronto

W. B. Saunders Company: West Washington Square
Philadelphia, Pa.   19105

12 Dyott Street
London, WC1A   1DB

833 Oxford Street
Toronto 18, Ontario

Physiological Basis of Rehabilitation Medicine   ISBN 0-7216-3180-0

Print No.:   9   8   7   6   5   4   3   2

DEDICATION

*To our wives, Elsie and Esther, and to
our valued colleague and friend, Ursula.*

A set of one hundred 35 mm slides selected from the illustrations of this work is available from the publisher.

CONTRIBUTORS

C. ANDREW L. BASSETT, M.D., Sc.D. (med.)

Professor of Orthopaedic Surgery, College of Physicians and Surgeons, Columbia University, New York, New York. Attending Orthopaedic Surgeon, New York Orthopaedic Hospital, Columbia Presbyterian Medical Center, New York, New York. Consultant, New York State Rehabilitation Hospital, West Haverstraw, New York.

LUIS E. BONILLA, M.D.

Formerly Chief Resident, Department of Rehabilitation Medicine, Columbia Presbyterian Medical Center, New York, New York. Currently practicing Neurosurgery and Rehabilitation Medicine, Armenia-Quindio, Colombia, S.A.

ELSWORTH R. BUSKIRK, Ph.D.

Professor of Applied Physiology, The Pennsylvania State University, University Park, Pennsylvania.

MALCOLM B. CARPENTER, M.D.

Professor of Anatomy, College of Physicians and Surgeons, Columbia University, New York, New York. Assistant Attending Neurologist, Neurological Institute of New York, Presbyterian Hospital, New York, New York.

W. CRAWFORD CLARK, Ph.D.

Associate Professor of Medical Psychology, College of Physicians and Surgeons, Columbia University, New York, New York. Associate Research Scientist (Psychology), New York State Psychiatric Institute and Hospital, New York, New York.

PAUL J. CORCORAN, M.D.

Assistant Professor of Rehabilitation Medicine, College of Physicians and Surgeons, Columbia University, New York, New York. Assistant Attending Rehabilitation Physician, Presbyterian Hospital, New York, New York.

BARD COSMAN, M.D.

Associate Clinical Professor of Surgery, College of Physicians and Surgeons, Columbia University, New York, New York. Assistant Attending Surgeon, Presbyterian Hospital, New York, New York. Associate Plastic Surgeon, St. Elizabeth's Hospital, New York, New York. Assistant Visiting Surgeon, Francis Delafield Hospital, New York, New York. Attending Surgeon, Valley Hospital, Ridgewood, New Jersey. Consulting Plastic Surgeon, Blythedale Children's Hospital, Valhalla, New York.

ROBERT C. DARLING, M.D.

Professor and Chairman of the Department of Rehabilitation Medicine, College of Physicians and Surgeons, Columbia University, New York, New York.

JOHN A. DOWNEY, M.D., D.Phil. (*Oxon.*)

Professor of Rehabilitation Medicine, College of Physicians and Surgeons, Columbia University, New York, New York. Consultant at Blythdale Rehabilitation Hospital for Children, Valhalla, New York.

HYMAN I. C. DUBO, M.D., F.R.C.P. (C)

Director, Spinal Unit, and Consultant in Physical Medicine, Manitoba Rehabilitation Hospital, Winnipeg, Manitoba. Director, Department of Physical Medicine and Rehabilitation, St. Boniface General Hospital, Winnipeg, Manitoba. Formerly Chief Resident, Department of Rehabilitation Medicine, Columbia Presbyterian Medical Center, New York, New York.

CHARLES E. HUCKABA, Ph.D.

Professor of Rehabilitation Medicine, College of Physicians and Surgeons, Columbia University, New York, New York.

HOWARD F. HUNT, Ph.D.

Professor of Psychology, Columbia University, New York, New York. Chief of Psychiatric Research (Psychology), New York State Psychiatric Institute and Hospital, New York, New York.

CALVIN L. LONG, Ph.D.

Research Associate, College of Physicians and Surgeons, Columbia University, New York, New York.

ROBERT E. LOVELACE, M.B. (Lond.), M.R.C.P. (Lond.). D.P.M. (Eng.)

Associate Professor of Neurology, College of Physicians and Surgeons, Columbia University, New York, New York. Associate Attending Neurologist, Presbyterian Hospital, New York, New York. Director of Neuromuscular Laboratories, Nerve Conduction and Electromyographic Laboratories, Muscle and Myasthenia Gravis Clinics, Columbia Presbyterian Medical Center, New York, New York. Consultant in Electrodiagnosis, Harlem Hospital Medical Center, New York, New York.

RICHARD C. MASON, Ph.D.

Assistant Professor of Physiology, College of Physicians and Surgeons, Columbia University, New York, New York.

JOHN M. MILLER, III, M.D.

Professor and Chairman, Department of Rehabilitation Medicine, University of Alabama in Birmingham, Alabama. Attending Physician, Spain Rehabilitation

Center, and Physiatrist-in-Chief, University Hospital, Birmingham, Alabama. Formerly Assistant Professor of Rehabilitation Medicine, College of Physicians and Surgeons, Columbia University, New York, New York.

STANLEY J. MYERS, M.D.

Assistant Professor, Department of Rehabilitation Medicine, College of Physicians and Surgeons, Columbia University, New York, New York. Assistant Attending Physician (Rehabilitation Medicine), Presbyterian Hospital, New York, New York. Director of Rehabilitation Medicine Clinics, Vanderbilt Clinic, Columbia Presbyterian Medical Center, New York, New York.

HELEN SCHUCMAN, Ph.D.

Associate Professor of Medical Psychology, Department of Psychiatry, College of Physicians and Surgeons, Columbia University, New York, New York. Chief Psychologist, Neurological Institute, New York, New York.

WILLIAM N. THETFORD, Ph.D.

Professor of Medical Psychology, Department of Psychiatry, College of Physicians and Surgeons, Columbia University, New York, New York. Director, Division of Clinical Psychology, Presbyterian Hospital, New York, New York.

PREFACE

Rehabilitation medicine is the area of specialty concerned with the management of patients with impairments of function due to disease or trauma. A careful distinction should be made between impairments, which are the physical losses themselves, and disabilities, which are the effects of impairments on overall function of the individual. Understanding and utilization of this distinction require knowledge of the manner in which the human body adapts to and compensates for the peculiar forms of stress which the original injury has produced. In this way, physiology is the parent basic science in this area of medicine.

This book is a compilation of essays on selected physiological topics most pertinent to adaptation and compensatory adjustments in patients with musculoskeletal and circulatory impairments. In some instances these physiological topics pertain to reduction of the impairments themselves, but more often they relate to the principles of compensatory adaptations which can reduce the resulting disability. The chapters are not designed to be directly applicable to immediate practice; they are compendia of background knowledge upon which the practitioner can build.

The range of topics has been chosen by criteria not wholly logical nor comprehensive. An encyclopedic approach would have been obviously impossible in a single volume of modest dimensions. There is an insufficient body of basic knowledge in some topics of importance to justify a chapter. For other topics on which there may be sufficient knowledge in scattered sources, the editors could not discover an appropriate author. Selectivity also resulted from the editors' bias, which favors the areas of their personal experiences. We have chosen, when possible, topics on which there is important new evidence and data, but we have avoided areas in which the evidence is so recent that it is likely to be modified or possibly disproved in the near future. In this way, we may have missed some exciting and useful frontiers of knowledge, but hopefully our book will have more than fleeting validity.

In this volume physiology is interpreted broadly. Where structure and functions are closely linked, as in studies of the central nervous system, we have considered neuroanatomy as a physiological topic. Where function is not associated with any local definite structure as in psychology, we have still considered human motivation as a physiological subject, as long as it is based on sound observation, in a system in which stimulus leads to a predictable response.

The contributors were asked to cover thoroughly their assigned areas and not to oversimplify. Yet the result of their efforts, and of the efforts of the editors, is a presentation of material that is easily understandable by physicians and other health professionals with a scientific background. Bibliographies at the conclusion of each chapter are designed to allow the student or practitioner to explore the topic in greater depth if he so desires. Exhaustive reference lists, which would not enhance the value of the volume, have been avoided.

Another reason for a book on physiology for practitioners in rehabilitation medicine lies in the nature of therapy in this area of medicine. Treatment by drugs and diet lends itself to controlled therapeutic trials with carefully constructed controls. Treatment by exercise devices, physical agents and environmental manipulation, since these require active participation and knowledge on the part of the patient, presents greater difficulties to construction of controls, although efforts along these lines are being made and should be continued. Rehabilitation medicine depends heavily for its scientific base on knowledge of normal responses to physiological stimuli and deduction therefrom as to the likely response of patients. A variety of efforts is necessary to reduce the excessive empiricism now operating in rehabilitation medicine, to discard traditions not in accord with modern scientific fact and to build up a body of validated knowledge peculiar to this growing area of medical need.

The editors, as professors in the Department of Rehabilitation Medicine, have emphasized the physiological approach in their teaching of medical students and young physicians. To solidify this interest and emphasis, several of the chapters were authored or coauthored by young specialists, currently or formerly of this department, who are trained in this tradition.

JOHN A. DOWNEY
ROBERT C. DARLING

ACKNOWLEDGMENTS

The editors wish to acknowledge their indebtedness to many former colleagues and students. One of us (J.A.D.) wishes particularly to mention his first teacher and tutor in physiology, Dr. John B. Armstrong, FRCP(C), currently Executive Director (Medical) of the Canadian Heart Foundation; also Dr. E. C. Eppinger, Professor of Medicine (now emeritus) at the Peter Bent Brigham Hospital, Boston, with whom so many of us were able to observe the practice of superb and humane medicine; and, most recently, Professor Sir George Pickering, FRS, formerly Regius Professor of Medicine at Oxford and currently Master of Pembroke College, with whom, during a most happy and profitable two years, this editor learned that good medicine and research are not only inseparable but fun. Many of the ideas expressed in this book and much of our current research stems from Sir George and his laboratories.

The other editor (R.C.D.) is indebted to a series of distinguished teachers and mentors: to Doctors Dickinson W. Richards and André Cournand, who introduced him to physiology in medicine and to the values of precise measurements; to Dr. David Seegal, Professor of Medicine (now emeritus) at Columbia University, who directed a research medical service in which thought, work and imagination flourished; and to Dr. David Bruce Dill, who, as director of the Harvard Fatigue Laboratory, stimulated an environment uniquely productive of human physiological studies.

Both editors wish to acknowledge their appreciation to Professor R. F. Loeb, Bard Professor of Medicine (emeritus) at Columbia University, College of Physicians and Surgeons, for his encouragement in our work in rehabilitation and for his help in the early planning of this book.

We are also grateful for editorial help and advice from Mr. John L. Dusseau, Vice President and Editor, W. B. Saunders Company; Miss Marjorie Kellogg, M.S.S.; and Miss Margaret Richardson, B.A., M.T., of our department.

Many others, including secretaries, artists and librarians, provided invaluable assistance and to them all we extend our thanks.

J.A.D.
R.C.D.

CONTENTS

Basic Structure and Function

Chapter 1

UPPER AND LOWER MOTOR NEURONS*

by Malcolm B. Carpenter, M.D.

One of the most important concepts in neurological diagnosis rests upon distinguishing the abnormalities of motor function which result from pathological involvement of, or injury to, the upper or lower motor neuron. This relatively simple, yet frequently puzzling, distinction forms one of the corner stones of clinical neurology. The ability to distinguish upper and lower motor neuron lesions constitutes the first step in attempting to localize the site of a neural lesion that manifests itself by disturbances of normal motor function. Once the site of the neural lesion has been established, the clinician can begin to consider the pathological processes which might be responsible.

THE LOWER MOTOR NEURON

Anterior horn cells and their axons, which innervate striated muscle, constitute anatomical and physiological units referred to as the final common motor pathway, or the lower motor neuron. The concept of the lower motor neuron is not limited to the spinal cord, even though it is most frequently used in this context. Cells of the motor cranial nerve nuclei (nerves III, IV, V, VI, VII, IX, X, XI and XII), which provide innervation for muscles of the head and neck, also must be classified as lower motor neurons, even though these nuclei form discontinuous cell columns in the brain stem and some of the cell

*Aided by Research Grant NS-01538-11 from the National Institute of Neurological Diseases and Stroke of NIH, Bethesda, Maryland.

3

columns innervate muscles derived embryologically from the branchial arches (i.e., branchiomeric musculature).

Anterior horn cells, the prototype for all motor neurons, lie in cell columns in the anterior gray horn of the spinal cord. The medial cell column, extending throughout the length of the spinal cord, is divisible into posteromedial and anteromedial parts and innervates the short and long muscles of the axial skeleton. The lateral cell column innervates remaining body musculature. In thoracic spinal segments the lateral cell column is small and gives rise to fibers which innervate intercostal and anterolateral trunk musculature. In the cervical and lumbosacral enlargements the lateral cell column enlarges and consists of several subgroups of cells that extend for variable rostrocaudal distances. Anterior horn cells in the cord enlargements innervate the musculature of the extremities. Cells of the anterior horn, innervating muscles of extensor and abductor groups, tend to be located anteriorly and peripherally; cells innervating flexor and adductor muscle groups are dorsal and central. Cell groups of the anterior horn, which innervate striated muscle, constitute lamina IX of Rexed (1952, 1954; Fig. 1–1). These large multipolar neurons (30 to 100μ), characterized by coarse Nissl granules and large central nuclei, give rise to numerous dendrites, some of which extend for considerable distances within the spinal gray (i.e., beyond lamina IX). The axons of these cells emerge from the spinal cord via the ventral roots. Ventral root fibers become mixed with dorsal root fibers distal to the dorsal root ganglia (Fig. 1–2). Peripherally these motor fibers, forming components of mixed spinal nerves, divide into dorsal and ventral primary rami and ultimately innervate striated muscles (Fig. 1–3). In the spinal enlargements the primary rami participate in plexus formations, which result in the brachial and lumbosacral plexuses; the nerves given off by these plexuses provide the innervation for the muscles of the upper and lower extremities.

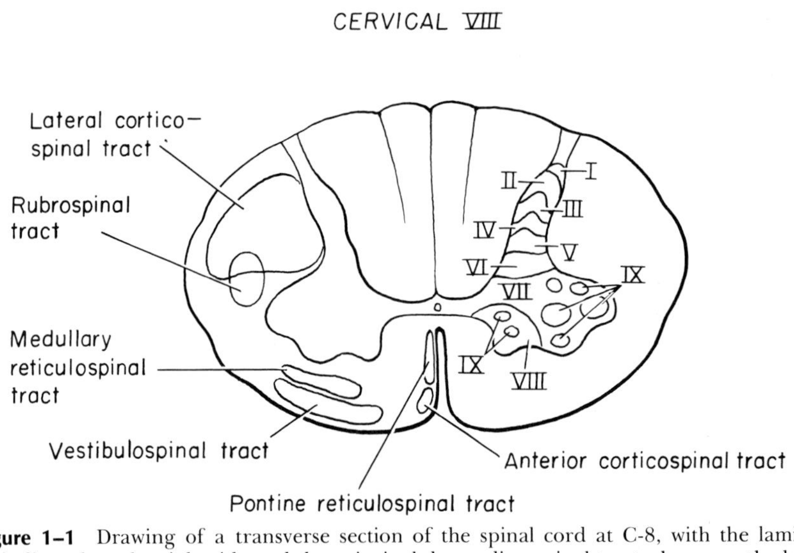

CERVICAL VIII

Figure 1–1 Drawing of a transverse section of the spinal cord at C-8, with the laminae of Rexed indicated on the right side and the principal descending spinal tracts shown on the left.

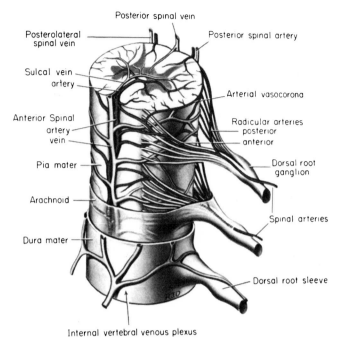

Posterior spinal vein

Posterolateral
spinal vein

Posterior spinal artery

Sulcal vein
artery

Arterial vasocorona

Anterior Spinal
artery
vein

Radicular arteries
posterior
anterior

Pia mater

Dorsal root
ganglion

Arachnoid

Spinal arteries

Dura mater

Dorsal root sleeve

Internal vertebral venous plexus

Figure 1–2 Drawing of the spinal cord, showing meninges, blood supply and spinal roots. (From Truex and Carpenter: *Human Neuroanatomy*, 1969. Reproduced by permission of the Williams and Wilkins Company, Baltimore, Md.)

Not all cells of the anterior horn give rise to fibers that innervate striated muscle. Cells in the anterior horn of the spinal cord may be divided into two basic groups: (a) root cells and (b) column cells. Column cells and their processes are confined to the central nervous system; these cells act as commissural, association and internuncial neurons. Root cells give rise to processes that emerge from the spinal cord and subserve effector functions. Root cells are of two types: (1) those giving rise to large fibers which innervate striated (extrafusal) muscle, known as *alpha* (α) *motor neurons* (Fig. 1-4), and (2) those giving rise to small motor fibers which innervate muscle spindles (intrafusal), known as *gamma* (γ) *motor neurons*. Examination of the myelinated fiber spectrum of a ventral root, or muscle nerve, indicates two distinct groups of fibers. Approximately 70 per cent of the fibers range between 8 and 13μ in diameter and are classified as alpha fibers, while the remaining 30 per cent of the fibers range from 3 to 8μ in diameter and are designated as gamma fibers. In addition the ventral roots in thoracic and upper lumbar segments (sympathetic) and certain sacral segments (parasympathetic) contain thinly myelinated preganglionic autonomic fibers destined for autonomic ganglia (Fig. 1-3).

Alpha fibers, which arise from regions of the spinal gray known as lamina IX (Rexed, 1952, 1954), terminate upon skeletal muscle fibers in small flattened expansions known as motor end plates, which constitute the so-called myoneural junction. Stimulation of a muscle nerve with graded shocks results in twitches of the muscle that are related directly to the strength of the stimulus, until the alpha spike reaches its full size. Further increases in shock

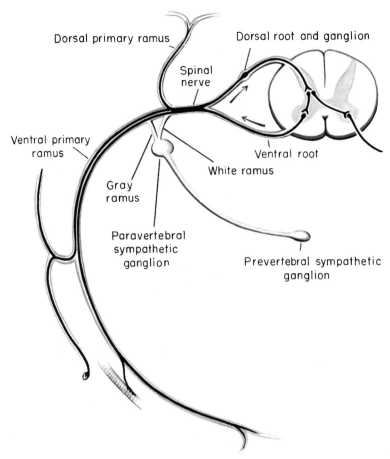

Dorsal primary ramus

Dorsal root and ganglion

Spinal nerve

Ventral primary ramus

Ventral root

White ramus

Gray ramus

Paravertebral sympathetic ganglion

Prevertebral sympathetic ganglion

Figure 1–3 Schematic diagram of a spinal nerve, indicating peripheral branches and central connections. (After Noback: *The Human Nervous System.* New York, McGraw-Hill Book Company, 1967. Reproduced with permission of the author and the McGraw-Hill Book Company.)

strength do not produce further increases in tension, even though such stimuli cause gamma fibers to discharge (Leksell, 1945). Hence it has been concluded that impulses conducted by alpha motor neurons are related to contractile tension in striated muscle, and gamma neurons do not contribute directly to muscle contraction. Gamma fibers are distributed exclusively to the contractile portions of the muscle spindles. While contractions of the polar parts of the muscle spindle may be sufficient to cause the discharge of spindle afferent fibers (group IA), these contractions cause no direct alteration of total muscle tension or of muscle length. However, afferent impulses from the muscle spindle pass centrally via group IA fibers, enter the spinal cord via the dorsal root and distribute collaterals to alpha motor neurons. This two-neuronal linkage constitutes the so-called gamma loop. Impulses passing via gamma efferent fibers can indirectly excite alpha motor neurons as a consequence of causing the muscle spindle to fire. Part of this mechanism underlies the myotatic or stretch reflex (Fig. 1-4).

The *myotatic reflex* is a monosynaptic reflex dependent upon two neurons, dorsal root ganglion cells, which receive impulses from the muscle spindle, and alpha motor neurons, which innervate striated muscle. A sudden stretching of a muscle produced by sharply tapping the muscle, or its tendon, results in a stretch of the muscle spindle and propagation of impulses that reach and excite

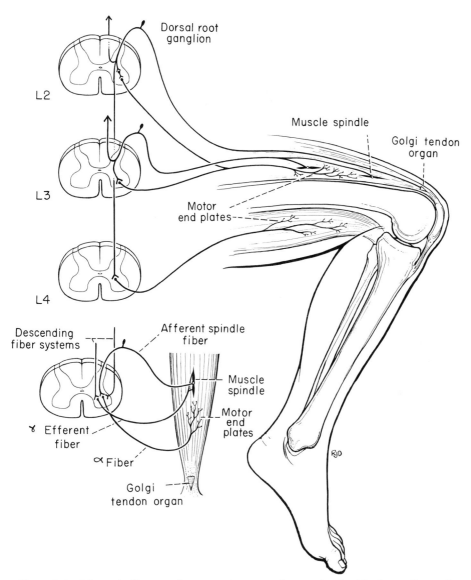

Figure 1–4 Schematic diagram of motor and sensory elements involved in the patellar tendon reflex. The muscle spindle afferents are shown entering only the L3 spinal segment, while afferents from the Golgi tendon organ are shown entering only the L2 spinal segment. In this monosynaptic reflex, afferent fibers enter L2, L3 and L4 spinal segments, and efferent fibers issue from the anterior horn cells of these levels and pass back to extrafusal muscle fibers in the quadriceps. Efferent fibers leaving the L4 spinal segment and passing to the hamstrings represent part of a pathway by which an antagonistic muscle group is inhibited. The small diagram on the left illustrates the gamma loop. Gamma efferent fibers pass to the polar portions of the muscle spindle. Contractions of the intrafusal fibers in the spindle stretch the nuclear bag region and cause an afferent impulse to be conducted centrally. Muscle spindle afferent fibers synapse upon alpha motor neurons. (From Truex and Carpenter: *Human Neuroanatomy*, 1969. Reproduced by permission of the Williams and Wilkins Company, Baltimore, Md.)

alpha motor neurons in the anterior horn. After a brief synaptic delay, impulses pass peripherally via the ventral root fibers back to the same muscle and produce a quick contraction of it. The myotatic reflex is a segmental reflex that usually involves two or three spinal segments. This reflex is localized to the muscle stimulated because (1) dorsal root afferents are distributed primarily to alpha motor neurons at their level of entrance into the spinal cord (Shriver, Stein and Carpenter, 1968; Carpenter, Stein and Shriver, 1968) and (2) particular muscles are innervated by alpha motor neurons in restricted regions of the spinal cord. A segment of somatic muscle innervated by efferent fibers from a single spinal segment constitutes a myotome. This unit is similar to the dermatome, defined as the cutaneous area supplied by sensory fibers which arise from cells in a single dorsal root ganglion. In both myotomes and dermatomes considerable overlapping innervation is provided by nerve fibers arising from adjacent spinal segments.

As the above description implies, afferent fibers, derived from the dorsal root ganglia, constitute one of the principal sources of input to the lower motor neuron. Dorsal root input conveys impulses from a wide variety of sensory receptors, both superficial and deep. Impulses conveyed centrally from the Golgi tendon organ by group IB fibers differ from those of group IA (muscle spindle afferents) in that they end upon interneurons, rather than directly upon alpha motor neurons, and thus form a disynaptic reflex arc (Fig. 1-4). The Golgi tendon organ exhibits a higher threshold than the muscle spindle, has no known efferent innervation and, unlike the muscle spindle, can be caused to discharge by either contracting or stretching the muscle. Fulton and Pi-Suñer (1928) regarded the Golgi tendon organ as being "in series" with extrafusal muscle fibers, while the muscle spindle appears to be arranged "in parallel". Electrophysiological evidence (McCouch, Deering and Stewart, 1950; Granit, 1950; Hunt, 1951) indicates that impulses conveyed by group IB fibers exert inhibitory influences upon monosynaptic reflex discharges of alpha motor neurons. This inhibition is of clinical importance in that it underlies the melting away of resistance to passive movement encountered in spasticity.

Impulses from skin and deep receptors concerned with noxious and painful sensations also reach the lower motor neuron as evidenced by the flexion reflex. The *flexion reflex*, elicited by noxious stimulation, consists of powerful contractions of ipsilateral flexor muscles so that an entire limb may be withdrawn from an offending stimulus. Since ipsilateral extensor muscles relax while flexor muscles contract, afferent fibers subserving this primitive reflex must have reciprocal connections with lower motor neurons, arranged so that impulses reaching flexor neurons are excitatory, while those to extensor neurons are inhibitory. Afferent impulses in this polysynaptic reflex come from broad receptive fields and are conveyed by the smaller fibers of groups II (secondary muscle spindle afferent), III and IV (cutaneous afferents). Centrally these afferent fibers convey impulses via multisynaptic articulations to both flexor and extensor motor neurons. This reflex is characterized by longer synaptic delays, diffuseness of the efferent discharge and afterdischarge phenomena due to recirculation and feedback of impulses among internuncial neurons. Thus, there is sustained firing of motor neurons so that muscle contractions may outlast the stimulus. Noxious stimuli applied to almost any place on the distal part of a limb can cause contractions of flexor muscle groups at all joints in the limb.

The crossed extension reflex is regarded as a part of the flexion reflex (Patton, 1965). Collateral fibers, subserving the flexion reflex, are believed to cross to the opposite side of the spinal cord where they establish reciprocal connections opposite to those prevailing on the ipsilateral side (Fig. 1-3). Contralaterally, excitatory impulses impinge upon extensor motor neurons, while inhibitory impulses reach the flexor motor neurons. In the case of the lower extremity, the crossed extension reflex serves to support the body when the ipsilateral lower limb is flexed.

The segmental input to the lower motor neuron is profuse, both direct and indirect, and largely, but not exclusively, ipsilateral. Muscle spindle afferents (group IA) project directly to the lower motor neuron, while afferents from most other receptors, including the Golgi tendon organ, influence the lower motor neuron indirectly via internuncial neurons. Afferent inputs from stretch receptors (i.e., muscle spindle and Golgi tendon organ) activate ipsilateral cell groups in the spinal cord, while afferent impulses from other sensory receptors are distributed by multisynaptic circuits to both sides of the spinal cord. The lower motor neuron also is under powerful suprasegmental control provided by impulses transmitted via descending spinal systems. These systems will be discussed in conjunction with the upper motor neuron.

Lesions of the Lower Motor Neuron

Lesions selectively involving the lower motor neuron result in weakness or paralysis, loss of muscle tone, loss of reflex activity and atrophy. All of these changes are confined to the affected muscles. *Weakness* or *complete paralysis*, occurring in affected muscles, bears a direct relationship to the extent and severity of the lesion. Since the anterior horn cells that innervate a single muscle extend longitudinally through several spinal segments, and since several such cell columns exist at each spinal level, a lesion confined to one spinal segment will cause weakness, but not complete paralysis, in all muscles innervated by this segment. Complete paralysis will occur only when the lesion involves the column of cells in several spinal segments that innervate a particular muscle, or the ventral root fibers that arise from these cells. Because most of the appendicular muscles are innervated by fibers arising from parts of three spinal segments, complete paralysis of a muscle resulting from a central lesion in the anterior horn indicates involvement of several spinal segments. Further, because neighboring cell columns are likely to be affected at each level, such a lesion usually produces paralysis in muscle groups, rather than individual muscles.

Since the lower motor neuron consists of the anterior horn cells and their axons, which innervate striated muscle, it becomes necessary to distinguish the motor deficits that occur as a consequence of lesions in spinal segments from those which occur in ventral roots, spinal nerves and peripheral nerves. A lesion in ventral root fibers usually produces motor deficits similar to those resulting from destruction of anterior horn cells. Complete severance of ventral root fibers produces the same somatic motor deficits as total destruction of anterior horn cells at the same level. However, at certain levels (i.e., thoraco-lumbar and sacral) section of the ventral root fibers would produce additional autonomic deficits which might not accompany anterior horn cell lesions at the same level. Section of a single ventral root, for example C-5, would produce weakness in the supraspinatus, infraspinatus, subscapularis, biceps brachii and brachioradialis muscles, but not complete paralysis of any of these muscles. This pattern of distribution is unique to the C-5 root and different from that of any single peripheral nerve.

Lesions of mixed spinal nerves produce motor and sensory deficits that correspond to those of combined dorsal and ventral root lesions. While the motor deficit corresponds almost exactly to that seen with pure lesions of the ventral root, sensory disturbances and loss follow a dermatomal distribution and tend to be less extensive because of overlapping innervation characteristic of dermatomes. If only one mixed spinal nerve were injured, for example C-5, the motor weakness would be the same as described above and no sensory loss would be detectable. The absence of detectable sensory loss in the C-5 dermatome is due to the extensive overlap of dorsal root fibers which arise from C-4 and C-6 dorsal root ganglia (Mott and Sherrington, 1895; Haymaker, 1956).

These findings are in sharp contrast to the motor and sensory deficits which occur as a consequence of a peripheral nerve lesion. With a peripheral nerve lesion the muscle paralysis and the sensory loss correspond to the peripheral distribution of the particular nerve. For example, a lesion of the ulnar nerve produces paralysis of the adductor pollicis, the deep head of flexor pollicis brevis, the interossei, the inner lumbrical muscles and the muscles of the hypothenar eminence, along with loss of all sensation in the little finger, the ulnar half of the ring finger and corresponding portions of the dorsal and volar surfaces of the hand.

Loss of muscle tone, *hypotonia*, is a characteristic and constant finding in lower motor neuron lesions. Flaccidity of the affected muscles is evidenced by greatly diminished resistance to passive movement. This reduction in muscle tone results from the withdrawal of streams of impulses transmitted to muscles that normally maintain a state of variable, but sometimes sustained, contraction in some of the muscle units.

Reflexes in the affected muscles are diminished or lost (areflexia) in lower motor neuron lesions because the reflex arc is interrupted. In this type of lesion the effector mechanism is destroyed.

Although paralysis, hypotonia and areflexia occur almost immediately following a lower motor neuron lesion, atrophy, or muscle wasting, does not become evident for two or three weeks. The *atrophy* develops gradually and in time is obvious on inspection. Why muscles deprived of their innervation atrophy and degenerate is not adequately understood and in a sense seems to contradict the neuron doctrine. It seems likely that the morphological and functional properties of muscle are dependent upon transmitter substances provided by the terminals of motor nerve fibers. Atrophy, of the type seen in lower motor neuron disease, does not result from depriving anterior horn cells of afferent impulses from either suprasegmental or segmental levels (Tower, 1937). However, some degree of muscle wasting does occur when muscles are not used (disuse atrophy). Disuse atrophy is seen in limbs immobilized in plaster casts for long periods of time, in muscles whose tendons have been resected and in upper motor neuron paralysis of long duration. Variable degrees of atrophy also are seen in old age, cachectic states, and in some myopathies.

In certain diseases of the lower motor neuron, the muscles exhibit small, localized spontaneous contractions known as *fasciculations*. These muscle twitches, visible through the skin, represent the discharge of squads of muscle fibers innervated by nerve fibers arising from a single lower motor neuron. Fasciculations occur asynchronously in different parts of various muscles and are thought to be due to a triggering of motor unit discharges that occur within the cell body of the motor neuron. Fasciculations of this type are interpreted as a disease process attacking the lower motor neurons in the anterior gray horn of the spinal cord. Fasciculations commonly are seen in amyotrophic lateral sclerosis, occasionally in acute inflammatory lesions of peripheral nerves and do not occur when anterior horn cells are rapidly injured or destroyed (i.e., in acute poliomyelitis).

The term *fibrillation*, frequently misused as the equivalent of the term fasciculation, refers to the small (10 to 200μV) potentials of 1 to 2 milliseconds duration that occur irregularly and asynchronously in electromyograms of denervated muscle. These spontaneous discharges cannot be observed through the skin and produce no detectable shortening of muscles. These potentials represent the spontaneous activation of single muscle fibers.

From this discussion it is obvious that the lower motor neuron exerts important trophic, metabolic, chemical and electrical influences upon muscle. One of the most striking effects of denervation upon muscle is the supersensitivity which it develops to acetylcholine.

THE UPPER MOTOR NEURON

All of the descending fiber systems that can influence and modify the activity of the lower motor neuron constitute the upper motor neuron (Fig. 1-1). This is a more inclusive definition than that used by many clinicians who equate the upper motor neuron solely with the corticospinal system. The narrower concept has become a rule of thumb because of the overwhelming clinical importance of the corticospinal system and the fact that information concerning the functional influences of descending non-pyramidal fiber systems has been poorly defined. Recent anatomical and physiological data concerning descending non-pyramidal fiber systems make it necessary to modify the venerable rule of thumb and to consider the concept of the upper motor neuron in its broadest sense.

Descending neural impulses, transmitted to spinal levels by a group of heterogenous tracts, are concerned mainly with (1) mediation of somatic motor activity, (2) control of muscle tone, (3) maintenance of posture and equilibrium, (4) suprasegmental control of reflex activity, (5) innervation of viscera and autonomic structures and (6) modification of sensory input. All of the descending spinal tracts, with one notable exception, arise from the three most caudal divisions of the brain stem. The exception is the corticospinal system.

Corticospinal System

This system consists of all fibers which (1) originate from cells within the cerebral cortex, (2) pass through the medullary pyramids and (3) enter the spinal cord (Fig. 1-5). These fibers constitute the largest and most important descending system in the human neuraxis. Each medullary pyramid contains approximately one million fibers which project to spinal levels via three separate tracts. The largest number of fibers, 75 to 90 per cent, cross in the pyramidal decussation and descend contralaterally as the *lateral corticospinal tract*. A smaller bundle of fibers (approximately 8 per cent) descend uncrossed in the anterior funiculus of the spinal cord (mainly to cervical segments) as the *anterior corticospinal tract*. Remaining fibers descend uncrossed in the ipsilateral lateral funiculus as the so-called uncrossed *anterolateral corticospinal tract*. Fibers of the corticospinal tract are considered to arise predominantly from the primary motor cortex (area 4), the premotor cortex (area 6) and the postcentral gyrus (Russell and DeMyer, 1961). Area 4 contains the gigantopyramidal cells of Betz, whose cell bodies reach a height of 120μ. These giant cells are not uniformly distributed in area 4; approximately 75 per cent are in the leg area, 18 per cent are in the arm area and 7 per cent are in the face area. According to Lassek (1940, 1947) there are about 34,000 giant pyramidal cells in each area 4 of the human brain. These cells give rise to the large diameter fibers of the corticospinal tract. Although the primary motor cortex is somatotopically* organized and electrical stimulations of localized regions in man give rise to motor responses interpreted by the patient (under local anesthesia) as "voluntary" in nature, corticospinal fibers are not distributed somatotopically at spinal levels (Nathan and Smith, 1955).

It has been estimated that 55 per cent of all pyramidal fibers terminate in cervical spinal segments, 20 per cent in thoracic segments and 25 per cent in lumbosacral segments. At spinal levels corticospinal fibers enter the gray matter and are distributed mainly to the zona intermedia (lamina VII of Rexed, 1952, 1954) and to adjacent regions at the base of the posterior horn (laminae IV, V and VI) (Fig. 1-1). A relatively small number of corticospinal fibers synapse directly upon anterior horn cells (lamina IX) of the lateral cell column in the cord enlargements (Kuypers, 1960; Liu and Chambers, 1964).

Phylogenetically the corticospinal tract is regarded as a relatively new tract; it is developed only in mammals. Myelinization of the tract begins at birth and is not complete until the end of the second year. The corticospinal tract is regarded universally as the tract most concerned with voluntary, somatic motor function. Impulses conveyed by this tract are thought to be concerned with highly discrete movements which display almost unlimited range and versatility and form the basis for acquired motor skills. This tract has the largest number of fibers conveying motor impulses, it has a length greater than that of any other tract, and either passes through, or lies adjacent to, every major division of the neuraxis except one, the cerebellum. Lesions of the corticospinal tract, usually in association with other neural structures, produce variable degrees of paralysis, alterations of muscle tone and modification of reflexes.

---

*The term somatotopic is employed here to mean that a relationship exists between particular areas of the motor cortex and specific parts of the body. Charts of the motor representation of various parts of the body have been furnished by a number of investigators (Foerster, 1936; Penfield and Boldrey, 1937; Scarff, 1940; Penfield and Rasmussen, 1950). In other parts of this chapter the term somatotopic is used with respect to organization of certain spinal tracts. In this usage the term indicates that cells from part of a particular nucleus, projecting fibers to selective spinal levels (i.e., to cervical levels), are capable of influencing motor activity only at that level.

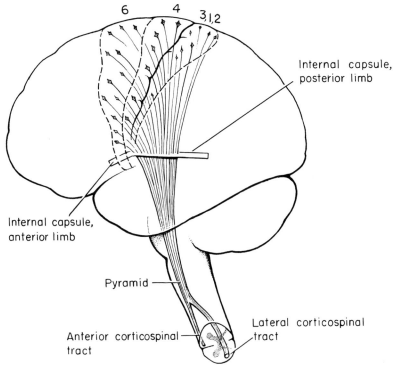

Figure 1–5 Schematic diagram of the origin and course of the fibers of the corticospinal tract. Approximate percentages of fibers arising from the indicated cortical areas are: area 4, 31 per cent; area 6, 29 per cent; postcentral gyrus and parietal lobe, 40 per cent.

The non-pyramidal descending spinal systems are small in comparison to the corticospinal system and arise from nuclei in the brain stem. These nuclei, the red nucleus in the mesencephalon and the vestibular nuclei and reticular formation in the pons and medulla, receive impulses from other parts of the neuraxis which they relay to spinal levels.

Rubrospinal Tract

This tract arises from cells in the red nucleus, crosses the midline at mesencephalic levels and descends to spinal levels where fibers of the tract lie anterior to, and partially intermingled with, those of the lateral corticospinal tract (Fig. 1-6). Fibers of the rubrospinal tract arise somatotopically from cells in caudal portions of the nucleus and are organized so that cells in dorsal and dorsomedial parts of the nucleus project fibers to cervical spinal segments, while ventral and ventromedial parts of the nucleus project to lumbosacral spinal segments (Pompeiano and Brodal, 1957). Fibers terminating in thoracic spinal segments arise from intermediate parts of the nucleus (Pompeiano and Brodal, 1957). Most of the information concerning the rubrospinal tract has been gathered from experimental studies in animals. In the cat cervical spinal segments receive the greatest number of fibers (Hinman and Carpenter, 1959;

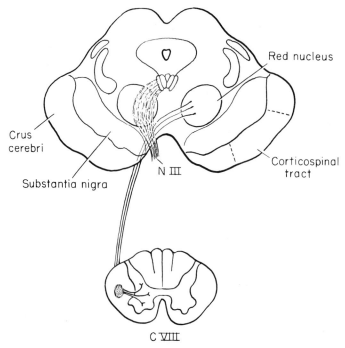

Figure 1–6   Schematic diagram of the rubrospinal tract.

Nyberg-Hansen and Brodal, 1964). Fibers of this tract enter the spinal gray matter laterally and terminate about cells in portions of laminae V, VI and VII of Rexed (Fig. 1–1).

The red nucleus receives afferent fibers from two principal sources, the cerebral cortex and certain deep cerebellar nuclei. Corticorubral fibers are uncrossed, arise from the primary motor cortex and are somatotopically organized with respect to origin and termination. Thus, corticorubral and corticospinal fibers together constitute a somatotopically organized non-pyramidal pathway linking particular regions of the motor cortex with specific spinal levels.

The red nucleus also receives a crossed somatotopic fiber projection from the anterior interposed nucleus (i.e., the emboliform nucleus in man). These fibers emerge from the cerebellum and cross in the superior cerebellar peduncle (Courville, 1966; Massion, 1967).

Stimulation of the red nucleus in the cat may produce flexion in either the opposite forelimb or hindlimb, depending upon which part of the nucleus is stimulated (Pompeiano, 1956, 1957). Microelectrode studies indicate that stimulation of cells in the red nucleus produces excitatory postsynaptic potentials in contralateral flexor alpha motor neurons and inhibitory postsynaptic potentials in extensor alpha motor neurons. The most important function of the rubrospinal tract concerns tone in flexor muscle groups (Massion, 1967). Facilitation of flexor muscle tone occurs contralateral to impulses descending from the motor cortex, because corticorubral fibers are uncrossed and rubrospinal fibers cross at midbrain levels. Flexor muscle tone is facilitated ipsilaterally by cerebellar inputs to the red nucleus, because both cerebellorubral and rubrospinal fibers cross at midbrain levels. Cerebellar influences upon flexor muscle tone are mediated by the red nucleus; thus, they involve two systems, both of which cross at midbrain levels (i.e., the so-called double-cross).

Vestibulospinal Tract

This uncrossed tract arises from the lateral vestibular nucleus, which receives inputs from the labyrinth (i.e., vestibular part of cranial nerve VIII) and from specific parts of the cerebellum (Fig. 1–7). The lateral vestibular nucleus is distinctive because it contains giant cells, larger than those found in any brain stem nucleus. The vestibulospinal tract arises somatotopically from cells of all sizes in the lateral vestibular nucleus. Cells in rostroventral parts of the nucleus project to cervical spinal segments, while cells in dorsocaudal parts of the nucleus project to lumbosacral spinal segments (Pompeiano and Brodal, 1957a).

The vestibulospinal tract descends in the anterior part of the lateral funiculus of the spinal cord relatively near the surface (Fig. 1–1). Fibers of the tract enter the gray matter and are distributed to all parts of lamina VIII and medial and central parts of lamina VII (Nyberg-Hansen and Mascitti, 1964). Terminal fibers form axodendritic and axosomatic synapses upon all types of cells within these laminae.* Few, if any, vestibulospinal fibers end directly upon motor neurons in lamina IX.

Vestibular influences upon spinal cord neurons are mediated largely by the vestibulospinal tract. Experimental studies (Pompeiano, 1960) indicate that

---

*The term axodendritic is used to designate axonal terminals that synapse upon the dendritic processes of another neuron. Axosomatic synapses are formed when the terminal boutons end directly upon the cell soma.

Figure 1–7 Schematic diagram of the brain stem and cervical spinal cord showing the course of the vestibulospinal tract. The vestibular nuclei are indicated (S, superior vestibular nucleus; L, lateral vestibular nucleus; M, medial vestibular nucleus; I, inferior vestibular nucleus). The vestibulospinal tract is somatotopically organized.

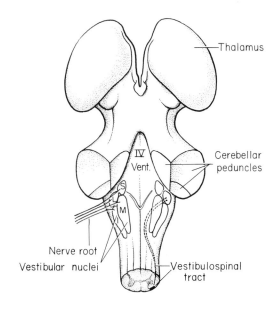

stimulation of the lateral vestibular nucleus produces increases in extensor muscle tone; microelectrode studies demonstrate that excitatory postsynaptic potentials can be recorded intracellularly from extensor alpha motor neurons. These effects must be mediated by interneurons in laminae VII and VIII.

Cerebellar impulses also are conveyed to the lateral vestibular nucleus from parts of the vermis and from the fastigial nuclei. These pathways show a somatotopic linkage (Walberg, Pompeiano, Brodal and Jansen, 1962). Thus, these parts of the cerebellum probably influence extensor muscle tone by impulses conducted along these pathways. No fibers from the cerebral cortex are known to project directly to the vestibular nuclei.

The only other nucleus of the vestibular complex that projects fibers to the spinal cord is the medial vestibular nucleus. In the spinal cord these fibers are not numerous, descend mainly to cervical segments and are predominantly uncrossed. These descending vestibular fibers form a component of the medial longitudinal fasciculus (abbreviated MLF). Recent evidence suggests that these vestibular fibers exert inhibitory influences mainly upon cervical motor neurons (Wilson, Wylie and Marco, 1968).

Reticulospinal Tracts

The reticular formation is the anatomical term used to designate the core of the brain stem, which is characterized by a wealth of cells of various sizes and shapes that lie enmeshed in a complex fiber network. The reticular formation is a phylogenetically old matrix surrounded by newer pathways and nuclei concerned with specific functions. In primitive forms the reticular formation may represent the largest part of the central nervous system. In higher vertebrates the reticular formation continues to develop and achieves considerable size owing to the process of encephalization. Although some authors regard the reticular formation as being diffusely organized, anatomical studies (Brodal, 1957; Scheibel and Scheibel, 1958) indicate that it can be subdivided into specific regions that possess distinctive cytoarchitecture, distinctive fiber connections and a unique internal organization. In spite of these features different regions of the reticular formation cannot always be regarded as entirely independent entities because complex fiber connections provide such numerous and diverse possibilities for interactions among subdivisions.

Spinal projections arise only from portions of the pontine and medullary reticular formation (Fig. 1-8). In the medulla reticulospinal fibers arise from a large nucleus which occupies the medial two-thirds of the reticular formation, known as the nucleus reticularis gigantocellularis, because of the characteristic large cells. These fibers are mostly uncrossed, descend in the anterior part of the lateral funiculus of the spinal cord and terminate chiefly upon cells in lamina VII, though some enter lamina IX. Fibers of the tract, referred to as the *medullary reticulospinal tract,* are present at all spinal levels (Fig. 1-1).

The *pontine reticulospinal tract* arises from the more extensive pontine reticular formation (i.e., nuclei reticularis pontis caudalis and oralis), which lies rostral to the medullary reticular formation. The nuclear mass constituting these subdivisions of the reticular formation extends rostrally into the caudal mesencephalon. Fibers from the pontine reticular formation are uncrossed and

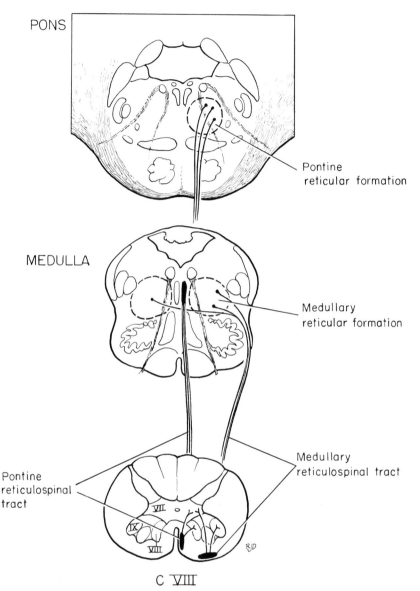

PONS

Pontine
reticular formation

MEDULLA

Medullary
reticular formation

Medullary
reticulospinal tract

Pontine
reticulospinal
tract

VII

IX

VIII

R/D

C VIII

Figure 1–8   Schematic diagram of the reticulospinal tracts, indicating their origin, course and regions of termination in the spinal gray.

descend in the medial part of the anterior funiculus near the anterior median sulcus (Fig. 1-8). Pontine reticulospinal fibers descend the entire length of the spinal cord, are not sharply segregated from those of the medullary reticulospinal tract and terminate in lamina VIII and adjacent parts of lamina VII.

Unlike the rubrospinal and vestibulospinal tracts, the reticulospinal tracts are not somatotopically organized with respect to either origin or termination. This anatomical finding suggests that descending impulses conducted by these fibers may produce effects that have broad influences upon large populations of spinal neurons. Portions of the reticular formation projecting fibers to the spinal cord do receive impulses from the cerebral cortex. Corticoreticular fibers originate from widespread regions of the cerebral cortex, are both crossed and uncrossed and, for the most part, terminate in regions of the reticular formation which project to spinal levels. One of the characteristic features of the brain stem reticular formation is that it receives afferent inputs from multiple sources. Other afferent fibers projecting to the brain stem reticular formation arise from the spinal cord (spinoreticular), the cerebellum and as collaterals of second order sensory neurons related to many cranial nerve nuclei. Collateral fibers from sensory cranial nerve nuclei project in an overlapping fashion to lateral parts of the medullary reticular formation, which do not give rise to either long ascending, or descending fiber systems. This portion of the reticular formation is referred to as the "sensory" part, not because it is related to any specific sensibility, but because it receives multiple sensory inputs. Axons of cells in the "sensory" part of the medullary reticular formation project medially to effector regions, which give rise to both ascending and descending projection systems.

Because information concerning the reticulospinal tracts in man is meager, almost all data are based upon experimental studies in animals. These studies demonstrate that stimulation of the brain stem reticular formation can (1) facilitate or inhibit voluntary movements, cortically induced movements and reflex activity, (2) modify muscle tone, (3) affect respiration, (4) exert pressor or depressor effects upon the circulatory system and (5) facilitate or inhibit the central transmission of sensory impulses. Areas of the medullary reticular formation from which inhibitory, inspiratory and depressor effects are obtained correspond closely to the regions from which medullary reticulospinal fibers arise. Electrical stimulation of this medullary region can inhibit (1) most forms of motor activity, (2) both the myotatic (stretch) and flexor reflexes and (3) muscle tone. Under these circumstances inhibitory effects are bilateral, but ipsilateral inhibition can be obtained at low thresholds. Reductions in muscle tone resulting from stimulation of this region of the medulla appear to be due to inhibitory effects exerted upon gamma motor neurons, which can influence alpha motor neurons via the gamma loop (Fig. 1-4).

A far larger region of the brain stem reticular formation facilitates, or augments, motor responses and somatic reflex activity. While the facilitatory region includes the pontine reticular formation, it extends rostrally beyond it into the mesencephalon and into parts of the diencephalon. Since the facilitatory region is extensive, and includes regions which do not contain cells projecting fibers to spinal levels, facilitatory effects must in part depend upon descending polysynaptic pathways connecting different regions of the brain stem. Since pontine reticulospinal fibers do not terminate upon alpha motor neurons, facilitating influences transmitted by this system must act upon internuncial neurons, such as gamma motor neurons, which can indirectly increase the firing rates of the alpha motor neurons.

Descending reticular fibers also are concerned with the transmission of impulses from the hypothalamus and other visceral centers to spinal levels. These fibers descend in anterior and anterolateral portions of the spinal cord close to the spinal gray matter and are believed to establish connections by which impulses can be conveyed to preganglionic cell groups in the thoraco-lumbar (sympathetic) and sacral (parasympathetic) spinal segments. Autonomic effects produced by stimulations of the reticular formation probably are mediated by these fiber systems.

Lastly, it should be mentioned that the influences of the brain stem reticular formation are not all directed toward the modification of spinal neuronal activities. Ascending reticular systems exert powerful, widespread influences upon the activity of the cerebral cortex. Ascending reticular systems serve to desynchronize and activate the cerebral cortex, and resulting changes recorded in the electroencephalogram can be correlated with behavioral arousal and the state of alertness.

Lesions of the Upper Motor Neuron

Lesions involving the upper motor neuron, at a wide variety of locations and resulting from many different kinds of pathological processes, produce paralysis, alterations of muscle tone and alterations of reflex activity. Lesions destroying the upper motor neuron are rarely selective, usually incomplete and frequently involve adjacent pathways and nuclear structures. The degree of paresis or paralysis does not bear a direct relationship to the size of the lesion or to the extent of involvement of the corticospinal tract (Lassek, 1954). Destruction of the upper motor neuron may result from vascular disease, trauma, neoplasm and infectious and degenerative diseases. Unilateral lesions in the cerebral hemisphere and brain stem produce contralateral paralysis, usually hemiplegia. Spinal lesions, most commonly the result of trauma, are usually bilateral and cause a paraplegia.

Because of its great clinical importance, it is worthwhile to consider first the most common lesion involving the upper motor neuron, namely, the so-called *cerebral vascular accident.* This vascular lesion usually involves variable portions of the corona radiata and internal capsule as a consequence of thrombosis of cerebral vessels, intracerebral hemorrhage or embolic phenomena. Cerebral thrombosis is the most common type of cerebral vascular lesion, and the middle cerebral artery (and its branches) or the main trunk of the carotid artery are involved with the greatest frequency. Sudden occlusion of a major cerebral vessel deprives local regions of neural tissue of blood and oxygen, causing the tissue to undergo necrosis. Tissue surrounding the infarcted area becomes congested and edematous.

In the majority of patients symptoms are of sudden onset. Initial symptoms are both focal and general in character. Generalized symptoms include headache, vomiting, convulsions and coma. Focal symptoms, such as paralysis, sensory loss or impairment of speech, are related to the site of the lesion and the structures involved. Immediately after the vascular lesion, the paralyzed limbs contralateral to the lesion usually are completely flaccid and the myotatic reflexes are depressed or absent. After the period of neural shock has passed, the myotatic reflexes reappear in an exaggerated form in the paralyzed limbs. The superficial abdominal reflexes, elicited by stroking the skin over the abdomen, and the cremasteric reflexes in the male disappear on the side of the paralysis. The plantar response, elicited by stroking the sole of the foot, becomes extensor. The latter response, known as the *sign of Babinski*, consists of extension of the great toe and fanning of the other toes. Although the sign of Babinski is of great clinical importance, the physiological mechanism underlying it is not understood.

After a variable period of time, usually two or three weeks, muscle tone gradually returns in the affected limb and ultimately exceeds that of the normal side. This exaggeration of muscle tone is referred to as *hypertonicity* or *spasticity*. The exaggeration of muscle tone is not exhibited by all muscles in the affected limbs. Spasticity involves the antigravity muscles. In the affected upper extremity spasticity is present particularly in the adductors and internal rotators of the shoulder, in the flexors of the elbow, wrist and digits and in the pronators of the forearm. In the affected lower extremity spasticity develops in the adductors of the hip, the extensors of the hip and knee and in the plantar-flexors of foot and toes. *Spasticity* is relatively easy to describe but extremely difficult to define. Descriptively spasticity is characterized by (1) increased resistance to passive movement, (2) extraordinarily hyperactive myotatic (deep tendon) reflexes that exhibit a low threshold, a large amplitude and an enlarged reflexogenous zone and have a briskness much greater than normal, and (3) the presence of clonus (Magoun and Rhines, 1947). *Clonus* is a manifestation of the exaggerated stretch reflex in which the contractions of one muscle group are sufficient to stretch antagonistic muscle groups and initiate myotatic responses in that muscle group. Clonus has a tendency to perpetuate itself in a synchronized manner. In some instances the threshold for this extreme exaggeration of the myotatic reflex is so low that passively moving a limb may initiate it.

The paralysis, which may appear complete at the onset of the cerebral vascular accident, tends to become less severe in time. Even the weakness tends ultimately to involve one limb more than the other. The motor functions that are affected most are those associated with fine, skilled movements; these movements show the smallest amount of recovery with time. The movements that are grosser and less skilled, and those which involve a whole limb, are least affected and show considerable restitution. Because of the distribution of muscular hypertonia, flexion movements tend to be stronger in the upper extremity, while extensor movements are strongest in the lower extremity. Atrophy of the type seen with lower motor neuron lesions does not occur with upper motor neuron lesions. However, after a period of years some atrophy of disuse becomes evident.

Many hemiplegics recover considerable motor function in time, in spite of the fact that there is great clumsiness in carrying out simple, skilled movements. Those that become ambulatory have a characteristic gait. The paralyzed leg is circumducted at the hip *en bloc* and swung forward because of the difficulty in flexing the knee. The foot is plantar flexed and the toe of the shoe is dragged in a circular fashion. The arm on the affected side is flexed at the elbow and wrist, the forearm is pronated, and the digits are flexed. The arm may be held close to the body, but if the arm is swung at all in walking, it moves primarily at the shoulder.

Upper motor neuron syndromes resulting from lesions in the brain stem produce disturbances of motor function similar to those described above, except that they usually involve particular cranial nerves and sometimes sensory pathways. Midbrain lesions frequently produce a contralateral hemiplegia and ipsilateral paralysis of the oculomotor nerve. Lesions in the ventral part of the pons may involve the corticospinal tract and fibers of the abducens and facial nerves, producing a contralateral hemiplegia and corresponding ipsilateral cranial nerve palsies. In the medulla lesions in, or near, the pyramid usually concomitantly involve emerging fibers of the hypoglossal nerve. This is the so-called hypoglossal alternating hemiplegia (Truex and Carpenter, 1969).

Complete spinal cord transection immediately produces, below the level of the lesion, loss of all (1) somatic sensation, (2) visceral sensation, (3) motor function, (4) muscle tone and (5) reflex activity. This state, referred to as *spinal shock*, is characterized by complete lack of neural function in the isolated spinal cord caudal to the lesion. Spinal shock occurs in all animals following complete transection of the spinal cord and is considered to be due to the sudden and abrupt interruption of descending excitatory influences. The period of spinal shock varies in different animals but in man ranges from one to six weeks and averages about three weeks. During this time there is no evidence of neural activity below the level of the lesion. The termination of the period of spinal shock is heralded by the appearance of the Babinski sign. A fairly orderly sequence of events follows which varies in duration. The various phases involved in the recovery of function in the isolated human spinal cord have been carefully analyzed by Kuhn (1950). These phases in recovery of neural function are (1) minimal reflex activity (three to six weeks), (2) flexor spasms (six to sixteen weeks), (3) alternate flexor and extensor spasms (after four months) and (4) predominant extensor spasms (after six months). The phase of minimal reflex activity is characterized by weak flexor responses to nociceptive stimuli, which begin distally and later involve proximal muscle groups in the extremities. During this period the Babinski sign can be obtained bilaterally, but the muscles are flaccid and the deep tendon reflexes cannot be elicited.

The phase of flexor muscle spasms is characterized by increasing tone in the flexor muscles and by stronger flexor responses to nociceptive stimuli, which progressively involve more proximal muscle groups. It is during this phase that the so-called *triple flexion response* is first seen. This involves flexion of the lower extremity at the hip, knee and ankle in response to a relatively mild nociceptive stimulus. The most exaggerated form of this reaction is the *mass reflex*, in which a relatively mild stimulus results in powerful bilateral triple flexion responses characterized by repeated discharge of motor units throughout the caudal part of the spinal cord. The mass reflex appears to be due to the spread of afferent impulses from one segment to the next and dispersion of impulses in such a manner as to cause motor units to continue to fire after the exciting stimulus has been withdrawn. The mass reflex is very distressing to the patient because it is almost impossible to control. This reflex becomes less severe about four months after spinal transection when extensor muscle tone gradually begins to increase. During this phase both flexor and extensor muscle spasms occur, but within a relatively short time extensor muscle tone may be so great that the patient can momentarily support his weight in a standing position (Kuhn, 1950).

Examination of the patient one year after complete spinal cord transection reveals the following: (1) complete paralysis below the level of the lesion, (2) loss of all sensation (somatic and visceral) below the lesion, (3) marked extensor muscle tone (spasticity) below the lesion, (4) hyperactive deep tendon (myotatic) reflexes below the lesion, (5) clonus in both lower extremities and (6) bilateral Babinski signs. Paralysis of bowel and bladder, present from the time of spinal transection, constitutes one of the major problems, but with good nursing care, reflex emptying of bowel and bladder can be established. In many patients there is reflex spinal sweating in response to noxious stimuli. This type of sweating is not under thermoregulatory control. In the male there is also disturbance of sexual activity (see Chapter 15).

Analysis of the Upper Motor Neuron Syndrome

For a long time it has been presumed that the upper motor neuron syndrome was due solely to the interruption of the fibers of the corticospinal tract at different locations. This concept appeared to be based on the thesis that impulses conveyed by this system directly and indirectly excited lower motor neurons and produced somatic movements of a voluntary nature. Thus, lesions involving corticospinal fibers deprived lower motor neurons of this input essential to so-called voluntary movement. The observation not adequately explained was the parallel assumption that spasticity occurring in association with hemiplegia and paraplegia was an expression of release phenomena due to injury of the corticospinal tract. The concept of release phenomena implies that the removal of inhibitory influences causes other intact neural structures to function in an abnormal manner. Thus, the intact corticospinal system was considered to possess excitatory properties with respect to voluntary movement, while interruption of this system was considered to cause release phenomena manifested by exaggerated muscle tone (i.e., spasticity).

From the descriptions of the locations and the kinds of lesions that produce the upper motor neuron syndrome, it is apparent that these lesions almost invariably involve other neural pathways. The only relatively pure corticospinal lesion is that which destroys the pyramid in the medulla. Experimental studies in the monkey and chimpanzee indicate that *section of the pyramids* produces a condition best characterized as hypotonic paresis (Tower, 1940, 1949). There is no paralysis, in the sense that no part of the body is rendered useless, but there is grave and general poverty of movement and impairment of what usage remains. The usage that survives bilateral section of the medullary pyramids, be it posture, progression, fighting or reach-grasping, is stripped of the finer qualities that endow these movements with aim, precision and versatility. In the chimpanzee paresis is more outstanding than hypotonia, the deep tendon reflexes are of large amplitude and not especially brisk, the superficial abdominal reflexes are abolished and the Babinski sign is invariably seen.

A recent study of bilateral pyramidal lesions in the monkey (Lawrence and Kuypers, 1968) confirms many of Tower's original observations and adds significant details. On the basis of long-term experiments these authors concluded that bilateral lesions of the medullary pyramid produce persistent slowness of movement, loss of individual finger movements and loss of ability to fractionate movements. They found that control of a wide range of movements of a grosser nature is recovered in time. In these animals there was never any gross evidence of loss of muscle bulk, nor any evidence of difficulty with bladder function. In animals in which some corticospinal fibers were preserved in different parts of the pyramid, return of dexterity and discrete finger movements was greater than in animals with complete lesions. These elegant studies suggest that the residual motor function seen following destruction of the corticospinal system must be due to impulses descending in subcorticospinal pathways* that are capable of initiating and guiding a limited range of motor functions, which include independent limb movements and total body-limb movements. The corticospinal system must therefore superimpose upon this subcortical mechanism functional qualities that provide speed, dexterity and the capacity to perform individual finger movements.

Further evidence of another type suggests that destruction of portions of the corticospinal tract does not cause spasticity. *Ablations of area 4* in the monkey produce a contralateral flaccid hemiparesis (Fulton, 1943; Mettler, 1948). While these lesions are not confined to the pyramidal elements, and only eliminate part of the origin of that system, they offer supporting evidence consistent with that obtained following lesions confined to the medullary pyramids.

The above observations and conclusions suggest that the non-pyramidal descending systems must make a significant contribution to total motor function. While these systems are capable of independent function, in the normal individual they would appear to form a basic mechanism upon which the activity of the corticospinal system is superimposed. Lawrence and Kuypers (1968a) have extended their important studies in this direction. They have divided the descending subcorticospinal (non-pyramidal) pathways into two groups on the basis of (1) the position of the tracts in the white matter of the spinal cord and (2) the distribution of terminal fibers within the spinal gray matter. From these criteria two fundamental subcorticospinal pathways, composed of various fiber systems, emerge. Fibers of the *ventromedial system* arise from ventromedial regions of the brain stem tegmentum, descend in the anterior funiculus, or in ventromedial parts of the lateral funiculus, and preferentially terminate upon internuncial neurons in lamina VIII or ventromedial parts of lamina VII. Spinal pathways of the ventromedial system include (1) the vestibulospinal tract, (2) the medial longitudinal fasciculus and (3) the reticulospinal tracts.

The *lateral system* of descending subcorticospinal fibers consists almost exclusively of the rubrospinal tract which descends in the dorsal part of the lateral funiculus and distributes fibers to internuncial neurons in dorsal and lateral parts of lamina VII. Both of these subcorticospinal systems differ from the corticospinal system in that they distribute only a few fibers that end directly upon alpha motor neurons in lamina IX.

In order to determine the functional contributions of the ventromedial and lateral systems to control of somatic motor activity, these systems were selectively interrupted at various levels in monkeys which had recovered from

---

*Subcorticospinal pathways include all pathways which arise from cell groups in the brain stem and project to spinal levels.

bilateral interruption of the medullary pyramids. This plan was necessary because corticospinal fibers terminate both on internuncial neurons and on alpha motor neurons (especially in the cord enlargements). Observations in these studies (Lawrence and Kuypers, 1968a) lead to the conclusion that the ventromedial descending subcorticospinal system is especially concerned with the maintenance of erect posture, the integration of body and limb movement and with directing the course of progression movements. The lateral descending subcorticospinal system appears to be concerned with control of the independent use of the extremities, particularly the hand. Deficits seen in animals with lesions of the lateral subcorticospinal system particularly involved impairment in ability to reach for and pick up food. Part of this motor deficit appeared to be due to impairment of the ability to flex the extended limb. In contrast to the above, affected limbs were used with minimal difficulty in standing and walking.

While these studies provide some insight into the contributions made by various components of the upper motor neuron, they do not provide information concerning the basic mechanisms that underlie spasticity. If spasticity does not occur with relatively pure lesions of the corticospinal system, or with lesions of subcorticospinal pathways, what systems are responsible for it? We have seen that spasticity is a regularly occurring phenomenon in association with most lesions of the upper motor neuron, yet its nature seems to elude even the most meticulous analysis. This raises the question as to whether spasticity might be due to involvement of a system not included in the above analysis. There is some evidence to support this suggestion, although it offers only a partial solution.

In man and monkey there is an additional motor area on the medial aspect of the hemisphere known as the supplementary motor area (Penfield and Rasmussen, 1950; Woolsey, 1958). The *supplementary motor area* is somatotopically organized in a sequential way somewhat similar to that of the primary motor area (Fig. 1–9). Stimulation of the supplementary motor area produces (1) bilateral synergic contractions of muscles of the trunk and legs, (2) complex patterned movements and (3) infrequent rapid incoordinated movements. Movements produced tend to be synergistic, tonic contractions of the postural type. These postural movements can be elicited after ablations of the primary motor cortex. Although no fibers from the supplementary motor area project directly to spinal levels, evoked responses can be recorded bilaterally at spinal levels in regions which contain corticospinal fibers (Bertrand, 1956). The outstanding feature appears to be the bilateral nature of the system.

Systematic studies in the monkey (Travis, 1955) indicate that bilateral simultaneous ablations of the supplementary motor area in the monkey produce disturbances of posture and muscle tone without producing paresis. Gradually increasing hypertonus develops in a period of two to four weeks in flexor muscle groups and ultimately produces flexion contractures. These ablations produce hyperactive myotatic reflexes and are associated with clonus. The significance of these observations lies in the suggestion that paresis and certain forms of spasticity can be dissociated.

Lesions involving the supplementary motor area and the primary motor area in the same hemisphere result in immediate contralateral hemiparesis

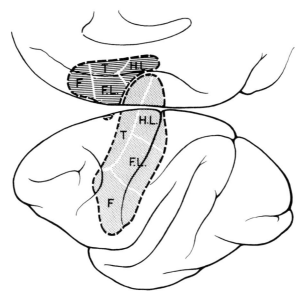

Figure 1–9 Diagram of the precentral and supplementary motor areas in the monkey. The precentral motor area, mainly on the lateral convexity, is stippled; the outlined area posterior to the central sulcus represents cortex hidden in the depths of the central sulcus. The supplementary motor area (lined) is on the medial aspect of the hemisphere. Abbreviations used indicate the somatotopic representation; *F*, face area; *T*, trunk; *FL*, forelimb; *HL*, hindlimb. (From Truex and Carpenter: *Human Neuroanatomy*, 1969. Reproduced by permission of the Williams and Wilkins Company, Baltimore, Md.)

associated with hypotonus and impaired myotatic reflexes. Within a relatively short time the hypotonus changes to hypertonus and the myotatic reflexes become exaggerated. The course of events thereafter resembles that seen in a classic capsular hemiplegia.

These observations suggest that the corticospinal system serves mainly to transmit impulses to segmental levels that are concerned with voluntary skilled movement and that other mechanisms probably are responsible for the release phenomenon, expressed as spasticity, that occurs in association with many lesions that involve this system.

REFERENCES

1. Bertrand, G.: Spinal efferent pathways from the supplementary motor area. Brain, 79:461–473, 1956.
2. Bing, R.: *Local Diagnosis in Neurological Diseases.* Translated, revised and enlarged from the 14th German edition by W. Haymaker. St. Louis, C. V. Mosby Co., 1956, pp. 57–62 and 105–112.
3. Brodal, A.: *The Reticular Formation of the Brain Stem: Anatomical Aspects and Functional Correlations.* Springfield, Ill., Charles C Thomas, 1957.
4. Carpenter, M. B., Stein, B. M. and Shriver, J. E.: Central projections of spinal dorsal roots in the monkey. II. Lower thoracic, lumbosacral and coccygeal dorsal roots. Am. J. Anat., 123:75–117, 1968.
5. Courville, J.: Somatotopical organization of the projection from the nucleus interpositus

anterior of the cerebellum to the red nucleus. An experimental study in the cat with silver impregnation methods. Exp. Brain Res. (Berlin), 2:191–215, 1966.

6. Foerster, O.: The motor cortex in man in the light of Hughlings Jackson's doctrines. Brain, 59:135–159, 1936.

7. Fulton, J. F.: *Physiology of the Nervous System,* 2nd ed. New York, Oxford University Press, 1943, pp. 369–393.

8. Fulton, J. F. and Pi-Suñer, J.: A note concerning the probable function of various afferent end-organs in skeletal muscle. Am. J. Physiol., 83:554–562, 1928.

9. Granit, R.: Reflex self-regulation of muscle contraction and autogenetic inhibition. J. Neurophysiol., 13:351–372, 1950.

10. Haymaker, W.: *Bing's Local Diagnosis in Neurological Diseases.* St. Louis, C. V. Mosby Co., 1956, pp. 57–62 and 105–112.

11. Hinman, A. and Carpenter, M. B.: Efferent fiber projections of the red nucleus in the cat. J. Comp. Neurol., 113:61–82, 1959.

12. Hunt, C. C.: The reflex activity of mammalian small-nerve fibers. J. Physiol. (London), 115:456–469, 1951.

13. Kuhn, R. A.: Functional capacity of the isolated human spinal cord. Brain, 7:1–51, 1950.

14. Kuypers, H. G. J. M.: Central cortical projections to motor and somatosensory cell groups. Brain, 83:161–184, 1960.

15. Lassek, A. M.: The human pyramidal tract. II. A numerical investigation of the Betz cells of the motor area. Arch. Neurol. Psychiat., 44:718–724, 1940.

16. Lassek, A. M.: The pyramidal tract: Basic considerations of cortico-spinal neurons. Res. Publ. Assoc. Nerv. Ment. Dis., 27:106–128, 1948.

17. Lassek, A. M.: *The Pyramidal Tract: Its Status in Medicine.* Springfield, Ill., Charles C Thomas, 1954.

18. Lawrence, D. G. and Kypers, H. G. J. M.: The functional organization of the motor system in the monkey. I. The effects of bilateral pyramidal lesions. Brain, 91:1–14, 1968.

19. Lawrence, D. G. and Kuypers, H. G. J. M.: The functional organization of the motor system in the monkey. II. The effects of lesions of the descending brain-stem pathways. Brain, 91:15–36, 1968a.

20. Leksell, L.: The action potential and excitatory effects of the small ventral root fibers to skeletal muscle. Acta Physiol. Scand., 10 (Suppl. 31):1–84, 1945.

21. Liu, C. N. and Chambers, W. W.: An experimental study of the cortico-spinal system in the monkey (Macaca mulatta). The spinal pathways and preterminal distribution of degenerating fibers following discrete lesions of the pre- and postcentral gyri and bulbar pyramid. J. comp. Neurol., 123:257–283, 1964.

22. McCough, G. P., Derring, I. D. and Stewart, W. B.: Inhibition of knee jerk from tendon spindles of crureus. J. Neurophysiol., 13:343–350, 1950.

23. Magoun, H. W. and Rhines, R.: *Spasticity; the Stretch-Reflex and Extrapyramidal Systems.* Springfield, Ill., Charles C Thomas, 1948.

24. Massion, J.: The mammalian red nucleus. Physiol. Rev., 47:383–436, 1967.

25. Mettler, F. A.: The nonpyramidal motor projections from the frontal cerebral cortex. Res. Publ. Assoc. Nerv. Ment. Dis. 27:162–199, 1948.

26. Mott, F. W. and Sherrington, C. S.: Experiments upon the influence of sensory nerves upon movement and nutrition of the limbs. Proc. Roy. Soc. (London), 57:481–488, 1895.

27. Nathan, P. W. and Smith, M. C.: Long descending tracts in man. I. Review of present knowledge. Brain, 78:248–303, 1955.

28. Nyberg-Hansen, R. and Brodal, A.: Sites and mode of termination of rubrospinal fibres in the cat. An experimental study with silver impregnation methods. J. Anat., 98:235–253, 1964.

29. Nyberg-Hansen, R. and Mascitti, T. A.: Sites and mode of termination of fibers of the vestibulospinal tract in the cat: An experimental study with silver impregnation methods. J. Comp. Neurol., 122:369–387, 1964.

30. Patton, H. D.: Reflex regulation of movement and posture. *In* Ruch, T. C. and Patton, H. D. (eds.): *Physiology and Biophysics,* 19th ed. Philadelphia, W. B. Saunders Company, 1965, pp. 181–206.

31. Penfield, W. and Boldrey, E.: Somatic motor and sensory representation in the cerebral cortex of man as studied by electrical stimulation. Brain, 60:389–443, 1937.

32. Penfield, W. and Rasmussen, T.: *The Cerebral Cortex of Man: A Clinical Study of Localization of Function.* New York, Macmillan Company, 1950.

33. Pompeiano, O.: Sulle risposte, posturali alla stimolazione elettrica del nucieo rosso nel gatto decerebrato. Boll. Soc. Ital. Biol. Sper., 32:1450–1451, 1956.

34. Pompeiano, O.: Analisi degli effetti della stimolazione elettrica del nucleo rosso nel gatto decerebrato. Atti Accad. Naz. Lincei. Rend. Cl. Sci. Fis. Mat. Nat., 22:100–103, 1957.

35. Pompeiano, O.: Organizzazione somatotopica delle riposte postulari stimolazione elettrica del nucleo di Deiters nel gatto decerebrato. Arch. Si. Biol., *44*:497–511, 1960.

36. Pompeiano, O. and Brodal, A.: Experimental demonstration of a somatotopical origin of rubrospinal fibers in the cat. J. Comp. Neurol., *108*:225–251, 1957.

37. Pompeiano, O. and Brodal, A.: The origin of vestibulospinal fibres in the cat. An experimental-anatomical study, with comments on the descending medial longitudinal fasciculus. Arch. Ital. Biol., *95*:166–195, 1957a.

38. Rexed, B.: The cytoarchitectonic organization of the spinal cord in the cat. J. Comp. Neurol., *96*:415–495, 1952.

39. Rexed, B.: A cytoarchitectonic atlas of the spinal cord in the cat. J. Comp. Neurol., *100*:297–379, 1954.

40. Russell, J. R. and DeMyer, W.: The quantitative cortical origin of pyramidal axons of Macaca rhesus; with some remarks on the slow rate of axolysis. Neurology, *11*:96–108, 1961.

41. Scarff, J. E.: Primary cortical centers for movements of upper and lower limbs in man; observations based on electrical stimulation. Arch. Neurol. Psychiat., *44*:243–299, 1940.

42. Scheibel, M. E. and Scheibel, A. N.: Structural substrates for integrative patterns in the brain stem reticular core. *In: Reticular Formation of the Brain.* Proceedings of the Henry Ford Hospital International Symposium, Detroit, 1957. Boston, Little, Brown & Co., 1958, pp. 31–55.

43. Shriver, J. E., Stein, B. M. and Carpenter, M. B.: Central projections of spinal dorsal roots in the monkey. I. Cervical and upper thoracic dorsal roots. Am. J. Anat., *123*:27–73, 1968.

44. Tower, S. S.: Function and structure in the chronically isolated lumbosacral spinal cord of the dog. J. Comp. Neurol., *67*:109–131, 1937.

45. Tower, S. S.: Pyramidal lesion in the monkey. Brain, *63*:36–90, 1940.

46. Tower, S. S.: Pyramidal tract. *In*: Bucy, P. C. (ed.): *The Precentral Motor Cortex*, 2nd ed. Urbana, University of Illinois Press, 1949, pp. 149–172.

47. Travis, A. M.: Neurological deficiencies following supplementary motor area lesions in Macaca mulatta. Brain, *78*:174–198, 1955.

48. Truex, R. C. and Carpenter, M. B.: *Human Neuroanatomy*, 6th ed. Baltimore, Williams and Wilkins Company, 1969.

49. Walberg, F., Pompeiano, O., Brodal, A. and Jansen, J.: The fastigiovestibular projection in the cat. An experimental study with silver impregnation methods. J. Comp. Neurol., *118*:49–75, 1962.

50. Wilson, V. J., Wylie, R. M. and Marco, L. A.: Organization of the medial vestibular nucleus. J. Neurophysiol., *31*:166–175, 1968.

51. Woolsey, C. N.: Organization of somatic sensory and motor area of the cerebral cortex. *In*: Harlow, H. F. and Woolsey, C. N. (eds.): *Biological and Biochemical Bases of Behavior*. Madison, University of Wisconsin Press, 1958, pp. 63–81.

Chapter 2

CEREBELLUM AND BASAL GANGLIA*

by Malcolm B. Carpenter, M.D.

Two large neural complexes considered to play major roles in suprasegmental control of motor function are the cerebellum and basal ganglia. While the disturbances associated with diseases of these structures are distinctive and highly characteristic, it is not possible to provide a complete physiological explanation of the underlying neural mechanisms. The influences of both of these neural complexes upon segmental parts of the nervous system are indirect, that is, impulses are relayed through complex neuronal circuits which ultimately modify neural activity in segmental parts of the neuraxis.

THE CEREBELLUM

The cerebellum, a derivative of the brain stem, lies posterior to the medulla and pons and extends laterally beyond these structures. Grossly, the cerebellum consists of a median portion, the cerebellar vermis and two lateral lobes, referred to as the cerebellar hemispheres. This structure consists of (1) a superficial gray mantle, the cerebellar cortex, (2) an internal white substance, composed of nerve fibers, and (3) four pairs of intrinsic nuclei. The cerebellar cortex, unlike the cerebral cortex, is composed of numerous narrow laminae or folia, most of which are oriented in various transverse planes. Three paired peduncles connect the cerebellum with the three infratentorial segments of the brain stem—the medulla, the pons and the mesencephalon.

Three distinctive parts of the cerebellum are recognized (Fig. 2-1). The

---

*Aided by Research Grant NS-04082-07 from the National Institute of Neurological Diseases and Stroke of NIH, Bethesda, Maryland.

phylogenetically oldest part, the *archicerebellum,* is small and consists of the *nodulus* and the paired *flocculi.* This part of the cerebellum is mainly connected with the vestibular apparatus and is concerned with the maintenance of equilibrium. Parts of the cerebellum rostral to the primary fissure constitute the *anterior lobe* or the *paleocerebellum;* this division of the cerebellum receives impulses from stretch receptors (via spinocerebellar tracts) and appears to be concerned with mechanisms that regulate muscle tone. The newest and largest part of the cerebellum lies between the flocculonodular and anterior lobes and is referred to as the *neocerebellum.* This part of the cerebellum receives impulses indirectly from the cerebral cortex and is considered to be related primarily to the coordination of skilled movements initiated at cortical levels.

Cerebellar Cortex

The cerebellar cortex is uniform in structure, consists of three well-defined cell layers, and its structural elements have intricate geometric relationships (Fig. 2-2). The three layers of the cerebellar cortex are: (1) a superficial *molecular layer,* (2) a deep *granular layer* and (3) between these a ganglionic or *Purkinje cell layer.* The granular layer is composed of a prodigious number of closely packed chromatic nuclei, between which are irregular spaces containing the "cerebellar glomeruli." Granule cells give rise to four or five short dendrites that enter the glomeruli. The axons of granule cells ascend vertically into the

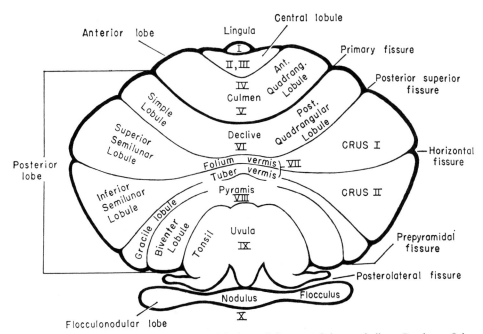

Figure 2-1 Schematic diagram of the lobules and fissures of the cerebellum. Portions of the cerebellum caudal to the posterolateral fissure represent the flocculonodular lobule, also known as the *archicerebellum.* The anterior lobe of the cerebellum lies rostral to the primary fissure; this is the *paleocerebellum.* The *neocerebellum* lies between the primary and posterolateral fissures. (From Truex and Carpenter: *Human Neuroanatomy,* 1969. Reproduced by permission of the Williams and Wilkins Company, Baltimore, Md.)

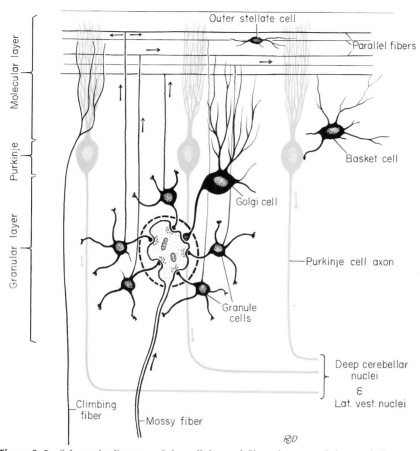

Figure 2–2 Schematic diagram of the cellular and fiber elements of the cerebellar cortex as seen in the longitudinal axis of a folium. The layers of the cerebellar cortex are indicated on the left. Excitatory inputs to the cerebellar cortex are conveyed by mossy and climbing fibers. The broken line represents a glial lamella surrounding a glomerulus. Granule cell axons ascend to the molecular layer, bifurcate and form an extensive system of parallel fibers which synapse on the dendrites of Purkinje cells. Climbing fibers ascend the dendrites of Purkinje cells (blue). Outer stellate, basket and Golgi cells are inhibitory. Arrows indicate the directions of impulse conduction. (From Truex and Carpenter: *Human Neuroanatomy*, 1969. Reproduced by permission of the Williams and Wilkins Company, Baltimore, Md.)

molecular layer where they bifurcate and run parallel to the long axis of the folia.

The Purkinje cell layer consists of a single sheet of large flask-shaped cells arranged uniformly along the upper margin of the granular layer. Each Purkinje cell gives rise to an elaborate dendritic tree which arborizes in a flattened fanlike expansion in the molecular layer at right angles to the long axis of the folia. Purkinje cell axons project to the intrinsic cerebellar nuclei and to the vestibular nuclei.

The molecular layer contains the axons of granule cells which course through the dendritic expansions of the Purkinje cells, like telegraph wires strung through the branches of a tree. These granule cell axons are referred to as "parallel fibers" and establish synaptic contacts with Purkinje cell dendrites.

In addition, the molecular layer contains so-called basket cells, whose axons arborize about numerous Purkinje cell bodies, and outer stellate cells, whose processes establish contacts with Purkinje cell dendrites. All fibers in the molecular layer are unmyelinated.

All afferent fibers entering the cerebellar cortex lose their myelin sheath and terminate as either mossy fibers or climbing fibers. Mossy fibers, constituting the most abundant cerebellar afferents, terminate in the granule cell layer where their endings form the core of the cerebellar glomeruli. A cerebellar glomerulus consists of (1) a mossy fiber terminal (rosette), (2) numerous dendrites from granule cells and (3) axons of Golgi cells. This complex synaptic junction controls a large part of the afferent input to the cerebellar cortex. The mossy fiber–granule cell relay is excitatory and can cause Purkinje cells to discharge. However, the axons of the Golgi cells that enter the glomeruli can inhibit synaptic transmission at this junction. Climbing fibers pass from the white matter through the granular layer and past the cell bodies of Purkinje cells to reach the dendrites of these cells. These fibers climb the dendritic branches of the Purkinje cells as these branches extend into the molecular layer. Synaptic contacts between the climbing fibers and Purkinje cell dendrites are secure, and climbing fiber discharges produce an all-or-none excitatory effect upon Purkinje cells.

Mossy fibers appear to represent the terminals of the principal cerebellar afferent systems (i.e., the spinocerebellar tracts, the pontocerebellar tracts and primary and secondary vestibulocerebellar fibers) (Mettler and Lubin, 1942; Brodal, 1954; Brodal and Høivik, 1964). Climbing fibers are now considered to represent the terminals of olivocerebellar fibers (Hámori and Szentágothai, 1966).

Recent advances in physiology indicate that the climbing fiber has an extremely powerful excitatory synaptic action on the primary and secondary dendrites of the Purkinje cell. The parallel fibers, representing the axons of granule cells, also excite Purkinje cells via cross-over synapses with Purkinje cell dendrites. The outer stellate cells, the basket cells and the Golgi cells are inhibitory neurons in the cerebellar cortex. Outer stellate cells exert inhibitory influences upon the dendrites of Purkinje cells in the molecular layer. Basket cells inhibit Purkinje cells via axosomatic synapses on the cell bodies. Golgi cells, found in the granular cell layer, project axons, which form a part of the cerebellar glomeruli; these cells inhibit afferent input to the cerebellar cortex at the mossy fiber–granule cell relay (Eccles, Ito and Szentágothai, 1967).

Although the cerebellar cortex is relatively simple, it has an elaborate structural and functional organization in which multiple interactions influence conduction of impulses, synaptic articulations and the output which passes via Purkinje cell axons to the deep cerebellar nuclei and parts of the vestibular nuclei. The most puzzling finding is that the entire output of the cerebellar cortex is inhibitory (Ito and Yoshida, 1964; Ito, Yoshida and Obata, 1964; Eccles, Ito and Szentágothai, 1967).

Afferent Fibers

Cerebellar afferent fibers are nearly three times as numerous as efferent fibers (Snider, 1950) and, with some exceptions, terminate mostly in the cerebellar cortex. These pathways convey impulses from peripheral receptors and from various levels of the neuraxis via relay nuclei in the brain stem. The largest number of these fibers enter the cerebellum via the inferior and middle cerebellar peduncles (Fig. 2-3).

The *inferior cerebellar peduncle* (restiform body) conveys impulses from the spinal cord and from relay nuclei in the medulla. The principal fibers composing the inferior cerebellar peduncle are (1) the posterior spinocerebellar tract (PSCT), (2) the cuneocerebellar tract (CCT), (3) reticulocerebellar fibers and (4) olivocerebellar fibers. The *posterior spinocerebellar tract* conveys impulses from stretch receptors which enter the spinal cord via group Ia and Ib muscle afferents and exteroceptive impulses from touch and pressure receptors in skin. These impulses are projected to the anterior lobe of the cerebellum ipsilaterally, and are concerned mainly with the lower extremity (Oscarsson,

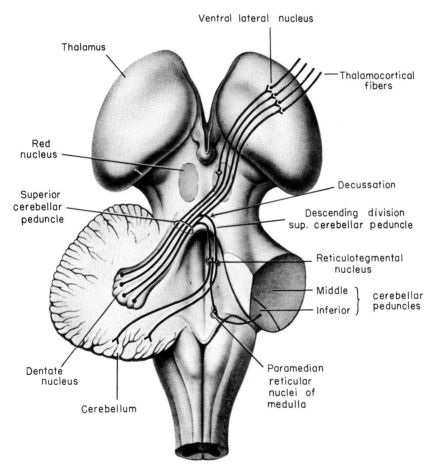

Figure 2-3 Diagram of the cerebellum and brain stem showing the cerebellar peduncles and some of the relay nuclei in the brain stem. Efferent fibers from the dentate nucleus form the principal part of the superior cerebellar peduncle, which decussates completely in the caudal midbrain. Most of the fibers of this peduncle project to the ventral lateral nucleus of the thalamus. (From Truex and Carpenter: *Human Neuroanatomy*, 1969. Reproduced by permission of the Williams and Wilkins Company, Baltimore, Md.)

1965; Truex and Carpenter, 1969). The *cuneocerebellar tract* conveys uncrossed impulses from muscle spindles to the anterior lobe of the cerebellum and is regarded as the forelimb equivalent of the PSCT. *Reticulocerebellar fibers* pass from the lateral reticular nucleus of the medulla to the anterior lobe and to parts of the cerebellar vermis. Impulses conveyed by this tract are related to tactile receptors (Combs, 1956). Olivocerebellar fibers, constituting the largest component of the inferior cerebellar peduncle, are all crossed (Fig. 2-4). These fibers are distributed to all parts of the cerebellar cortex in an orderly pattern, as well as to the intrinsic nuclei. Impulses from the spinal cord reaching the inferior olivary complex convey impulses from stretch receptors, so that in some respects the spinoolivary-olivocerebellar pathway resembles the PSCT.

A structure medial to the inferior cerebellar peduncle, known as the

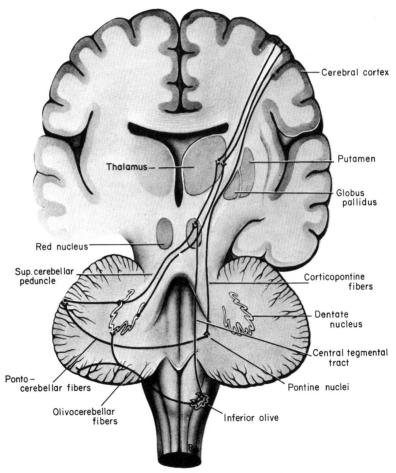

Figure 2–4 Diagram of some afferent and efferent cerebellar pathways. Fibers from the cerebral cortex pass to the pontine nuclei and to parts of the inferior olivary nucleus; both of these structures give rise to crossed cerebellar afferent fibers. Purkinje cell axons project to the deep cerebellar nuclei, which in turn give rise to cerebellar efferent fiber systems. (From Truex and Carpenter: *Human Neuroanatomy*, 1969. Reproduced by permission of the Williams and Wilkins Company, Baltimore, Md.)

Emboliform nucleus   Dentate nucleus

Cm

Fastigial nucleus   Globose nucleus

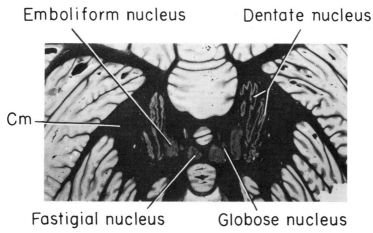

Figure 2–5 Section of the cerebellum showing portions of the deep cerebellar nuclei and the corpus medullare (Cm). (From Truex and Carpenter: *Human Neuroanatomy*, 1969. Reproduced by permission of the Williams and Wilkins Company, Baltimore, Md.)

juxtarestiform body, contains vestibulocerebellar and cerebellovestibular fibers. Vestibulocerebellar fibers project mainly to the nodulus and the flocculus.

The *middle cerebellar peduncle*, or brachium pontis, is part of a pathway that conveys impulses from the cerebral cortex to the cerebellum (Figs. 2-3 and 2-4). This pathway involves two links: (1) uncrossed fibers from the cerebral cortex which end upon pontine nuclei and (2) fibers from the pontine nuclei which cross and enter the lateral hemisphere of the cerebellum. This is a massive system that relates areas of cerebral cortex of one hemisphere with the lateral lobe of the cerebellum on the opposite side. Regions of cerebral cortex projecting corticopontine fibers include the motor area, the somatosensory area and the visual and auditory areas. It is apparent that the cerebellum receives impulses from a variety of different receptors, including those concerned with the special senses.

Deep Cerebellar Nuclei

Within the medullary core of the cerebellum four nuclear masses can be distinguished which are referred to as the deep cerebellar nuclei (Fig. 2–5). These nuclei give rise to the principal cerebellar efferent fiber systems. The four deep cerebellar nuclei are the dentate, emboliform, globose and fastigial. The *dentate nucleus* is a large, convoluted band of gray matter, having the shape of a folded bag with the opening directed dorsomedially. This nucleus lies in the white matter of the cerebellar hemisphere. The emboliform and globose nuclei are small gray masses located near the hilus of the dentate nucleus. The fastigial nuclei are located in the roof of the fourth ventricle, and are appropriately referred to as the roof nuclei. These deep cerebellar nuclei receive impulses from the cerebral cortex via Purkinje cell axons (Fig. 2-2). Purkinje cell axons project in an orderly fashion from the different parts of the cerebellar cortex. Cortex of the lateral hemispheres projects fibers to the dentate nucleus (Fig. 2-4). Cortex of the cerebellar vermis gives rise to fibers that pass to fastigial nuclei. Paravermal regions of the cortex project to the emboliform and globose nuclei. In addition to afferent fibers coming from the cerebellar cortex, the deep cerebellar nuclei receive fibers from the vestibular nuclei (i.e., from the fastigial nucleus), the red nuclei (i.e., from the emboliform nucleus) and from the inferior olivary nuclear complex. Impulses conveyed by these systems to the deep cerebellar nuclei are considered to be excitatory. The principal efferent fibers from the cerebellum arise from the deep cerebellar nuclei.

Efferent Fibers

Two separate efferent cerebellar systems are recognized on the basis of nuclei of origin, course of the fibers and terminal projection areas. The largest and most important bundle, the *superior cerebellar peduncle*, arises from the dentate, emboliform and globose nuclei (Figs. 2–3 and 2–4). Fibers of this large bundle sweep ventromedially into the pontine tegmentum and completely decussate in the caudal mesencephalon. Fibers from the emboliform nucleus largely terminate in the caudal two-thirds of the opposite red nucleus (Courville, 1966), while fibers from the dentate nucleus give collaterals to rostral parts of the red nucleus but primarily ascend to the contralateral thalamus. In the contralateral thalamus fibers of the superior cerebellar peduncle terminate in the ventrolateral nucleus, a relay nucleus that in turn projects upon the motor cortex. This connection thus brings impulses from the cerebellum to parts of the cerebral cortex that are concerned with motor function. Cerebellar impulses conveyed to the red nucleus can modify flexor muscle tone via the rubrospinal tract (Massion, 1967).

Cerebellar efferent fibers arising from the fastigial nuclei project mainly to the vestibular nuclei via the uncinate fasciculus and the juxtarestiform body. The uncinate fasciculus is a thin band of fibers that hooks around the superior cerebellar peduncle. Fastigial fibers passing to the vestibular nuclei convey excitatory impulses that facilitate extensor muscle tone via the vestibulospinal tracts (Walberg, Pompeiano, Brodal and Jansen, 1962).

Cerebellar Functions

Although the cerebellum receives a large part of its input from sensory systems, the cerebellum is not concerned with the conscious perception of sensation. The inputs to the cerebellum are concerned primarily with the coordination of complex reciprocal innervations that underlie motor activity. The cerebellum serves as a prime example of how important sensory information is to the regulation and control of coordinated motor performance. The cerebellum is one of the higher neural structures that automatically regulate muscle tone, both at rest and during movement, and plays an integral part in virtually all simple and complex muscle actions.

One of the simplest and best ways of demonstrating the importance of these regulating mechanisms is to describe the disturbances which occur with cerebellar lesions. There are several general principles concerning cerebellar lesions which are unique. These principles are: (1) disturbances occur ipsilateral to the lesion, (2) disturbances occur as a constellation of related phenomena, (3) disturbances due to non-progressive pathological conditions undergo attenuation with time and (4) disturbances probably are the physiological expression of intact neural structures deprived of controlling and regulating influences normally provided by the cerebellum.

Three distinct cerebellar syndromes are recognized in relation to lesions in different parts of the cerebellum. The most common is the *neocerebellar syndrome,* due to lesions involving the lateral lobes of the cerebellum, the dentate nucleus or the superior cerebellar peduncle. This syndrome is characterized by hypotonia and asynergic disturbances. The muscles show decreased resistance to passive movement, are soft and tire easily. The tendon reflexes are difficult to obtain and frequently exhibit a pendular quality. The precise explanation for the loss of muscle tone is unknown but is presumed to be related to interruption of pathways from stretch receptors.

Asynergic disturbances are expressed by faulty range, direction and force of muscular contractions. The impairment in the ability to gauge distances (dysmetria) is striking. These disturbances underlie the impairment of rapid successive movements, the breaking up of complex movement patterns into groups of simple movements performed serially (decomposition of movement) and impairment of abilities to hold particular positions. Perhaps the outstanding asynergic disturbances are tremor and ataxia.

The *tremor* classically associated with cerebellar lesions occurs only during voluntary and associated movements, has a coarse, irregular quality and particularly involves the limbs. This tremor is referred to as "intention tremor," but it is an involuntary motor activity which the patient cannot control, except by stopping all voluntary movement. Cerebellar tremor frequently is contrasted with the tremor of parkinsonism (paralysis agitans), which classically is present at rest, that is, when no voluntary or associated movements are in progress.

Ataxia is another form of asynergic disturbance which results in a bizarre, forceful distortion of basic movement patterns. This expression of asynergia involves especially the larger axial muscle masses and the muscles of the shoulder and pelvic girdles, and it produces disturbances in walking. The gait is broad-based and unsteady; the patient lurches, stumbles and reels. Frequently there is overstepping and a tendency to veer to one side, usually the side of the largest lesion.

Speech disturbances, common with neocerebellar lesions, are characterized by slow, unnatural separation of syllables uttered in a slurred and explosive manner. *Nystagmus* may be seen in association with cerebellar lesions and is most pronounced when the eyes are directed laterally to the side of the lesion.

Lesions involving the nodulus and the uvula relatively selectively produce the so-called *archicerebellar syndrome.* These lesions affect the axial musculature used for the maintenance of equilibrium and for locomotion. This syndrome, seen mainly in children with midline cerebellar tumors (medulloblastoma), is characterized by unsteadiness in standing, a tendency to fall backwards and a generally ataxic gait. Muscle tone is affected very little and tremor and incoordination in the extremities usually are absent.

Lesions of the anterior lobe of the cerebellum (paleocerebellum) in the dog produce severe disturbances of posture and greatly increased extensor muscle tone. Animals with such lesions exhibit opisthotonos, hyperactive deep tendon reflexes, increased positive supporting mechanisms and periodic tonic seizures. In time most of these disturbances disappear (Fulton, 1949). A corresponding paleocerebellar syndrome has not been described in man, but similar tonic seizures do occur as a consequence of brain stem compression. Since the classic experiments of Sherrington (1898) it has been known that ablations of the anterior lobe of the cerebellum cause an exaggeration of extensor muscle tone in decerebrate animals.

Although recent advances concerning the functional properties of the systematically organized elements of the cerebellar cortex provide certain insights concerning cortical functions, we still do not have a complete understanding of how the cerebellum provides its controlling influence. Present evidence suggests that the cerebellum integrates and organizes information flowing to it and participates in the control of motor function by transmitting impulses to (1) certain brain stem nuclei (i.e., the vestibular and red nuclei), which in turn project to spinal levels, and (2) thalamic nuclei, which can modify activity in cortical regions concerned with motor function. Most of the cerebellar input projects indirectly to the cortex. The only output of the cerebellar cortex, conveyed by Purkinje cell axons, is inhibitory. These inhibitory influences are exerted upon the deep cerebellar nuclei and the lateral vestibular nucleus. The fact that the cerebellar cortex transforms all input into inhibitory activity precludes the possibility of dynamic storage of information. These data suggest that the cerebellar cortex may function as a special kind of computer that can provide a quick response to a particular kind of input, convey impulses promptly to other parts of the nervous system and has virtually no short-term dynamic memory.

THE BASAL GANGLIA

The basal ganglia represent large subcortical nuclear masses derived from the telencephalon, considered to constitute a phylogenetically ancient motor mechanism. In submammalian forms with poorly developed cerebral cortices the basal ganglia are thought to be responsible for most motor activities. In these lower forms the motor activities are highly stereotyped, repetitive, and resemble well-patterned reflex movements. With the evolution of the cerebral cortex in mammals the basal ganglia play a less important role in motor function but continue to be utilized for more or less automatic movements concerned with locomotion, posture and defensive reactions. According to Wilson (1928), the basal ganglia provide a postural background for voluntary skilled movements and in this way contribute a steadying and reinforcing influence. Even though the basal ganglia may become subordinate to motor centers in the cerebral cortex in the process of evolution, the basal ganglia are structures of considerable size and clinical importance.

Clinical interest in the basal ganglia centers on the unique kinds of disturbances associated with disease processes affecting these nuclear masses. Two basic types of disturbances are seen: (1) various types of abnormal involuntary activity, referred to as dyskinesia, and (2) disturbances of muscle tone.

Structures forming the basal ganglia are the *caudate nucleus,* the *putamen,* the *globus pallidus* and the *amygdaloid nuclear complex* (Fig. 2-6). The amygdaloid nuclear complex, phylogenetically the oldest part of the basal ganglia, is known as the *archistriatum.* This complex nuclear mass lies in the medial part of the temporal lobe and has important connections with the olfactory system. The *paleostriatum* is represented by the two segments of the globus pallidus which lie lateral to the internal capsule. The *neostriatum,* the largest and newest component of the basal ganglia, consists of two structures which have partial continuity, the caudate nucleus and the putamen.

The *amygdaloid nuclear complex* receives fibers from the olfactory bulb and indirect impulses from the olfactory cortex. Efferent fibers from this complex project to the septal region and the hypothalamus via complex pathways. In spite of the rich olfactory connections, the amygdaloid complex does not seem to be closely related to olfactory sense or discrimination (Swann, 1934; Allen, 1941). Electrical stimulation of the amygdaloid complex in animals consistently produces visceral, somatic, behavioral and endocrine changes (Gloor, 1960). The most pronounced behavioral changes elicited in unanesthetized animals are reactions of fear and rage. Bilateral lesions confined to the amygdaloid complex mainly alter emotional behavior. Previously dominant and aggressive animals become tame, placid, and do not display reactions of fear, rage or hostility.

The *corpus striatum* is a large nuclear complex partially divided by fibers of the internal capsule into two cellular masses, the caudate nucleus and the lentiform nucleus. The *caudate nucleus* is an elongated C-shaped structure related throughout its extent to the surface of the lateral ventricle (Fig. 2–7). An enlarged anterior part of the caudate nucleus bulges into the anterior horn

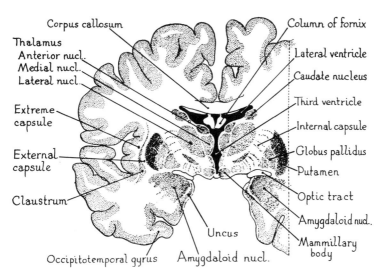

Figure 2–6 Drawing of a transverse section of the brain passing through the basal ganglia and diencephalon. The caudate nucleus lies lateral to the lateral ventricle, while the putamen and globus pallidus are lateral to the internal capsule. The amygdaloid nuclear complex underlies the uncus in the temporal lobe. (From Truex and Carpenter: *Human Neuroanatomy,* 1969. Reproduced by permission of the Williams and Wilkins Company, Baltimore, Md.)

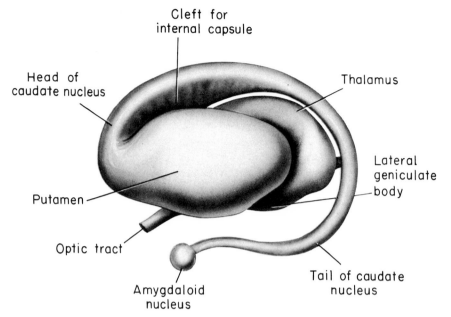

Figure 2–7 Schematic drawing of the isolated neostriatum showing relationships between the putamen and caudate nucleus, thalamus and caudate nucleus, and caudate nucleus and amygdaloid nucleus. (From Truex and Carpenter: *Human Neuroanatomy*, 1969. Reproduced by permission of the Williams and Wilkins Company, Baltimore, Md.)

of the lateral ventricle, while the body and tail of the caudate nucleus arch posteriorly to lie in the roof of the inferior horn of the lateral ventricle. The tail of the caudate nucleus is in continuity with the amygdaloid nuclear complex in the temporal lobe.

The *lentiform nucleus*, consisting of two separate parts, lies lateral to the internal capsule. The lateral part of the lentiform nucleus is the putamen, a large nuclear mass that is in continuity with the head of the caudate nucleus. The caudate nucleus and putamen are histologically the same and have similar connections. The medial part of the lentiform nucleus, formed by the globus pallidus, is grossly and microscopically distinctive from the neostriatum (i.e., the caudate nucleus and the putamen). The globus pallidus is smaller than the putamen, appears wedge-shaped in cross-section and consists of two parts, designated as the medial and lateral segments (Fig. 2-6).

Connections of the Neostriatum and Paleostriatum

The neostriatum receives projections from nearly all cortical areas, which are distributed in a systematic manner. Anterior regions of the cortex project to anterior parts of the neostriatum, and posterior regions show a similar correspondence. These fibers are referred to as *corticostriate fibers* (Webster, 1961, 1965; Carman, Cowan and Powell, 1963). There is no evidence that the globus pallidus receives fibers from the cortex. In addition to this large cortical projection, the neostriatum receives a large number of fibers from the intralaminar thalamic nuclei, designated as *thalamostriate fibers* (Fig. 2-8). Thalamostriate fibers are topographically organized (Powell and Cowan, 1956) and come from thalamic nuclei which have no cortical projection.

The neostriatum projects fibers medially and caudally to two structures, the globus pallidus and the substantia nigra. *Striopallidal fibers* from the putamen radiate into both pallidal segments like the spokes of a wheel (Nauta and Mehler, 1966; Szabo, 1967). Strionigral fibers pass caudally into the reticular zone of the substantia nigra, a large nuclear mass situated dorsal to the crus cerebri in the midbrain. The substantia nigra contains heavily pigmented cells and appears to be involved with great consistency in Parkinson's disease.

It is apparent from the preceding description that impulses from both the cerebral cortex and the thalamus are funneled into the neostriatum and then transmitted to the globus pallidus. The striatum appears to serve as the principal receptive center, while the globus pallidus gives rise to efferent fibers, most of which project back to specific relay thalamic nuclei.

Pallidofugal fibers are arranged in three principal bundles (Fig. 2-8). Fibers from the lateral pallidal segment project exclusively to the subthalamic nucleus, a small lens-shaped structure medial to the internal capsule and beneath the thalamus. Fibers from the medial pallidal segment primarily project to thalamic relay nuclei (i.e., the ventral lateral and ventral anterior thalamic nuclei). Because the globus pallidus borders on the lateral surface of the internal capsule, efferent fibers passing to the thalamus must either pass through or around the internal capsule to enter the thalamus. Different fiber bundles follow both of these courses. Fibers from dorsal parts of the medial pallidal segment traverse the internal capsule rostral to the subthalamic nucleus; this

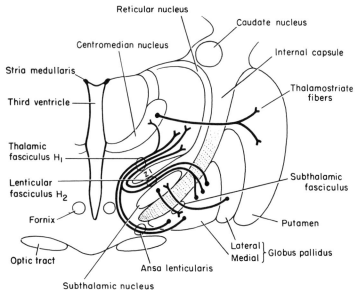

Figure 2-8 Schematic drawing in a transverse plane of pallidofugal fiber systems. Fibers of the lenticular fasciculus and ansa lenticularis arise from the medial pallidal segment and merge; these fibers pass in the thalamic fasciculus to the ventral anterior, ventrolateral and centromedian thalamic nuclei. Thalamostriate fibers also are indicated. (From Truex and Carpenter: *Human Neuroanatomy*, 1969. Reproduced by permission of the Williams and Wilkins Company, Baltimore, Md.)

bundle is referred to as the *lenticular fasciculus.* Fibers from ventral parts of the medial pallidal segment loop around the medial margin of the internal capsule; these fibers form the *ansa lenticularis.* Medial to the subthalamic nucleus fibers of the lenticular fasciculus and the ansa lenticularis merge and then pass laterally and rostrally to thalamic nuclei, as a component of the thalamic fasciculus. Most of these fibers pass to the lateral thalamic relay nuclei (i.e., the ventral lateral and ventral anterior thalamic nuclei), but a small number pass to the largest of the intralaminar thalamic nuclei (i.e., the centromedian nucleus).

From the above description it is apparent that the major output from the basal ganglia passes back to the thalamus (Fig. 2-9). Part of the thalamic input from the basal ganglia is in turn projected upon the motor cortex. A small part of the output of the globus pallidus projects downward to reach a small region in the midbrain reticular formation (i.e., the pedunculopontine nucleus). Except for this small descending bundle, there are no fibers that project to nuclei of the lower brain stem (Fig. 2-9).

Two other nuclear masses closely associated with the basal ganglia are of great importance. These nuclei are the subthalamic nucleus and the substantia nigra (Figs. 2-8 and 2-9). The *subthalamic nucleus* is a relatively small structure ventral to the thalamus, which lies next to the internal capsule. This nucleus receives fibers from the lateral pallidal segment and projects most of its fibers back through the internal capsule to the medial pallidal segment (Carpenter and Strominger, 1967; Carpenter, Fraser and Shriver, 1968).

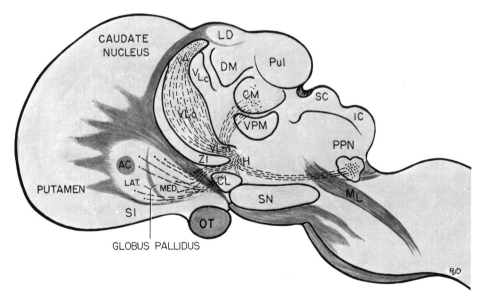

Figure 2–9 Schematic diagram of pallidofugal fibers in a sagittal plane. The principal pallidofugal fibers pass to the ventral anterior (VA), ventral lateral (VLo), and centromedian (CM) thalamic nuclei. Pallidotegmental fibers descend to terminate in the pedunculopontine nucleus (PPN). AC, anterior commissure; CL, subthalamic nucleus; DM, dorsomedial nucleus, thalamus; H, field H of Forel; IC, inferior colliculus; LD, laterodorsal nucleus, thalamus; ML, medial lemniscus; OT, optic tract; Pul, pulvinar; SC, superior colliculus; SI, substantia innominata; SN, substantia nigra; VLc, ventral lateral nucleus thalamus, pars caudalis; VLm, ventral lateral nucleus thalamus, pars medialis; VPM, ventral posterior medial nucleus thalamus; ZI, zona incerta. (From Truex and Carpenter: *Human Neuroanatomy,* 1969. Reproduced by permission of the Williams and Wilkins Company, Baltimore, Md.)

The *substantia nigra* is the largest single nuclear mass in the midbrain. It lies along the inner surface of the crus cerebri (Fig. 2-6). This nucleus consists of a *pars compacta*, located dorsally and containing large cells with melanin pigment. Beneath the pars compacta is the *pars reticularis*, which is rich in iron. The substantia nigra receives strionigral fibers, projects fibers to the thalamus and is rich in catecholamines. Biochemical data suggest that a biogenic amine, dopamine, may be transmitted to the putamen via nerve terminals (Andén, Carlsson, Dahlström, Fuxe, Hillarp and Larsson, 1964; Fuxe and Andén, 1966).

Neural Mechanisms of the Basal Ganglia

The physiological mechanisms involved in the contributions of the basal ganglia to motor functions are not known. While there is evidence suggesting that the neostriatum is concerned with inhibitory activities and the globus pallidus with excitatory functions, considerable data are fragmentary, inconclusive and sometimes contradictory. With one notable exception it has not been possible to reproduce the same kinds of dyskinesia in animals as occur in man as a consequence of disease processes (Carpenter, 1961). This may be because most of the disease processes that affect the basal ganglia are widespread. The types of dyskinesia occurring with these diseases are categorized as tremor, athetosis, dystonia, chorea and ballism.

Tremor is a rhythmical, alternating, abnormal, involuntary activity of relatively regular frequency and amplitude. The kind of tremor associated with diseases of the basal ganglia is typified by that present in Parkinson's disease. This is a fine, small amplitude tremor present at rest, which disappears during voluntary movements. The tremor is present in the digits, the lips and sometimes in the head. This tremor, like all abnormal involuntary movements, is exaggerated by situations in which the patient becomes self-conscious, anxious or emotionally excited.

Athetosis is a term used to designate a form of dyskinesia characterized by slow, writhing, vermicular, involuntary movements that involve particularly the extremities, the face and the cervical musculature. These movements give the appearance of a mobile spasm. *Dystonia* is considered as a form of athetosis (Jakob, 1925; Alexander, 1942), which involves primarily the axial musculature. Involuntary contractions of axial muscle masses result in torsion spasms and bizarre distortions of the trunk. Athetosis and dystonia usually occur together (Carpenter, 1950).

Chorea is an abnormal involuntary activity characterized by brisk graceful movements that resemble fragments of purposeful movements. Choreoid movements involve primarily the distal portions of the extremities, the facial muscles and the muscles of the tongue. While choreoid activity occurs as a consequence of a number of different disease processes, it is most commonly seen as a sequel to acute rheumatic fever (i.e., Sydenham's chorea) or in a hereditary form (Huntington's chorea).

Ballism is the term used to designate violent, forceful, flinging movements involving primarily the proximal appendicular musculature and muscles about the shoulder and pelvic girdles. This form of dyskinesia, usually unilateral, is referred to as hemiballism. This is the only form of dyskinesia commonly associated with a small, discrete lesion. The lesion most commonly present is hemorrhagic destruction of the subthalamic nucleus contralateral to the dyskinesia.

While athetosis, chorea and ballism each possess distinctive features, their common characteristics suggest that they may form a spectrum of choreoid activity in which athetosis and ballism represent the extreme forms. The slow, writhing character of athetosis may be due to the fact that it occurs in association with varying degrees of paresis and spasticity. In chorea and ballism the forceful, brisk nature of the dyskinesia may in part be due to the marked hypotonus that is almost invariably present.

Tremor of the type seen in parkinsonism is distinctive and may bear close relationship to the tremor present in cerebellar disease. The major clinical criterion used to distinguish cerebellar tremor from the tremor commonly seen in parkinsonism is based upon whether the tremor occurs "at rest" or "during movement." While great importance is attached to this difference, it may not always be clear-cut, because tremor "at rest" and tremor "during movement" sometimes occur together, in association with pathological processes involving either the basal ganglia or the cerebellum. One other feature of parkinsonism that is of great importance is the rigidity of the muscles, which frequently is the initial symptom and which gradually increases over a period of years. This increase in muscle tone is not selective but involves both flexor and extensor muscle groups. This rigidity can be easily demonstrated by passively flexing and extending the extremities or by attempting to rotate the hand at the wrist in a circular fashion. These movements are interrupted by a series of jerks, referred to as cog-wheel phenomena. Parkinsonism also is characterized by what have been called negative symptoms. These symptoms, regarded as neural deficits, largely concern postural fixation, locomotion, phonation and speech. Patients with parkinsonism exhibit a masklike face, infrequent blinking of the eyes, a stooped posture with flexion of the neck and knees, a slow shuffling gait, loss of associated movements in walking and slow dysarthric speech.

The various types of dyskinesia and excesses of muscle tone associated with diseases of the basal ganglia are regarded as positive disturbances because their existence must depend upon excess neural activity and the expenditure of energy (Martin, 1959). Since disturbances of this nature cannot be due to neural structures which are destroyed, they must represent functional properties of intact neural structures operating in an abnormal or excessive manner. It has been suggested that the excessive function probably results from the removal of controlling or inhibitory influences. Thus, a lesion in one neural structure may lead to overactivity in another by removing the normal restraining influences. This relatively simple thesis suggests that most forms of dyskinesia are the physiological expression of release phenomena. This thesis forms the basis of most neurosurgical attempts to alleviate or abolish dyskinesia and excesses of muscle tone.

The circuitry described earlier would suggest that lesions produced in either the globus pallidus or particular relay nuclei of the thalamus could prevent impulses from the basal ganglia from reaching the motor cortex.

Experimental studies (Carpenter, 1961) and clinical experience (Spiegel and Wycis, 1954, 1958; Martin and McCaul, 1959; Cooper, 1960) have substantiated this concept. Lesions produced in either the medial segment of the globus pallidus or the ventral lateral nucleus of the thalamus can ameliorate most forms of dyskinesia contralaterally. Lesions in the ventral lateral nucleus of the thalamus appear to be most successful in reducing tremor, while lesions in the globus pallidus are particularly effective in relieving contralateral rigidity in parkinsonism. The fact that most forms of dyskinesia can also be abolished by lesions of the motor cortex or the corticospinal tract suggests that the outflow from the basal ganglia must ultimately reach the motor cortex and that impulses concerned with various forms of dyskinesia must be transmitted to spinal levels via the corticospinal tract. The fact that the corticospinal tract is largely crossed probably explains why these disturbances occur contralaterally.

Recent studies (Hornykiewicz, 1966) suggest that parkinsonism may be due to a deficiency of brain dopamine. Dopamine is an intermediate product in the metabolic pathway leading to the biosynthesis of norepinephrine. Most of the dopamine of the brain is found in the neostriatum and in the substantia nigra. Biochemical analysis of the brains of patients with parkinsonism has revealed the virtual absence of dopamine in both the striatum and substantia nigra. This finding suggests that in parkinsonism a decreased ability of the affected tissues to form dopamine probably exists. It is assumed that the striatal dopamine is contained mainly in nigrostriatal nerve fiber terminals. This thesis is consistent with neuropathological observations which indicate that degeneration of the large cells of the substantia nigra is commonly found in parkinsonism, particularly in the postencephalitic type. Neurophysiological observations suggest that the most consistent effect of dopamine upon the activity of single brain neurons is one of inhibition. Biochemical and clinical evidence suggests that a close relationship exists between the dopamine deficiency and the clinical symptomatology of parkinsonism. Because dopamine cannot pass the blood-brain barrier, artificial replacement of dopamine is accomplished by giving its immediate precursor, L-dopa. L-Dopa can cross the blood-brain barrier and is converted to dopamine within the brain. There is considerable evidence suggesting that L-dopa can bring about a reversal of many of the disturbances associated with parkinsonism (Yahr, Duvoisin, Schear, Barrett and Hoehn, 1969).

It is of interest that in other diseases of the basal ganglia characterized by different forms of dyskinesia the concentrations of dopamine in the striatum and substantia nigra are within normal limits. If these distinctive syndromes have a biochemical basis, it would seem to be different from that underlying parkinsonism.

REFERENCES

1. Alexander, L.: The fundamental types of histopathologic changes encountered in cases of athetosis and paralysis agitans. Res. Publ. Assoc. Nerv. Ment. Dis., *21*:334–493, 1942.
2. Allen, W. F.: Effect of ablating the pyriform-amygdaloid areas and hippocampi on positive and negative olfactory conditioned reflexes and on conditioned olfactory differentiation. Am. J. Physiol., *132*:81–92, 1941.
3. Andén, N.-E., Carlsson, A., Dahlström, A., Fuxe, K., Hillarp, N.-Å. and Larsson, K.: Demonstration and mapping out of nigro-neostriatal dopamine neurons. Life Sci., *3*:523–530, 1964.

4. Brodal, A.: Afferent cerebellar connections. *In:* Jansen, J. and Brodal, A. (eds.): *Aspects of Cerebellar Anatomy.* Oslo, J. G. Tanum, 1954, pp. 82–188.
5. Brodal, A. and Høivik, B.: Site and mode of termination of primary vestibulocerebellar fibres in the cat. An experimental study with silver impregnation methods. Arch. Ital. Biol., *102*:1-21, 1964.
6. Carman, J. B., Cowan, W. M. and Powell, T. P. S.: The organization of cortico-striate connexions in the rabbit. Brain, *86*:525-562, 1963.
7. Carpenter, M. B.: Athetosis and the basal ganglia. Arch. Neurol. Psychiat., *63*:875-901, 1950.
8. Carpenter, M. B.: Brain stem and infratentorial neuraxis in experimental dyskinesia. Arch. Neurol., *5*:504-524, 1961.
9. Carpenter, M. B., Fraser, R. A. R. and Shriver, J. E.: The organization of pallidosubthalamic fibers in the monkey. Brain Res., *11*:522-559, 1968.
10. Carpenter, M. B. and Strominger, N. L.: Efferent fibers of the subthalamic nucleus in the monkey; a comparison of the efferent projections of the subthalamic nucleus, substantia nigra and globus pallidus. Am. J. Anat., *121*:41-72, 1967.
11. Combs, C. M.: Bulbar regions related to localized cerebellar afferent impulses. J. Neurophysiol., *19*:285-300, 1956.
12. Cooper, I. S.: Results of 1,000 consecutive basal ganglia operations for parkinsonism. Ann. Intern. Med., *52*:483-499, 1960.
13. Courville, J.: Somatotopical organization of the projection from the nucleus interpositus anterior of the cerebellum to the red nucleus. An experimental study in the cat with silver impregnation methods. Exp. Brain Res. (Berlin), *2*:191-215, 1966.
14. Eccles, J. C., Ito, M. and Szentágothai, J.: *The Cerebellum as a Neuronal Machine.* New York, Springer-Verlag, 1967.
15. Fulton, J. F.: *Functional Localization in the Frontal Lobes and Cerebellum.* Oxford, Clarendon Press, 1949.
16. Fuxe, K. and Andén, N.-E.: Studies on central monoamine neurons with special reference to the nigro-neostriatal dopamine neuron system. *In:* Costa E., Côté, L. J. and Yahr, M. D. (eds.): *Biochemistry and Pharmacology of the Basal Ganglia.* Proceedings of the Second Symposium of the Parkinson's Disease Information and Research Center, College of Physicians and Surgeons, Columbia University, 1965. Hewlett, N.Y., Raven Press, 1966, pp. 123–129.
17. Gloor, P.: Amygdala. *In:* J. Field (ed.): *Handbook of Physiology.* Washington, American Physiological Society, 1960, Sect. 1, Vol. 2, pp. 1395-1420.
18. Hámori, J. and Szentágothai, J.: Identification under the electron microscope of climbing fibers and their synaptic contacts. Exp. Brain Res. (Berlin), *1*:65-81, 1966.
19. Hornykiewicz, O.: Metabolism of brain dopamine in human parkinsonism: neurochemical and clinical aspects. *In:* Costa, E., Côté, L. J. and Yahr, M. D. (eds.): *Biochemistry and Pharmacology of the Basal Ganglia.* Proceedings of the Second Symposium of the Parkinson's Disease Information and Research Center, College of Physicians and Surgeons, Columbia University, 1965. Hewlett, N.Y., Raven Press, 1966, pp. 171-185.
20. Ito, M. and Yoshida, M.: The cerebellar-evoked monosynaptic inhibition of Deiters' neurones. Experientia, *20*:515-516, 1964.
21. Ito, M., Yoshida, M. and Obata. K.: Monosynaptic inhibition of the intracerebellar nuclei induced from the cerebellar cortex. Experientia, *20*:575-576, 1964.
22. Jakob, A.: The anatomy, clinical syndromes and physiology of the extrapyramidal system. Arch. Neurol. Psychiat., *13*:596-620, 1925.
23. Martin, J. P.: Remarks on the functions of the basal ganglia. Lancet, *1*:999-1005, 1959.
24. Martin, J. P. and McCaul, I. R.: Acute hemiballismus treated by ventrolateral thalamolysis. Brain, *82*:104-108, 1959.
25. Massion, J.: The mammalian red nucleus. Physiol. Rev., *47*:383-436, 1967.
26. Mettler, F. A. and Lubin, A. J.: Termination of the brachium pontis. J. Comp. Neurol., *77*:391-397, 1942.
27. Nauta, W. J. H. and Mehler, W. R.: Projections of the lentiform nucleus in the monkey. Brain Res., *1*:3-42, 1966.
28. Oscarsson, O.: Functional organization of the spino- and cuneocerebellar tracts. Physiol. Rev., *45*:495-522, 1965.
29. Powell, T. P. S. and Cowan, W. M.: A study of thalamo-striate relations in the monkey. Brain, *79*:364-390, 1956.
30. Sherrington, C. S.: Decerebrate rigidity and reflex coordination of movements. J. Physiol. (London), *22*:319-332, 1898.
31. Snider, R. S.: Recent contributions to the anatomy and physiology of the cerebellum. Arch. Neurol. Psychiat., *64*:196-219, 1950.

32. Spiegel, E. A. and Wycis, H. T.: Ansotomy in paralysis agitans. Arch. Neurol. Psychiat., *71*:598-614, 1954.
33. Spiegel, E. A. and Wycis, H. T.: Pallido-ansotomy: anatomic-physiologic foundation and histopathologic control. *In*: Fields, W. S. (ed.): *Pathogenesis and Treatment of Parkinsonism.* Springfield, Ill., Charles C Thomas, 1958, pp. 86-105.
34. Swann, H. G.: The function of the brain in olfaction. II. The results of destruction of olfactory and nervous structures upon the discrimination of odors. J. Comp. Neurol., *59*:175-201, 1934.
35. Szabo, J.: The efferent projections of the putamen in the monkey. Exp. Neurol., *19*:463-476, 1967.
36. Truex, R. C. and Carpenter, M. B.: *Human Neuroanatomy*, 6th ed. Baltimore, Williams and Wilkins Company, 1969.
37. Walberg, F., Pompeiano, O., Brodal, A. and Jansen, J.: The fastigiovestibular projection in the cat; an experimental study with silver impregnation methods. J. Comp. Neurol., *118*:49-75, 1962.
38. Webster, K. E.: Cortico-striate interrelations in the albino rat. J. Anat. (London), *95*:532-544, 1961.
39. Webster, K. E.: The cortico-striatal projection in the cat. J. Anat. (London), *99*:329-337, 1965.
40. Wilson, S. A. K. *Modern Problems in Neurology.* London, Edward Arnold & Co., 1928.
41. Yahr, M. D., Duvoisin, R. C., Schear, M. J., Barrett, R. E. and Hoehn, M. M.: Treatment of parkinsonism with levodopa. Arch. Neurol., *21*:343-354, 1969.

Chapter 3

GAMMA NERVOUS SYSTEM AND MUSCLE SPINDLES

by Hyman I. C. Dubo, M.D., and Robert C. Darling, M.D.

HISTORICAL REVIEW

Voluminous literature has accumulated regarding the mammalian muscle spindle and its nervous control.[28] This chapter will trace the highlights of the discoveries which have led to an ever increasing knowledge of the anatomical and functional significance of that structure, which Hassall first described in 1851 as "groups of little muscle fibers situated within skeletal muscle."[22] Kuhne coined the term "muscle spindle" in 1861, in recognition of its shape. The muscle spindle was thought to be a center of muscle regeneration until 1888, when Kirschner suggested that the spindles functioned as sensory endings. The first histologic proof of this was established by Ruffini in 1892, when he demonstrated the presence of nerve endings of two distinct types arising from the muscle spindle.[30] In 1894, Sherrington traced the fibers into the dorsal roots and proved that the muscle spindle was a sensory end organ with an afferent nerve supply.[35] Over the next 40 years, Sherrington and others developed the concept of the stretch reflex,[34] and in 1930, Eccles and Sherrington demonstrated that the muscle spindle also had a motor component. The significance of this innervation was unknown until Leksell in 1945 studied the gamma motor innervation to the spindle by stimulating the small motor fibers in the ventral root of the spinal cord, and observed a consequent afferent discharge from the spindle.[26] It became clear that the spindle is a sensory structure and also that its underdeveloped contractile elements (intrafusal muscle fibers) respond to gamma motor nerve stimulus, which in turn stimulates, by stretch, the sensory elements.

In 1956, Boyd, working with the cat,[3] and Cooper and Daniel, working with man,[7] described two morphologically distinct types of intrafusal muscle fibers within the spindle. Boyd and others proposed the presence of separate sensory and motor fibers innervating each type of intrafusal muscle fiber in the spindle.[3,7] In 1962, Jansen and Matthews provided a physiological basis for this morphological dual arrangement when they showed one system to have dynamic and the other static properties.[23]

STRUCTURE OF THE MUSCLE SPINDLE

Muscle spindles are small, fusiform, intramuscular structures distributed parallel to skeletal muscle fibers in the interfascicular connective tissue. They have an independent innervation and an independent vascular supply.

Spindle counts, which have been made in various muscles, range from 43 to 57 spindles per muscle. The soleus of the cat has 50 spindles, 45 Golgi tendon organs and 25,000 extrafusal muscle fibers. There are no spindles in the extrinsic eye muscles of the cat, dog, rabbit or horse, but they are present in man and in the ape, goat, and sheep. Respiratory muscle spindles are of special interest functionally and will be discussed later.

The muscle spindle has a thick outer connective tissue sheath, which expands at the equator of the spindle into a fluid-filled sac, called the lymph space.

As seen in Figure 3-1, two types of intrafusal muscle fibers are found in a typical mammalian muscle spindle,[3,7] a nuclear bag fiber and a nuclear chain fiber. These are differentiated by the arrangement of their nuclei, by the

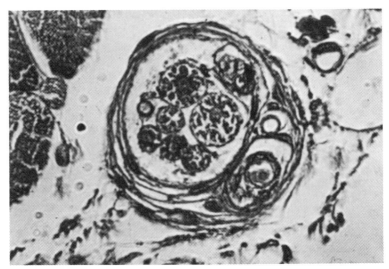

Figure 3–1 Cross section of a muscle spindle of the cat near the end of the lymph space. Within the sheath there are two large nuclear bag intrafusal muscle fibers, four small nuclear chain intrafusal fibers and several axons. Extrafusal muscle fibers can be seen in the left upper corner of the photograph. (From Boyd, I. A., Eyzaguirre, C., Matthews, P. B. C. and Rushworth, G.: The role of the gamma system in movement and posture. Association For The Aid of Crippled Children, New York, 1968.

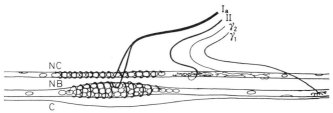

Figure 3–2 Schematic diagram of a muscle spindle, showing nuclear bag and nuclear chain intrafusal muscle fibers and their innervation. *C*, capsule of muscle spindle; *NC*, nuclear chain intrafusal muscle fiber with its single chain of nuclei; *NB*, nuclear bag intrafusal muscle fiber with its dilated bag of nuclei. Group Ia afferent nerve fiber, with its primary ending, divides to innervate both nuclear bag and nuclear chain intrafusal muscle fibers. Group II afferent nerve fiber, with its secondary ending, innervates the nuclear chain intrafusal and rarely the nuclear bag type. A gamma 1 fusimotor fiber is shown innervating the nuclear bag intrafusal. A gamma 2 fusimotor fiber is shown innervating the nuclear chain intrafusal. (From Rushworth, G.: The nature and management of spasticity. Proc. Roy. Soc. Med., 57:715, 1964.)

differences in size and length of the intrafusal fibers and by the degree of atrophy following denervation.

In the nuclear chain type, the nuclei are present in linear arrangement, forming a single row at the equatorial region. In the nuclear bag type, the nuclei are bunched together at the equatorial region, forming a dilated clump or bag (Fig. 3-2). Nuclear bag intrafusals are approximately twice the diameter (25 microns versus 12 microns) and twice the length (8 mm versus 4 mm) of nuclear chain intrafusal fibers. Typically, there are two nuclear bag fibers and four nuclear chain fibers in each cat spindle, but there may be considerable variation from spindle to spindle. In man, there are as many as 10 intrafusal fibers, the ratio of nuclear chain to nuclear bag being 2:1. The total length of a spindle is 7 or 8 mm, with the smaller nuclear chain fibers tapering out on the surface of the nuclear bag fibers. The nuclear bag intrafusal fibers are arranged parallel to the extrafusal muscle fibers. This is important in order to understand function; it contrasts with the Golgi tendon organs, which lie in series with the extrafusal muscle fibers. During active contraction of the extrafusal muscle fibers, the muscle spindle is unloaded and "silenced" because it lies parallel to the contracting fibers, while the Golgi tendon organ is activated because it lies in series.

Following denervation of the muscle spindle by cutting the ventral roots, atrophy of the nuclear chain and nuclear bag intrafusal fibers occurs at different rates.[3] Within three months of denervation, the nuclear bag fibers undergo slight atrophy, compared to severe atrophy of the nuclear chain fibers. The reason for the difference is not clear, but it is further evidence in support of the separation of intrafusal muscle fibers into two distinct morphological entities.

Histochemical studies of the intrafusal fibers in man have not demonstrated distinct enzymatic differences between the nuclear chain and nuclear bag types.[36] The histochemical reactions for oxidative enzymes, glycogen, phosphorylase and lipids in both the nuclear bag and nuclear chain fibers are similar. A difference between the two types of fibers is shown only with the

ATPase reaction; the chain fibers stain darkly, and the bag fibers stain lightly. The intrafusal fiber histochemical reactions are not the same as those of either the Type I or Type II extrafusal fibers, and this may indicate differences in the metabolic mechanisms.

Microscopically, striations are evident along the entire length of the intrafusal muscle fibers of both types, except in the noncontractile equatorial region (nuclear region). Electron microscopic studies of mammalian (including human) spindles have demonstrated a miniature A-I band pattern similar to extrafusal skeletal muscle.[21]

INNERVATION OF THE MUSCLE SPINDLE

The spindle is richly endowed with nerves, which can be divided into two distinct types.

Afferent or Sensory Innervation

The sensory endings arising from the spindle are of two types, primary and secondary.[3, 7, 25] Each spindle has only one primary sensory ending, which is found at the equatorial region and which is wound around the intrafusal fibers in the form of a spiral, hence the old term of "annulospiral ending" (Fig. 3-2). There is one spiral around each intrafusal fiber of both the bag and chain types. A branch from each spiral connects the ending to the stem axon. All the axons leading from the primary endings come together to form the Group Ia sensory afferent nerve, which passes through the dorsal root to the spinal cord.

The secondary endings are situated primarily on nuclear chain intrafusal muscle fibers and lie close to the primary ending, but spread out on either side of it in a ramification resembling a flower spray (Fig. 3-2). It is not always easy to distinguish primary and secondary endings by shape alone, especially in man; also, the location on the intrafusal fiber has to be considered. There are from one to five secondary endings per muscle spindle, and these combine to form Group II afferent nerve fibers, which enter the spinal cord via the dorsal root.

The classification of dorsal root fibers into Group Ia and Group II is based upon fiber size and stimulation threshold. Group Ia fibers are larger, conduct more rapidly and have a lower threshold to stimulation than do Group II fibers.

Motor or Efferent Innervation

One-third of the motor fibers in the ventral root of the spinal cord are small motor fibers destined for the muscle spindles. These fibers are of the gamma subgroup of A group motor axons and are smaller and conduct more slowly than do the axons to extrafusal muscle fibers, which are of the alpha subgroup. The fusimotor axons or gamma fibers can be further subdivided into two groups (gamma 1 and gamma 2) on the basis of nerve cross-sectional size, type of motor terminal ending, threshold stimulation and conduction velocity differences.[3, 4] Gamma 1 fusimotor fibers, as they approach the spindle, are larger (3–4 microns) in diameter than gamma 2 fibers (0.5 to 1 micron). Gamma 1 fibers end in discrete motor end plates and appear to be miniature replicas of motor end plates of alpha nerve fibers ending on extrafusal muscle fibers. Gamma 2 fiber endings terminate in a more diffuse ramification of nerve strands, trailing along the surface of the intrafusal muscle fiber. Thus, gamma 1 fibers are often called "plate endings," and gamma 2, "trail endings."

Initially it was believed that the gamma 1 plate endings terminated only on nuclear bag intrafusals and gamma 2 trail endings on nuclear chain intrafusal muscle fibers. However, it is now known that gamma 1 plate endings may innervate nuclear chain intrafusals and gamma 2 trail endings may innervate nuclear bag intrafusals. In some cases, both gamma 1 and gamma 2 endings may innervate the same intrafusal type of fiber. Some motor axons have been found to branch and innervate both the extrafusal and intrafusal muscle fibers. These have been termed beta fibers.[2, 25] Not all spindles show the beta fiber type of motor innervation, and its functional significance is unknown.

The similarity of the gamma nerves to other motor nerves is emphasized by the fact that cholinesterase activity is found along the length of the intrafusal fibers, except for the sensory equatorial region.

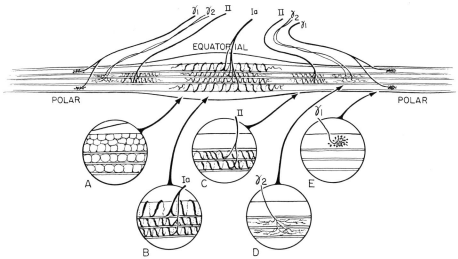

Figure 3–3 Schematic summary of the dual structure and innervation of the mammalian muscle spindle. Inset A (from above downwards): capsule, lymph space, one nuclear bag fiber, two nuclear chain fibers (in a typical spindle there is a ratio of two chain fibers to one bag fiber). Inset B: Sensory nerve fibers originating from intrafusal fibers of both bag and chain type unite to form a single primary sensory ending of the Group Ia afferent nerve. (Each spindle is innervated by only one primary ending which is located at the equatorial region.) Inset C: Secondary sensory endings originate predominantly from nuclear chain intrafusals and unite to form Group II afferent nerves. There may be up to five secondary endings per spindle. They are located on either side of the primary ending between the equatorial and polar regions of the intrafusal muscle fibers. Inset D: Trail endings of a Gamma 2 fusimotor fiber innervating a nuclear chain intrafusal muscle fiber. Inset E.: Plate ending of a Gamma 1 fusimotor fiber innervating a nuclear bag intrafusal. There may be many fusimotor gamma fibers located along the polar regions of each muscle spindle. (Modified from: Roberts, T. D. M.: Neurophysiology of Postural Mechanisms, page 82. Butterworths, London, 1967.)

In summary, the muscle spindle and its nervous innervation can be divided into two distinct systems, consisting of two types of intrafusal muscle fibers, nuclear chain and nuclear bag; two types of sensory endings, primary and secondary; two types of sensory nerves, Group Ia and Group II; two types of motor nerves, gamma 1 and gamma 2; and two types of motor endings, plate and trail. Figure 3-3 is a schematic summary of the dual structure and innervation of the muscle spindle.

Teleologically, one might expect that each component of this dual system would have a different function, and physiological evidence has been accumulating to support this concept.

CORRELATION OF SPINDLE STRUCTURE AND FUNCTION

There are two types of afferent discharges from the muscle spindle, dynamic (phasic) and static (tonic). A dynamic discharge is one which responds to a stimulus with a brief, unsustained, but rapidly conducting high frequency impulse. A static discharge is one which responds to a stimulus by sustained, repetitive impulses which long outlast the original stimulus.

The structural components of the muscle spindle can also be separated physiologically into a dynamic and a static system. The primary sensory ending gives both a dynamic and a static response to stretch.[23] The dynamic portion of the primary ending arises from the nuclear bag intrafusals and is sensitive to the rate of change of intrafusal muscle length during stretching. The static portion of the primary ending is located on nuclear chain intrafusals and is sensitive to change in length of the fiber, irrespective of the rate at which the length is changed. Both the dynamic and static discharges arising from the

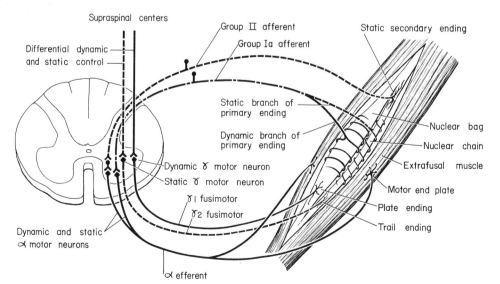

Figure 3—4 Structural separation of the muscle spindle and gamma system into dynamic and static components. The dynamic pathways through the spindle loop (alpha-gamma linkage) are depicted by the solid lines and the static pathways by the broken lines. The Group Ia afferent is shown with dots to emphasize that it is both a dynamic and a static pathway.

TABLE 3–1 THE DYNAMIC AND STATIC COMPONENTS OF THE
MUSCLE SPINDLE AND THE GAMMA SYSTEM

Dynamic	Static
Gamma 1 motoneuron	Gamma 2 motoneuron
Gamma 1 fusimotor fiber	Gamma 2 fusimotor fiber
Plate ending	Trail ending
Nuclear bag intrafusal fiber	Nuclear chain intrafusal fiber
Primary sensory ending	Primary sensory ending
(Portion arising from nuclear bag intrafusal fiber)	(Portion arising from nuclear chain intrafusal fiber)
	Secondary sensory ending
Group Ia afferent* fiber	Group Ia afferent* fiber
	Group II afferent fiber
Dynamic alpha motoneuron	Static alpha motoneuron

*Group Ia afferent fiber transmits both dynamic and static impulses from primary endings.

primary ending of each spindle are transmitted centrally along Group Ia afferent nerves.

Secondary endings situated on nuclear chain intrafusals, on the other hand, behave in a static fashion and, like the static primary ending, are sensitive only to changes in length.[8] The static discharges from secondary endings are transmitted centrally along Group II afferent nerves.

The dynamic and static sensitivity of the primary sensory ending and the static sensitivity of the secondary sensory ending may be controlled independently by the central nervous system via the gamma fusimotor fibers.[27]

The two functionally distinct fusimotor nerve fiber types provide separate dynamic and static motor pathways to the spindle; the dynamic fusimotor fibers correspond to the gamma 1 fibers, and the static fusimotor fibers correspond to the gamma 2 fibers.[27]

Figure 3–4 and Table 3–1 illustrate the separate dynamic and static pathways that indirectly link alpha and gamma motoneurons through the spindle loop. It seems reasonable to make this separation on the basis of present evidence in order to simplify thinking on the subject, but it is certain that the two systems do not operate in isolation. Work is necessary to clarify further the integration of the dynamic and static components of the muscle spindle and gamma system and their influence on the alpha motoneuron.

The gamma 1 and gamma 2 motoneurons are under the influence of higher supraspinal centers. Specific pathways have not yet been elucidated, but there is evidence that the dynamic and static gamma fusimotor fibers are influenced differentially by various centers in the brain. For example, stimulation of the red nucleus facilitates the dynamic and inhibits the static discharge response of a primary sensory nerve ending.

ALPHA-GAMMA LINKAGE

The neurons of the gamma motor fibers lie in the grey matter of the spinal cord in close proximity to the alpha motoneurons innervating the same skeletal muscle, although no direct synapse exists between them in the spinal cord. The alpha-gamma linkage is indirect, occurring around the muscle spindle loop (Fig. 3-4).

Unlike the alpha motoneurons, the gamma motoneurons do not have direct monosynaptic connections from dorsal root fibers but can be reflexly facilitated or inhibited by complex polysynaptic pathways, which have not as yet been clearly elucidated. The threshold for excitation of gamma motoneurons is usually lower than for alpha motoneurons. With naturally occurring contractions of the extrafusal fibers, the gamma motoneurons are activated first, followed by the muscle spindle afferent discharge and, finally, by activation of the alpha motoneurons.

The beliefs that voluntary movements are primarily under alpha motoneuron control via direct connections with higher centers and that gamma motoneurons are involved mainly in slow postural activities are no longer valid. Much evidence has accumulated to show that the indirect route of the gamma system and muscle spindle plays a definite, it not prime, role in motor function.[5, 16, 17, 18, 28]

The gamma system acts as an ignition mechanism in initiating voluntary movement, as well as working to maintain reflex muscle tone and posture. In addition, it improves the performance of the spindle afferents as a sense organ by increasing the sensitivity of the primary and secondary endings to stretch.

The linkage of the alpha and gamma motoneurons via the muscle spindle loop acts as a servomechanism. A servomechanism is defined as an automatic control system that is activated by an error signal occurring in a closed loop control cycle, and which possesses power amplification. Thus, the gamma fusimotor impulses cause the intrafusals of the spindle to contract to a definite desired length, and the extrafusal fibers are forced to follow suit by the subsequent stretch reflex. The spindle is also a sense organ, able to detect differences in both the length and rate of change in length, between the intrafusal and extrafusal muscles. Thus, a length setting or gamma bias exists, making the spindle a zero point recorder of extrafusal length. Activation of the gamma system to the spindle facilitates an afferent discharge from the muscle spindle, which activates alpha motoneurons to initiate an extrafusal muscle contraction. When the desired shortening is achieved, the spindle becomes silent. In this manner, extrafusal muscle length will oscillate around the zero point set by the gamma bias. By means of automatic servomechanism adjustments within the stretch reflex loop, the central nervous system is relieved of much of the work of continuous precise involvement in producing or modifying a desired motor response.

It seems reasonable to discuss further the function of the muscle spindle and gamma system in terms of dynamic and static components. It must be understood, however, that the dynamic and static systems are not divorced from each other or from central control mechanisms.

ROLE OF MUSCLE SPINDLE PRIMARY ENDINGS

Primary endings (dynamic and static portions) have monosynaptic connections with alpha motoneurons of the same muscle via Group Ia sensory fibers and also with the alpha motoneurons of the synergist and antagonist muscles. These interconnections provide a mechanism for the facilitation of the agonist and synergist muscles, with simultaneous inhibition of the antagonist muscles at the moment when this is necessary to provide a smooth, coordinated voluntary movement. This coordinating mechanism, present at the spinal cord level, is not available if the alpha motoneuron is stimulated by any other means than Group Ia afferent fibers from the primary endings of the muscle spindles.

Another function of the primary ending is to provide a damping mechanism for the stretch reflex. The dynamic primary ending senses the rate of muscle length change by means of the fast conducting impulses, which reach the spinal cord and higher centers before the stretch is completed. This enables a prediction of the length change of the muscle after the delay time of the reflex, ensuring that future motor response will be appropriate to the time at which the reflex becomes effective, rather than to the time at which the reflex was initiated. This prevents oscillation of the stretch reflex and ensures smooth, voluntary motor control.

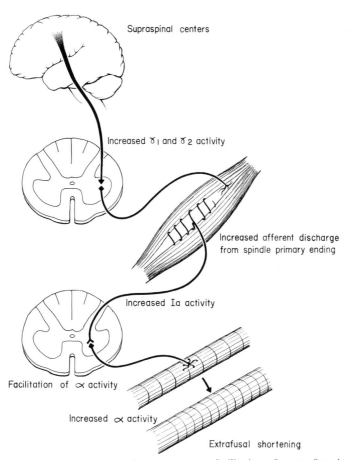

Figure 3−5 Schematic summary of gamma system facilitation of motor function. Control of extrafusal length is mediated through the spindle loop servomechanism. See text for discussion. (Modified from Eldred, E.: Functional implications of dynamic and static components of the spindle response to stretch. Am. J. Phys. Med., *46*:134, 1967.)

There is a large afferent projection of information to the cerebellum derived from the primary endings of the muscle spindles. In this way, the primary endings are capable of informing the central nervous system as to the length and rate of change in length of skeletal muscles at any given instant during steady-state contraction and voluntary movement.

The cerebellum has efferent connecting tracts through which the gamma system can be facilitated or inhibited. The cerebellum also has connecting tracts with the cerebral cortex and most other supraspinal centers, and it acts to integrate and regulate the sensory information it receives. This information is important in initiating and controlling the coordination of voluntary movement.

Some direct facilitation of alpha motoneurons occurs from supraspinal centers without involving the muscle spindle loop. The ratio of the direct alpha control to indirect gamma control of voluntary movement is controversial. However, there is no doubt that the gamma pathway does play an important role.

The primary ending innervates both nuclear bag and nuclear chain intrafusals, and is under the influence of both dynamic gamma 1 and static gamma

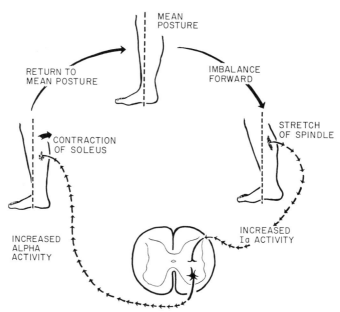

Figure 3−6   Illustration of a mechanism of maintaining body balance. Stretch of the muscle spindle elicits a stretch reflex which aids in regulation of posture. The role of the gastroc-soleus spindles is illustrated. In normal relaxed standing, the line of gravity passes behind the hip joint, in front of the knee joint and in front of the ankle joint. Electromyographic studies have shown that all extrafusal muscles of the lower extremities are silent during normal relaxed standing. The body is supported solely by ligaments and mechanical stabilization of joints. An imbalance forward leads to displacement of the line of gravity with resultant stretch of spindles in the gastroc-soleus muscle. This elicits a stretch reflex through the spindle loop with resultant contraction of the gastroc-soleus muscle group and return to the original posture. (From Eldred, E.: Functional implications of dynamic and static components of the spindle response to stretch. Am. J. Phys. Med., 46:130, 1967.)

2 fusimotor drives.[1, 24] The alpha-gamma linkage is monosynaptically completed along Group Ia afferents.

Figure 3-5 depicts the facilitation of movement initiated by the gamma system through changes in the servo loop mechanism. Supraspinal centers send impulses to the gamma motoneurons. These in turn send impulses down the gamma fusimotor fibers to the intrafusal muscle fibers of the spindle, initiating contraction. This puts tension on the primary ending, which discharges impulses along the Group Ia afferent fibers. The increased Group Ia activity monosynaptically facilitates the alpha motoneurons, producing increased alpha activity. This causes extrafusal muscle shortening. The gamma bias has in this way forced the extrafusal muscle to contract. Thus, extrafusal muscle length is controlled by gamma system drive. The ratio of dynamic to static involvement in this servo control mechanism requires further elucidation, as it is not known to what extent dynamic and static discharges traveling along Group Ia fibers are sorted out at spinal level.

The postural role of the stretch reflex as an aid in standing is illustrated in Figure 3-6.

Figures 3-5 and 3-6 are simplified examples of how the combination of dynamic and static influences on alpha motoneurons from the primary ending of the muscle spindle create a mechanism, under gamma system control, which can initiate and coordinate movement and regulate posture.[12, 13, 17]

The clinical manifestations of spasticity and decerebrate rigidity can be explained on the basis of gamma system release from supraspinal inhibition.[18, 31, 32] Similarly, the signs of cerebellar dyssynergias have been shown to result from disordered cerebellar control of the gamma system, producing abnormal alpha-gamma linkage.[15, 32]

ROLE OF MUSCLE SPINDLE SECONDARY ENDINGS

Less is known of the function of the spindle secondary endings. They are situated on nuclear chain intrafusals and give a static response to stretch. The firing frequency of secondary endings increases linearly with muscle length occurring in the form of slow, sustained discharges.

Information from secondary endings travels along Group II afferent fibers. Group II nerves are smaller and conduct more slowly than Group Ia afferents. They have a disynaptic or polysynaptic connection with alpha motoneurons by means of spinal interneurons. It is known that Group II afferents facilitate flexor and inhibit extensor alpha motoneurons, whether they originate from spindles situated in flexor muscles or from those in the extensor muscles. Thus, secondary endings may play a role in the regulation of posture. Another role of secondary endings is to feed back to supraspinal centers information regarding change in muscle length.

The secondary endings are under the control of slowly conducting, static gamma fusimotor fibers. The dynamic fusimotor fibers do not activate secondary endings. The static portion of the primary ending is also influenced by static gamma 2 fusimotor fibers. Its Group Ia connection provides a faster conducting static system. Much further work is necessary in order to elucidate the relative importance of each static pathway at both the spinal and the supraspinal level.

The role of secondary endings in the maintenance of body posture is supported by the effects that are seen to occur when function is disordered. Parkinson's disease has been related to the release from inhibition of those spinal interneurons that mediate activity of spindle secondary endings.[11] This produces an overactivity of the secondary ending via static gamma 2 facilitation, and most of the clinical signs of Parkinson's disease (rigidity, flexed posture and dyskinesia) stem from a hyperactive static gamma system, resulting, in turn, from release of inhibition or from facilitation from supraspinal centers.[32]

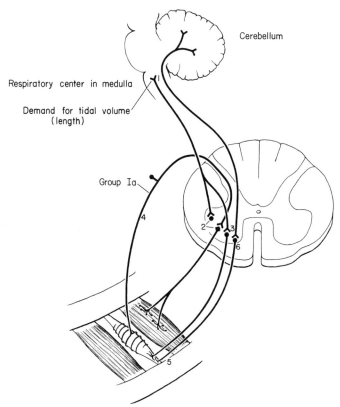

Cerebellum

Respiratory center in medulla

Demand for tidal volume (length)

Group Ia

Figure 3 – 7 Control of respiratory movement by the interaction of alpha and gamma linkage in a length follow-up servo system. (1) Descending signals (demand for tidal volume) are transmitted directly to alpha motoneurons as well as to gamma motoneurons (mainly rhythmic gamma motoneurons). Since the spindle afferent discharge is not unloaded (silenced) during the phase of active intercostal muscle contraction, it is believed that the gamma drive and not the alpha drive dominates in the control of respiratory movements. (2) Alpha motoneuron. (3) Rhythmic gamma motoneuron. (4) Group Ia afferent from spindle. (5) The spindle acts as a micro strain gauge, recording and relaying information regarding changes in intercostal extrafusal length (load). An increase in load may be interpreted as an increased demand for tidal volume and automatic adjustments can reflexly be made via the servo system. (6) The cerebellum can influence the alpha-gamma linkage via the tonic gamma motoneuron. (Modified from Euler, C. V.: The Control of Respiratory Movement. *In: Breathlessness* (Howell, J. B. L., and Campbell, E. J. M., eds.). Oxford, 1966, p. 27.)

ROLE OF THE GAMMA SYSTEM IN VENTILATION

The alpha-gamma linkage is important in the control of ventilation. The afferent fibers in the dorsal roots carrying impulses from the chest muscles facilitate ventilation.[10] The intercostal gamma motoneurons are of two types: rhythmic gamma motoneurons and tonic gamma motoneurons.[9] These two types of intercostal gamma neurons seem to have different functions.[14] The rhythmic gamma motoneurons are closely linked to intercostal alpha motoneurons and become coactivated with them and are under the control of the respiratory center in the medulla. Therefore, rhythmic gamma motoneurons can be said to be specific respiratory motoneurons, which under the influence of the medulla provide the drive that regulates ventilation.

The tonic gamma motoneuron discharge is not influenced by the respiratory rhythm or blood gas composition, but rather by postural reflexes from the chest and trunk, under cerebellar control.[9] Thus, there is a convergence on the intercostal muscle spindles of fusimotor fibers that mediate the different demands, postural and respiratory, which must be achieved by the same muscle. Figure 3-7 illustrates the gamma motoneuron control of respiration.

Cerebellar stimulation either increases or decreases intercostal spindle sensitivity to stretch, mainly via the tonic intercostal gamma motoneurons. These have shown firing patterns and modes of activation that resemble the fusimotor activity of limb muscles. In contrast, the rhythmic intercostal gamma motoneurons are controlled mainly by blood gas alterations acting at the respiratory center in the medulla and not by the cerebellum.[14]

After low cervical spinal cord transection in the cat, the activity of tonic intercostal gamma neurons continues, but the rhythmic gamma activity is abolished. Tonic gamma motoneuron reflex activity can still be elicited by passive movements of the chest wall and by other postural changes. In man, following cervical spinal cord injury, the respiratory vital capacity increases after spinal shock has passed and spinal reflex excitability has been re-established. It seems plausible that diaphragmatic excursion could provide a mechanism for eliciting passive stretch reflexes from paralyzed intercostal muscles by the activation of tonic gamma motoneurons, producing an increase in vital capacity. On the other hand, rhythmic gamma motoneurons below the level of the lesion are cut off from the medulla and are no longer capable of regulating respiration by sensitivity to changes in blood gases.

ROLE OF GAMMA SYSTEM IN SPEECH

Speech is closely linked with precise ventilatory muscle control. The respiratory system is the source of power for speech sounds. An increase in subglottal pressures produced by the action of ventilatory muscles is necessary for all stressed syllables and many pitch changes. There must be coordination of vocal cord movement with that of ventilatory muscles, which produce the pressure and flow of air needed to drive the larynx in the production of speech. The intercostal muscle spindle, via the primary ending, provides a reflex mechanism sensitive to changes in lung volume (length or load), as well as to rate of volume change. The voluntary activation of the intercostal muscles is dependent at least in part on the afferent discharge from the primary ending, which discharge is in turn driven by the activity of fusimotor neurons (servomechanism).

During phonation, the chest movements are controlled by the gamma system and the spindle loop. The phonating larynx constitutes an appreciable load that is continuously changing according to the utterances. As the dynamic primary ending provides a damping mechanism to prevent oscillation of the stretch reflex in limb muscles, so the dynamic intercostal primary endings respond to variations in load during speech to produce a phased activation of intercostal fusimotor and alpha motoneurons.[33] Thus, the concept of a servomechanism under gamma system drive seems valid for ventilatory muscle function and control of speech, as well as for limb-muscle motor function.

Much more information regarding the intricate workings of the gamma system and muscle spindle is needed to complete our understanding of both normal and disordered functioning. The study of the pathology[6] and pathophysiology[32] of the muscle spindle and gamma system may provide important clues regarding the etiology and pathogenesis of certain neurological disorders. In addition, the development of therapeutic techniques should take into account the functional importance of the muscle spindle and gamma system in motor performance.

REFERENCES

1. Appelberg, B., Bessou, P., and Laporte, Y.: Action of static and dynamic fusimotor fibres on secondary endings of cat's spindles. J. Physiol. (Paris), *185*:160–171, 1966.
2. Barker, D. (ed.): *Symposium on Muscle Receptors, 1961.* New York, Oxford University Press, 1962.
3. Boyd, I. A.: The structure and innervation of the nuclear bag muscle fiber system and the nuclear chain muscle fiber system in mammalian muscle spindles. Roy. Soc. Lond. Phil. Trans., Series B, *245*:81–136, 1962.
4. Boyd, I. A., and Eccles, J. C.: Fast and slow conducting small motor fibers in nerves to mammalian skeletal muscle. J. Physiol., *165*:29–30P, 1963.
5. Boyd, I. A., Eyzaguirre, C., Matthews, P. B. C., and Rushworth, G.: *The Role of the Gamma System in Movement and Posture.* New York, Association for the Aid of Crippled Children, 1968.
6. Cazzato, G., and Walton, J. N.: The pathology of the muscle spindle: a study of biopsy material in various muscular and neuromuscular diseases. J. Neurol. Sci., 7:15–70, 1968.
7. Cooper, S., and Daniel, P. M.: Muscle spindles in man: their morphology in the lumbricals and the deep muscles of the neck. Brain, *86*:563–583, 1963.
8. Cooper, S.: The responses of the primary and secondary endings of muscle spindle with intact motor innervation during applied stretch. Quart. J. Exp. Physiol., *46*:389–398, 1961.
9. Corda, M., Euler, C. V., and Lennerstrand, G.: Reflex and cerebellar influences on alpha and on rhythmic and tonic gamma activity in the intercostal muscle. J. Physiol. (London), *184*:898–923, 1966.
10. Critchlow, V., and Euler, C. V.: Intercostal muscle spindle activity and its gamma motor control. J. Physiol. (London), *168*:820–847, 1963.
11. Eccles, R. M., and Lundberg, A.: Supraspinal control of interneurons mediating spinal reflexes. J. Physiol. (London), *147*:565–584, 1959.
12. Eldred, E.: The dual sensory role of muscle spindles. J. Physical Therapy, *45*:290–313, 1965.
13. Eldred, E.: Functional implications of dynamic and static components of the spindle response to stretch. Am. J. Physical Med., *46*:129–140, 1967.
14. Euler, C. V.: The control of respiratory movement. *In* Howell, J. B. L., and Campbell, E. J. M. (eds.): *Breathlessness.* Philadelphia, F. A. Davis, 1966.
15. Gilman, S.: The nature of cerebellar dyssynergia. *In* Williams, D. (ed.): *Modern Trends in Neurology,* 5th ed. London, Butterworths, 1970.

16. Granit, R. (ed.): *Muscular Afferents and Motor Control.* Proceedings of the First Nobel Symposium, June, 1965. New York, John Wiley & Sons, 1966.
17. Granit, R.: The functional role of the muscle spindle's primary end organs. Proc. Roy. Soc. Med., *61*:69-78, 1968.
18. Granit, R.: The gamma loop in the mediation of muscle tone. Clin. Pharm. Ther., 5:837-847, 1964.
19. Granit, R.: *Receptors and Sensory Perception.* New Haven, Yale University Press, 1955.
20. Granit, R., Henatsch, H. D., and Steg, G.: Tonic and phasic ventral horn cells differentiated by post tetanic potentiation in cat extensors. Acta Physiol. Scand., *37*:114–126, 1956.
21. Gruner, J. E.: La structure fine du fuseau neuromusculaire humain. Rev. Neurol., *104*:490-507, 1961.
22. Hassall, A. H., quoted from Sherrington, C. S.: The Muscular Sense. *In* Schafer's Textbook of Physiology. Pentland, London and Edinburgh, 1900 b, 2, pages 1002-1025.
23. Jansen, J. K. S., and Matthews, P. B. C.: The central control of dynamic response of muscle spindle receptors. J. Physiol., *161*:357-378, 1962.
24. Jansen, J. K. S., Nicolaysen, K., and Rudjord, T.: The firing pattern of spinal neurons activated from the secondary endings of muscle spindles. Acta Physiol. Scand., *70*:188-193, 1967.
25. Kennedy, W. R.: Innervation of normal human muscle spindle. Neurology, *20*:463-475, 1970.
26. Leksell, L.: The action potential and excitatory effects of the small ventral root fibers to skeletal muscle. Acta Physiol. Scand., 10 (suppl.) *31*, 84 pages, 1945.
27. Matthews, P. B. C.: The differentiation of two types of fusimotor fibre by their effects on the dynamic response of muscle spindle primary endings. Quart. J. Exp. Physiol., *47*:324-333, 1962.
28. Matthews, P. B. C.: Muscle spindles. Physiol. Rev., *44*:219-288, 1964.
29. Roberts, T. D. M.: *Neurophysiology of Postural Mechanisms.* London, Butterworths, 1967.
30. Ruffini, A. quoted from: Les dispositifs anatomiques de la sensibilitie cutanee: sur les expansions nerveuses de la peau chez l'homme et quelques autres mammiferes. Rev. Gen. Histol., *1*:421-540, 1905.
31. Rushworth, G.: Spasticity and rigidity: an experimental study and review. J. Neurol. Neurosurg. Psychiat., *23*:99-117, 1960.
32. Rushworth, G.: Some aspects of the pathophysiology of spasticity and rigidity. J. Clin. Pharm. Ther., 6, Part 2:828-836, 1964.
33. Sears, T. A., and Davis, J. N.: The control of respiratory muscles during voluntary breathing. Ann. N. Y. Acad. Sci. *155*:183-190, 1968.
34. Sherrington, C. S.: Man on his nature. The Gifford Lectures, Edinburgh, 1937-38. New York, Macmillan, 1941.
35. Sherrington, C. S.: On the anatomical constitution of nerves of skeletal muscles; with remarks on recurrent fibers in the ventral spinal nerve root. J. Physiol. *17*:211-258, 1894.
36. Spiro, A. J., and Beilin, R. L.: Human muscle spindle histochemistry. Arch. Neurol. *20*:271-275, 1969.

Chapter 4

MUSCLE: MICRO-STRUCTURE AND CHEMISTRY

by Hyman I. C. Dubo, M.D., and Robert C. Darling, M.D.

INTRODUCTION

The electron microscope has revealed many of the secrets of muscle structure at the cellular level. Since it is beyond the scope of a single chapter to discuss all aspects of the available knowledge, structure will be emphasized only where it can be directly correlated with function. Physiological and biochemical processes will be stressed where existing knowledge leads to functional interpretation.

Skeletal muscle fibers are multinucleated cylindrical cells, each from 10 to 100 microns in diameter and as long as 40 cm. The muscle fiber is composed of many myofibrils, arranged parallel to one another. Each myofibril, 1 to 2 microns in diameter and 1 to 40 mm. in length, is composed of protein myofilaments of two types: actin and myosin; each is arranged structurally to produce the striated appearance of the cell. A loosely woven tubular network, called the sarcoplasmic reticulum, encloses each myofibril. The aqueous sarcoplasm fills the space surrounding the myofibrils and the sarcoplasmic reticulum, and contains soluble enzymes, lipid and glycogen granules, mitochondria, and myoglobin. The entire muscle fiber structure is enclosed within a surface membrane called the sarcolemma. Figure 4-1 illustrates the structural organization of the human skeletal muscle fiber.

Each aspect of the ultrastructure of the muscle fiber will be described and immediately correlated with function wherever possible.

65

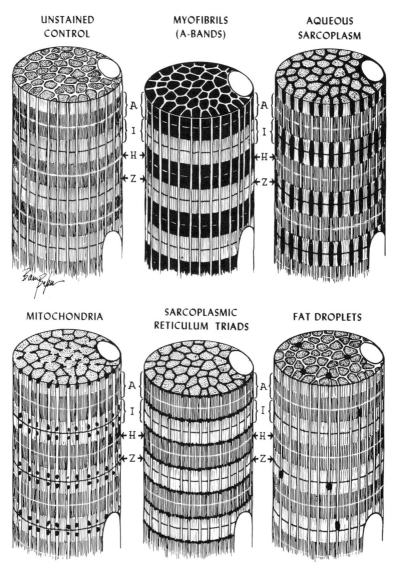

Figure 4–1 Structural organization of the human muscle fiber. Superimposed on the diagram of the unstained control are various components of the fiber in black. The oval-shaped structure at the periphery of the fiber is the nucleus. Note that the triads of the sarcoplasmic reticulum occur at the junctions of A and I bands. The appearance of the bands is due to the arrangement of thick and thin myofilaments. (From Engel, W. K. (ed.): *Current Concepts of Myopathies.* Philadelphia, J. B. Lippincott Co., 1965. Reprinted from Clinical Orthopaedics and Related Research, Number 39.)

ULTRASTRUCTURE AND FUNCTION

Sarcolemma

The sarcolemma is the surface membrane of the muscle fiber. It can be differentiated into an outer basement membrane and an inner plasma membrane (Fig. 4-2, inset B).[23, 27] The basement portion is much thicker than the plasma membrane, it has no defined structure and serves as a stabilizing membrane.

The plasma membrane is intimately related to the inner surface of the basement membrane. It is a three-layered complex of polysaccharide, mucoprotein and lipoprotein, measuring about 100 Å in thickness. In the resting muscle there is an electrical potential difference of about −90 mv between the inside and outside of the cell, owing to the ionic arrangement across the plasma membrane (sodium outside and potassium inside).

Depolarization of the plasma membrane is the initial activating process leading to muscular contraction. Conduction along the sarcolemma is about 5 meters per second. Invaginations from the sarcolemma form transverse tubular systems (T-systems), which connect the plasma membrane and extracellular space with the interior of the muscle.

T-System and Sarcoplasmic Reticulum

An interfibrillary membranous system, present throughout the skeletal muscle fiber, forms a complex tubular network, or reticulum, of delicate strands interwoven around the myofibrils. Two functionally distinct components of this membranous tubular complex are recognized: (1) a transverse tubular system, or, as it is commonly called, the T-system, and (2) the sarcoplasmic reticulum (Fig. 4-2).[24, 26, 27, 30] Structurally the T-system and sarcoplasmic reticulum have an important functional relationship.

Tubules of the sarcoplasmic reticulum are longitudinally arranged between the myofibrils and are closely aligned to each myofibril over its full length. The same tubules form a loosely woven network and interconnect laterally with the tubular systems of adjacent myofibrils.

In contrast, the tubular elements of the T-system are transversely oriented between the myofibrils (Fig. 4-2) and interrupt the tubules of the sarcoplasmic reticulum at regular intervals. The terminal segments of the sarcoplasmic reticulum become transversely oriented to the T-system, forming a structural unit called a triad.[9, 28]

A triad is two dilated terminal transverse segments, or cisternae, of the sarcoplasmic reticulum separated by the T-system tubule (Fig. 4-3). In birds, reptiles, man and other mammals, the triads are located near the junction of the A and I bands. There are two triads per sarcomere. In the frog and fish skeletal muscles, the triad is located at the Z line region and only one triad per sarcomere is present. In skeletal muscle fibers of the fish, tadpole, adult frog, birds and rat the T-system has been shown to be continuous with the sarcolemma. Thus the T-system, as an invagination of the sarcolemma, is continuous

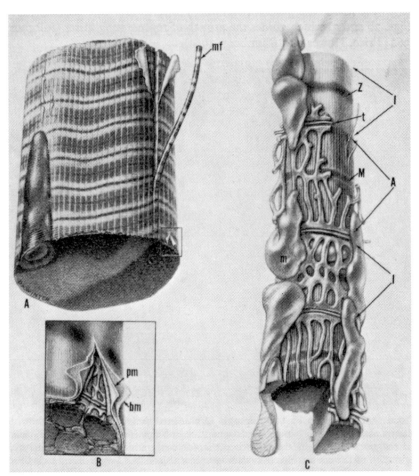

Figure 4 – 2   Ultrastructure of the skeletal muscle fiber. (A) Longitudinal segment of a muscle fiber as seen with a light microscope; *mf*, myofibril. (B) Membranous components of the sarcolemma as seen with an electron microscope; *bm*, basement membrane, *pm*, plasma membrane. (C) The isolated myofibril. The sarcoplasmic reticulum forms a tubular network interwoven around the myofibril and arranged longitudinally throughout its length. The tubular elements of the T-system are transversely oriented between the myofibril. Near the junction of the A and I bands the components of these two tubular systems form a complex called the triad, which is composed of an intermediate transverse tubule of the T-system bounded on each side by a transverse cisterna of the sarcoplasmic reticulum; *t*, transverse tubule of T-system; *I*, I band; *A*, A band; *M*, M-line; *Z*, Z-line; *m*, mitochondrion. (From Price, H. M.: Ultrastructure of the skeletal muscle fiber. *In* Walton, John N., ed.: *Disorders of Voluntary Muscle*, 2nd ed. London, J & A Churchill, Ltd., 1969.)

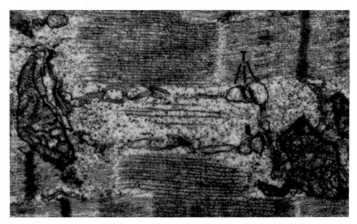

Figure 4 — 3   Electron micrograph of a triad (× 32,000). Longitudinal section of human skeletal muscle, showing tubular components of the sarcoplasmic reticulum and T-system at triad level. *T*, triad, with sarcoplasmic reticulum transverse tubules on either side of the central T-system tubule. (From Price, H. M., E. L. Howes, Jr., D. B. Sheldon, O. D. Hutson, R. T. Fitzgerald, J. M. Blumberg and C. M. Pearson: An improved biopsy technique for light and electron microscopic studies of human skeletal muscle. Lab. Invest., *14*:197, 1965.)

with the extracellular fluid. The sarcoplasmic reticulum (unlike the T-system) has no connection with the sarcolemma or extracellular fluid.[10, 19, 32]

At the triad level the tubules of the T-system are separated from the apposed terminal tubules of the sarcoplasmic reticulum (approximately 100 Å).[31] Membranelike connections between the T-system and terminal cisternae of the sarcoplasmic reticulum have been shown to occupy this space. The correlation of structure and function of the T-system and the sarcoplasmic reticulum is described in a discussion of excitation-contraction-coupling.

Excitation-Contraction-Coupling

The mechanism of muscular contraction involves the interaction of electrophysiological, biochemical and mechanical sequences at the cellular level.[16, 18, 21] The initial event leading to muscular contraction is depolarization of the plasma membrane. Since the T-system is an invagination of the sarcolemma and continuous with it, a route is provided whereby excitation can spread from the surface membrane to the interior of the muscle. The exact mode of excitation along the T-system tubules is not known, but the sodium ion distribution in the tubules is consistent with the ability for self-propagation. The action potential precedes the onset of tension development in the isometric twitch of single frog muscle fibers,[29] and thus must be the initial and initiating step in muscular contraction.

How excitation spreads from the T-system tubule to the terminal tubules of the sarcoplasmic reticulum has not been determined. At triad level, the gap separating the surface membranes of the T-system and sarcoplasmic reticulum is small enough so that it may be a site of ion transfer. The triad structural relationship is important functionally because it is known that calcium ions are stored in the terminal tubules of the sarcoplasmic reticulum[3] at this level, and calcium plays an important role in excitation-contraction-coupling.[17] Small concentrations of calcium chloride placed on exposed frog muscle fiber produces contraction, but no other ion — neither sodium, potassium, nor magnesium — produces contraction if calcium is not present.[15] As a result of spread of excitation from the sarcolemma along the T-system to the triad in the interior of the muscle, calcium is released from the terminal tubules of the sarcoplasmic reticulum. The calcium diffuses through the sarcoplasm to the myofibril, completing the coupling between excitation and contraction.

There is evidence that the contractile response to calcium is due to the interaction of thick (myosin) and thin (actin) filaments where they overlap.[20] When calcium is applied to muscle fibers from which the sarcolemma has been removed, and when sarcomere length is short enough to insure myofilament overlap, a contractile response is elicited. There is no response to added calcium when the sarcomere length is greater than the sum of the thin filament length and the thick filament length (i.e., when there is no overlap). The critical sarcomere length for contraction in response to added calcium is very close to the critical length for activation by electrical stimulation. This is further support for the concept that electrical excitation and calcium release are intimately related.

The mechanism by which this chemical reaction initiates a mechanical response in terms of muscle contraction and the development of tension will be discussed in detail later.

Contraction-Relaxation

Following the completion of muscular contraction, relaxation occurs. Relaxation is due to repolarization of the conducting membranes with subsequent cessation of calcium release from the sarcoplasmic reticulum. A substance known as "relaxing factor" is closely associated with the sarcoplasmic reticulum. The "relaxing factor" seems to act as a calcium pump, causing the removal of calcium from the sarcoplasm and its reaccumulation in the sarcoplasmic reticulum.[6, 14] When the calcium is removed from the sarcoplasm and its effect on the myofibrils is eliminated, relaxation occurs. In relaxed frog muscle fibers, calcium has been found to be localized in the sarcoplasmic reticulum but not in the sarcoplasm.[25] Within a few milliseconds after contraction is over, calcium ions become bound to the sarcoplasmic reticulum again, indicating that the rate of calcium uptake by the reticulum is sufficiently rapid to remove the calcium liberated into the sarcoplasm during excitation.[14]

Recent evidence indicates that the physiological contracture which occurs in McArdle's syndrome (myophosphorylase deficiency) after exercise is in fact due to defective reaccumulation of calcium by the sarcoplasmic reticulum, and hence, failure of relaxation.[12]

Figure 4-4 is a schematic summary of the various stages of excitation-contraction-coupling and the contraction-relaxation sequence.

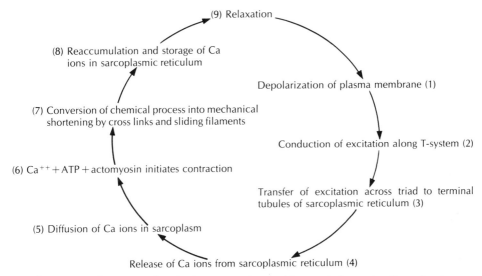

(9) Relaxation

(8) Reaccumulation and storage of Ca ions in sarcoplasmic reticulum

Depolarization of plasma membrane (1)

(7) Conversion of chemical process into mechanical shortening by cross links and sliding filaments

Conduction of excitation along T-system (2)

(6) Ca^{++} + ATP + actomyosin initiates contraction

Transfer of excitation across triad to terminal tubules of sarcoplasmic reticulum (3)

(5) Diffusion of Ca ions in sarcoplasm

Release of Ca ions from sarcoplasmic reticulum (4)

Figure 4 – 4 Summary of excitation-contraction-coupling and the contraction-relaxation sequence in muscle.

Contractile Proteins

Actin and myosin are the two contractile proteins found in each myofibril. Myosin filaments are thick, measuring about 100 Å in diameter and 1.5 microns in length. Actin filaments are thin, measuring about 50 Å in diameter and 1 micron in length. The arrangement of thick myosin filaments and thin actin filaments produces the horizontal or transverse bands or striated appearance of skeletal muscle as seen microscopically[20, 21] (Fig. 4-5). The alternate dark and light bands are called A and I bands respectively. The A bands, which are anisotropic and appear dense (dark), consist of overlapping thick and thin filaments. The I bands, which are isotropic and less dense (light), are composed only of thin actin filaments. The actin filaments of adjacent bands are attached at a line called the Z line. Thus, the Z line bisects the I band.

The functional unit of the muscle fiber in relation to the contractile process is the sarcomere, which is the material between two Z lines (Fig. 4-5). In a relaxed muscle the sarcomere length is such that one half of the length of a thin filament and two-thirds of the length of an adjacent thick filament overlap. In this region of overlap there are twice as many thin filaments (actin) as thick ones (myosin).

The actin filaments extend from the Z line and end at the edge of a lighter zone within the A band called the H zone. This H zone appears lighter because it consists of thick filaments only, with no overlap. A so-called pseudo-H zone lies in the center of the H zone (absence of cross bridges). An M line in the center of the myosin filaments is believed to be caused by a bulge in the filaments.

Electron microscopy has demonstrated cross bridges between thick and thin filaments,[21] appearing at regular intervals every 400 Å. To understand the function of these cross bridges, it is necessary to describe the structure of actin and myosin molecules.

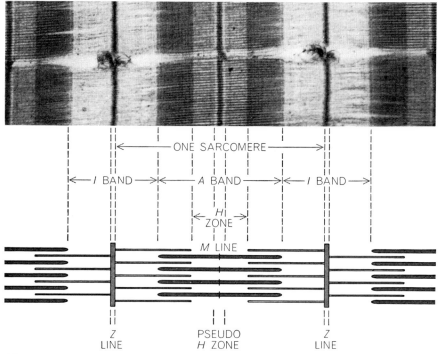

Figure 4 – 5   Striated muscle from the leg of a frog is shown in longitudinal section in an electron micrograph (top); the overlap of filaments that gives rise to its band pattern is illustrated schematically (bottom). Parts of two myofibrils (long parallel strands organized into muscle fiber) are enlarged some 23,000 diameters in the micrograph. The myofibrils are separated by a gap that runs horizontally across the micrograph. The major features of the sarcomere (a functional unit enclosed by two membranes, the Z lines) are labeled. The I band is light because it consists only of thin filaments. The A band is dense (and thus dark) where it consists of overlapping thick and thin filaments; it is lighter in the H zone, where it consists solely of thick filaments. The M line is caused by a bulge in the center of each thick filament, and the pseudo H zone by a bare region immediately surrounding the bulge. (From The Mechanisms of Muscular Contraction, by H. E. Huxley. Copyright © 1965 by Scientific American, Inc. All rights reserved.)

The myosin molecule has a molecular weight of 400,000 and is about 1500 Å in length and between 20 and 40 Å in diameter. Each myosin molecule can be split into two fragments, termed light meromyosin and heavy meromyosin. The heavy meromyosin fragment has an affinity for actin, with which it easily combines. Also, it can split an energy-rich phosphate group from ATP (adenosine triphosphate). Thus, myosin is capable of acting as an ATPase (in the presence of calcium ions), providing the energy-producing chemical reaction for muscular contraction.[21]

Isolated myosin molecules are linear structures, each with a head and a tail[20] (Fig. 4-6). The heads contain the sites responsible for the enzymatic

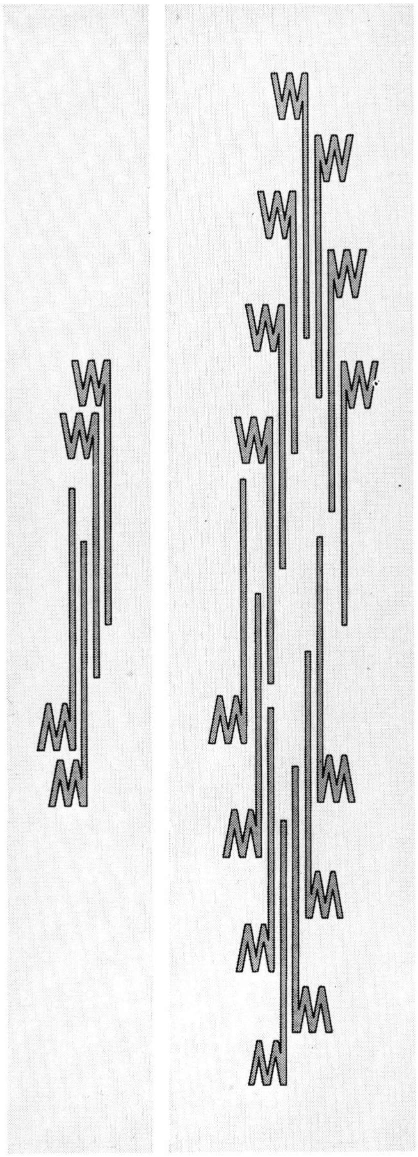

Figure 4—6 Schematic representation of myosin molecule. The head of the molecule is represented by zigzag line, and the tail by a straight line. Myosin molecules are oriented so that the tails are joined in the center, while the heads are oppositely pointed at each end. (From The Mechanism of Muscular Contraction, by H. E. Huxley. Copyright © 1965 by Scientific American, Inc. All rights reserved.)

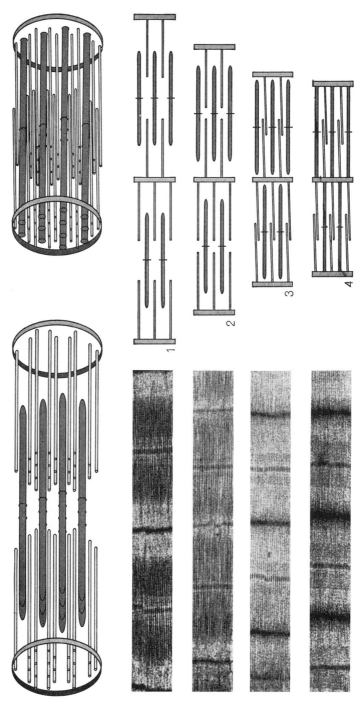

Figure 4—7   *See opposite page for legend.*

activity of myosin (ATPase) as well as for its affinity for actin. The tail portion contains the sites for its affinity with other myosin molecules. Cross bridges have been assumed to have ATPase and actin binding properties. Since the heads of the myosin molecules have these properties, it would seem that they actually are the cross bridges.

The molecular weight of the actin molecule is 70,000. Thin filaments consist of two chains of globular subunits of actin twisted around each other in the form of a double helix.[13] The actin molecules interact with myosin cross bridges at regular intervals.

Sliding Filament Theory

Huxley first hypothesized that muscular contraction occurred by means of the myofilaments sliding past one another.[20] Accordingly, the cross bridges between thick and thin filaments serve as a mechanical link and the cross bridges initiate and maintain the tension developed during muscular contraction. Thus the filaments do not change length, but slide past one another; the thin filaments (actin) slide farther into the A bands during shortening and farther out of the A band during stretching, causing shortening or lengthening of the sarcomere (Fig. 4–7).

The initial chemical reaction between myosin ATPase and ATP (in the presence of calcium) occurs at the cross bridges between thick and thin filaments. The release of energy from this dephosphorylation of ATP is somehow then converted into a mechanical force that causes the thick and thin filaments to slide past one another. Huxley also suggested that the cross bridges are attached to one site on the filament for part of a contraction and then detach and reattach themselves at new sites further along during the shortening of the sarcomere.

Length-Tension Relationship

A direct correlation exists between structure and function, to explain the relationship between length and tension of a muscle. There are six stages of muscular contraction during which changes occur in the relations between thick and thin filaments and the Z lines,[11] as a sarcomere shortens and the

Figure 4—7 Muscular contraction by sliding filaments. Contraction of muscle entails change in relative position of the thick and thin filaments that comprise the myofibril (top left and right). The effect of contraction on the band pattern of muscle is indicated by four electron micrographs and accompanying schematic illustrations of muscle in longitudinal section, fixed at consecutive stages of contraction. First the H zone closes (1), then a new dense zone develops in the center of the A band (2, 3, and 4) as thin filaments from each end of the sarcomere overlap. (From The Mechanism of Muscular Contraction, by H. E. Huxley. Copyright © 1965 by Scientific American, Inc. All rights reserved.)

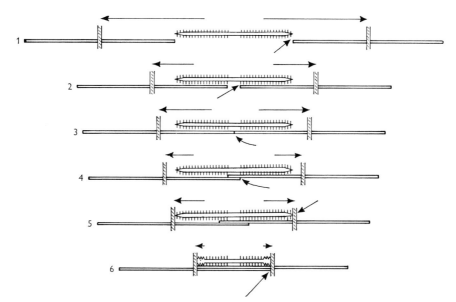

Figure 4–8 Schematic diagram of the six stages in the increase of overlap between thick and thin filaments as a sarcomere shortens during the sliding process. Stage 1—no overlap; Stage 2—maximum single overlap of thin filaments with bridges on thick filaments; Stage 3—meeting of thin filaments at M line; Stage 4—beginning of double overlap of thin filaments with bridges on thick filaments; Stage 5—collision of thick filaments with Z lines; Stage 6—completion of double overlap of thin filaments. (From Gordon, A. M., A. F. Huxley, and F. J. Julian: The variation in isometric tension with sarcomere length in vertebrate muscle fibres. J. Physiol., *184*:186, 1966.)

overlap between thick and thin filaments increases. Figure 4-8 presents these six stages and will be referred to repeatedly in the ensuing discussion.

Figure 4-9 shows the relationship between tetanus tension and sarcomere lengths in frog skeletal muscle fibers (length-tension curve).[11] The tension developed during an isometric tetanus decreases as the length of the muscle is altered (lengthened or shortened) in either direction from an optimum value. This relationship between length and tension can be explained with reference to the sliding filament theory of muscular contraction. No tension occurs in a sarcomere when there is no overlap between thick and thin filaments (stage 1, Fig. 8; Fig. 9, point A). Maximum tension occurs at the sarcomere length at which maximum single overlap of thin filaments with bridges on thick filaments occurs (stage 2, Fig. 8; Fig. 9, points B and C). Tension falls off rapidly when there is double overlap of the filaments (stages 4, 5 and 6, Fig. 8; Fig. 9, points D and E). The double overlap region interferes with the functioning of cross bridges between myosin and actin filaments and disrupts the normal orientation between them. Thus, sarcomere length and tension development shows a quantitative relationship between the number of cross bridges in the single overlap zone and the amount of tension developed. In summary, tension is proportional to the amount of single overlap between the thick and thin filaments. If there is no overlap (excessive length), or if there is double overlap (excessive shortening), tension is minimal.

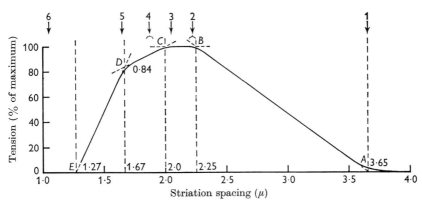

Figure 4—9 Length-tension curve of frog skeletal muscle fiber during tetanus. Tetanus tension is shown along ordinate and sarcomere lengths along abscissa. A, B, C, D, and E represent "corners" of the length tension curve. The six stages in the process of contraction are indicated by numbers 1 through 6 at the top of the diagram and correspond to the stages described in Figure 4–8. (From Gordon, A. M., A. F. Huxley, and F. J. Julian: The variation in isometric tension with sarcomere length in vertebrate muscle fibers. J. Physiol., *184*:185, 1966.)

It is probable that the greater tension developed in a tetanic contraction, as opposed to a twitch contraction, can be explained by the degree of single overlap during the sliding of the filaments. In a tetanus, greater single overlap would occur than in a twitch contraction.

HISTOCHEMISTRY

Types of Fibers

Two major types of muscle fibers,[4, 7] termed type I and type II, are distinguished by histochemical techniques. In animals, whole muscles are composed of either type I (red) or type II (white) fibers, but in man all muscles contain both types of fibers. Type I fibers are smaller and appear darker than type II fibers. Further divisions of type II into subgroups on the basis of differences in the ATPase reaction are of interest but do not affect the discussion of functional differences which follows.

There are important differences between the two types of fibers with respect to their content of oxidative enzymes, glycogenolytic enzymes, number of mitochondria, sarcoplasm and myoglobin. These basic differences between type I and II fibers reflect their different metabolic and functional properties, which are summarized in Table 4-1.

Type I fibers are rich in the mitochondrial oxidative enzymes utilized in metabolism of carbohydrates (Krebs cycle) and fatty acid oxidation, and they have a much higher concentration of mitochondria than type II fibers. Type II fibers, in contrast, are poor in oxidative enzymes, but have a high concentration of glycogen, phosphorylase and other glycogenolytic enzymes. Thus, the

TABLE 4–1 DIFFERENTIATION OF SKELETAL MUSCLE FIBERS INTO TWO DISTINCT TYPES

	TYPE I	TYPE II
Diameter	smaller	larger
Color	red, dark, opaque	white, light, translucent
Myoglobin	high	low
Sarcoplasm	high	low
Mitochondria	numerous	sparse
Oxidative enzymes	high	low
Phosphorylase	low	high
Myosin ATPase	low	high
Glycogen	low	high
Energy source	Krebs cycle	glycolysis
Function	sustained activity (tonic)	rapid activity (phasic)
Speed of contraction	slow	fast

two types of fibers are suited for different metabolic acitivities. Type I relies on aerobic metabolism within the mitochondria for its energy source, whereas energy requirements of type II fibers are primarily produced by anaerobic glycolysis within the aqueous sarcoplasm.

Functionally, type I fibers have slower contraction times than type II fibers.[2] Type I fiber activity predominates when muscles are used primarily for sustained work, and type II fiber activity predominates during rapid, unsustained muscular contraction.

Cross-innervation experiments in animals have shown that the contraction

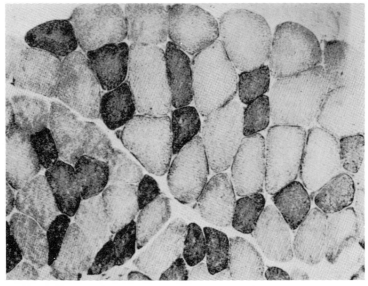

Figure 4–10 Histochemistry of normal human muscle. Small dark fibers, type I, stain strongly for lactate dehydrogenase. Large, type II, fibers stain poorly for lactate dehydrogenase. (From Dubowitz, V.: Histochemical aspects of muscle disease. *In* Walton, John N., ed.: Disorders of Voluntary Muscle, 2nd ed., London, J & A Churchill, Ltd., 1969.

time of fast (type II) and slow (type I) muscles can be reversed, and in the process the characteristic enzyme patterns of type I and type II fibers are also reversed,[5] indicating that metabolic and physiologic properties of muscle fiber are influenced by their innervation.

The reciprocal relationship between oxidative enzymes and phosphorylase in each muscle fiber produces a checkerboard appearance in stained microscopic preparations. If a phosphorylase stain is used, type II fibers will appear dark, owing to a high concentration of phosphorylase, and type I fibers will appear light. When the fiber is stained for oxidative enzymes, i.e., lactic dehydrogenase, the reverse pattern will occur[4] (Fig. 4-10).

Myoglobin

Myoglobin is evenly distributed throughout the sarcoplasm. Histochemical staining for myoglobin shows type I fibers to be rich in myoglobin, whereas type II fibers are deficient. Myoglobin serves to store and transport oxygen within the muscle cell; thus the fiber type which depends primarily upon aerobic metabolism has the higher myoglobin content. Myoglobin is believed to speed the inward diffusion of oxygen into the muscle fiber.[33] Myoglobin functions in a state of partial oxygenation and is believed to produce a gradient of myoglobin-bound oxygen from the periphery to the center of the fiber.

Myoglobin acts as a store of oxygen that is called upon during sudden changes in oxygen demand. During a tetanic contraction, myoglobin is deoxygenated within seconds, and as the store is depleted at the mitochondria, it is replenished at the periphery of the muscle fiber by oxygen diffusing from the capillaries.

Sarcoplasm and Mitochondria

The sarcoplasm is the aqueous matrix of the skeletal muscle fiber that corresponds to the cytoplasm of other living cells. It lies between the myofibrils and surrounds the tubular elements of the sarcoplasmic reticulum.

Glycogen granules are abundant in the sarcoplasm and in electron microscopic views they can be seen lying in the intermyofibrillar spaces. The glycogen stores are sources for anaerobic glycolysis within the sarcoplasm and produce rapidly a small amount of ATP for muscular contraction (anaerobic breakdown of one glucose unit of glycogen yields three molecules of ATP). The glycolytic pathway is the metabolism of carbohydrates to the level of pyruvate. On the other hand, the aerobic metabolism, via the Krebs cycle, is the prime source of ATP regeneration and occurs within the mitochondria.[22] Glycogen is important for metabolism and this is emphasized by a recent study[1] of prolonged physical exercise to exhaustion. Glycogen content of muscles decreased with exercise, proportional to both the total energy developed and to the duration of the exercise. The results suggest that the capacity for prolonged and exhausting work is related to the glycogen storage in the working muscle.

The mitochondria are membranous compartmentalized sacs, specialized and complicated in structure and function. Mitochondria are found in the sarcoplasm, at the level of the Z lines, encircling each myofibril (Figs. 4–1 and

4-2) as well as in long columns regularly arranged in the spaces between the myofibrils. They are also found in aggregates in the subsarcolemmal region. The mitochondria are the site of aerobic metabolism within the muscle cell. The Krebs cycle (aerobic metabolism of carbohydrates), fatty acid oxidation, electron transport and oxidative phosphorylation all occur within the mitochondria.[22]

Creatine phosphate reacts with ADP (adenosine diphosphate) in the sarcoplasm to form creatine and ATP. This, along with anaerobic glycolysis, provides a rapid and readily available supply of ATP for muscular contraction, whereas the greater yield of ATP from aerobic metabolism via the Krebs cycle requires more time.

CONCLUSION

Although there are still gaps in knowledge of the mechanism of muscular contraction, the preceding discussion of recent studies develops a fairly clear picture. The muscle cell as a chemical engine to convert chemical to mechanical energy depends both on a finely attuned chemical system and an elaborate structural arrangement. The fine steric arrangement of the chemical ingredients is necessary to explain the more general characteristics of muscular contraction. Activation of contraction, speeds of contraction and relaxation and supply of fuels for aerobic and anaerobic metabolism are among the properties now explainable.

REFERENCES

1. Ahlborg, B., Bergstrom, J., Ekelund, L. G., and Hultman, E.: Muscle glycogen and muscle-electrolytes during prolonged physical exercise. Acta Physiol. Scand., 70:129-142, 1967.
2. Buller, A. J., Eccles, J. C., and Eccles, R. M.: Interactions between motoneurons and muscles in respect of the characteristic speeds of their responses. J. Physiol. (London), 150:417-439, 1960.
3. Constantin, L. L., Franzini-Armstrong, C., and Podolsky, R. J.: Localization of calcium-accumulating structures in striated muscle fibers. Science, 147:158-160, 1965.
4. Dubowitz, V.: Histochemical Aspects of Muscle Disease. In Walton, J. (ed.): Disorders of Voluntary Muscle, 2nd edition. London, J. & A. Churchill Ltd., 1969.
5. Dubowitz, V., and Newman, D. L.: Change in enzyme pattern after cross innervation of fast and slow skeletal muscle. Nature (London), 214:840-841, 1967.
6. Ebashi, S.: Calcium binding activity of vesicular relaxing factor. J. Biochem. (Tokyo), 50:236-244, 1961.
7. Engel, W. K.: The essentiality of histo- and cytochemical studies of skeletal muscle in the investigation of neuromuscular disease. Neurology, 12:778-794, 1962.
8. Engel, W. K. (ed.): Current Concepts of Myopathies. Philadelphia, J. B. Lippincott Co., 1965. Reprinted from Clinical Orthopaedics and Related Research, no. 39.
9. Fahrenbach, W. H.: Sarcoplasmic reticulum: ultrastructure of the triadic junction. Science, 147:1308, 1965.
10. Franzini-Armstrong, C., and Porter, K. R.: Sarcolemmal invaginations constituting the T-system in fish muscle fiber. J. Cell Biol., 22:675-696, 1964.
11. Gordon, A. M., Huxley, A. F., and Julian, F. J.: The variation in isometric tension with sarcomere length in vertebrate muscle fibers. J. Physiol., 184:170-192, 1966.
12. Gruener, R., McArdle, B., Ryman, B. E., and Weller, R. O.: Contracture of phosphorylase deficient muscle. J. Neurol., Neurosurg., Psychiat., 31:268-283, 1968.
13. Hanson, J., and Lowy, J.: The structure of F-actin and of actin filaments isolated from muscle. J. Molec. Biol., 6:46-60, 1963.

14. Hasselbach, W.: Relaxation and the sarcotubular calcium pump. Fed. Proc., *23*:909–912, 1964.
15. Heilbrunn, L. V., and Wiercinski, F. J.: The action of various cations on muscle protoplasm. J. Cell. Comp. Physiol., *29*:15-32, 1947.
16. Huxley, A. F.: Muscle structure and theories of contraction. Prog. Biophys., 7:255-318, 1957.
17. Huxley, A. F.: The links between excitation and contraction. Proc. Roy. Soc. (London), *160*:486-488, 1964.
18. Huxley, A. F., and Taylor, R. E.: Local activation of striated muscle fibers. J. Physiol., *144*:426-441, 1958.
19. Huxley, H. E.: Evidence for continuity between central elements of the triads and extracellular space in frog sartorius muscle. Nature (London), *202*:1067–1071, 1964.
20. Huxley, H. E., and Hanson, J.: Changes in the cross-striations of muscle during contraction and stretch and their structural interpretation. Nature (London), *173*:973-976, 1954.
21. Huxley, H. E.: The mechanism of muscular contraction. Scient. Amer., *213*:18-27, 1965.
22. Lehninger, A. L.: Cell Organelles: The Mitochondrion. *In* Quarton, G. C., Melnechuk, T., and Schmitt, F. O. (eds.): *The Neurosciences.* New York, Rockefeller University Press, 1967.
23. Mauro, A., and Adams, R.: The structure of the sarcolemma of the frog skeletal muscle fiber. J. Biophys., Biochem., Cytol., *10*(suppl.):177, 1961.
24. Peachey, L. D.: The sarcoplasmic reticulum and transverse tubules of the frog's sartorius. J. Cell Biol., *25*:209-231, 1965.
25. Podolsky, R. J., and Constantin, L. L.: Regulation by calcium of the contraction and relaxation of muscle fibers. Fed. Proc., *23*:933-939, 1964.
26. Porter, R. R., and Palade, G. E.: Studies on the endoplasmic reticulum—III. Its form and distribution in striated muscle cells. J. Biophys., Biochem., Cytol., *3*:269-300, 1957.
27. Price, H. M.: Ultrastructure of the Skeletal Muscle Fibre. *In* Walton, J. N. (ed.): *Disorders of Voluntary Muscle*, 2nd edition. London, J. & A. Churchill Ltd., 1969.
28. Price, H. M., Howes, E. L., Jr., Sheldon, D. B., Hutson, O. D., Fitzgerald, R. T., Blumberg, J. M., and Pearson, C. M.: An improved biopsy technique for light and electron microscopic studies of human skeletal muscle. Lab. Invest., *14*:194-199, 1965.
29. Sandow, A., Taylor, S. R., and Preisser, H.: The role of the action potential in excitation contraction coupling. Fed. Proc., *24*:1116-1123, 1965.
30. Smith, D. S.: The organization and function of the sarcoplasmic reticulum and T-system of muscle cells. Prog. Biophys. & Mol. Biol., *16*:109-142, 1966.
31. Walker, S. M., Schrodt, G. R.: Connections between the T-system and sarcoplasmic reticulum. Anat. Rec., *155*:1-10, 1966.
32. Walker, S. M., and Schrodt, G. R.: Continuity of the T-system with the sarcolemma in rat skeletal muscle. J. Cell Biol., *27*:671-677, 1965.
33. Wittenberg, J. B.: Myoglobin-facilitated oxygen diffusion: role of myoglobin in oxygen entry into muscle. Physiol. Revs., *50*:559-636, 1970.

Electrophysiology

Chapter 5

NERVE CONDUCTION AND SYNAPTIC TRANSMISSION

by Robert E. Lovelace, M.B. (Lond.), M.R.C.P. (Lond.),
and Stanley J. Myers, M.D.

A consideration of the anatomical and chemical composition of the nerve fiber is important in order to understand the physiological processes involved in transmission of the nerve impulse.[28, 53] The nerve fiber consists of a rodlike structure surrounded by a membrane composed of lipid-protein dipoles, with an internal medium containing predominantly K^+ cations and an external medium comprising principally Na^+ cations. Divalent cations (Ca^{++} and Mg^{++}) are also present, in much smaller concentrations, in the external medium. The anions are principally Cl^- and HCO_3^- externally; internally, there are mainly complex organic anions of protein type and a very low concentration of Cl^-. By means of these concentration differences, and because of the biological activity of the membrane, with its variable permeability and ion extrusion pump, a negative charge is maintained on the inside of the membrane relative to the outside, giving rise to the membrane potential. This axonal membrane, of thickness between 50 and 100 Å (5 to 10 nanometers), occupies only 0.1 per cent of the total volume of the neuron, but it is of predominant importance in conduction.

During excitation, the resting equilibrium is disturbed by depolarization of the membrane, during which the internal negativity is reduced towards zero. When this depolarization reaches a critical level—i.e., a threshold—an action potential is produced in the nerve, and the internal potential overshoots past zero to a positive value. Upon repolarization, the internal potential returns to its negative value. Unless conductivity is blocked, the action potential is self-propagating in either direction along the nerve, and is followed

85

by an electrical and chemical recovery phase. This electrical manifestation of the action potential can be explained by postulating potential-dependent changes (condensor/battery system) in a selectively permeable membrane (pore or aperture theory) along with extrusion pumps.[23] An alternative explanation considers the resting and active states of the membrane in terms of variation of its cation exchange properties.[51] Certainly, the axonal protoplasm is completely unnecessary for conduction.[4] Removal of the divalent cations from the external medium leads to loss of excitability, whereas, under proper conditions, complete elimination of univalent cations may not result in total loss of excitability,[4] although the amplitude of the action potential is markedly diminished.[52] In the normal state, a depolarizing stimulus coursing outward through the membrane will drive the internal univalent (K^+) ions by electrophoresis into the inner layers of the membrane and finally into the outer layer, thereby displacing the divalent cations (i.e., Ca^{++}).[51] Abrupt depolarization occurs at a critical level, as is shown by a sudden change in the relationship of univalent membrane cation concentration to membrane conductance.

Our knowledge of these various aspects of nerve conduction derives either from voltage clamp experiments, in which the internal potential is kept at constant voltage, or from perfusion experiments, in which internal and external electrolytic concentrations are varied. Turbidity, birefringence of nerves and intensity of fluorescence of stained nerves also vary during excitation, and these changes have been explained by postulating alterations in orientation of the membrane macromolecules during the active state.[50]

Intracellular potentials are measured with glass micropipettes filled with hypertonic electrolytic solution ($3M$ KCl)[33] (Fig. 5–1). With a balanced bridge, the same setup can be used for stimulation and for recording events.[55] In most

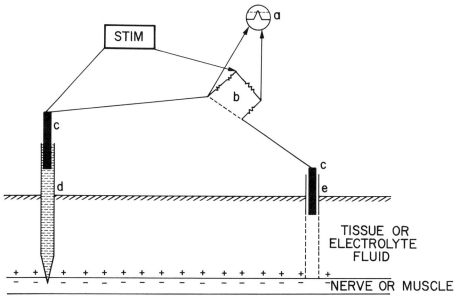

Figure 5–1   Microelectrode recording (intracellular). STIM = stimulator; a = oscilloscope recording; b = balanced Wheatstone bridge; c = anodized silver electrodes; d = recording electrode: glass micropipette (3 Molar KCL filled); e = indifferent or reference electrode.

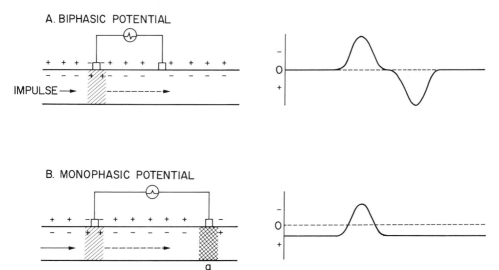

Figure 5–2 Surface recording (extracellular). (A) The derivation of a biphasic potential with surface active and reference electrodes is shown. Second phase is produced by impulse travelling to and activating reference electrode. (B) Demonstration of a monophasic potential using an injury or crushed end reference electrode which cannot be activated by the transmitted impulse. a = crushed nerve end (reference).

animal muscle and nervous tissue, the resting potential value is about −90 mv and varies slightly according to whether the readings are made in vitro on excised tissue,[10] in situ with an open pool method,[25] or in situ with a closed (percutaneous) method.[40] In the percutaneous technique, so far applied only to muscle, a microelectrode is passed through a hollow insertional electrode placed in a muscle belly.[2, 19, 48] Recordings from single nerve fibers are achieved easily only in crustaceans and some other invertebrates, with particular success using the giant axon of the squid, but recent studies by Eliasson with a voltage clamp applied to a mammalian single fiber have confirmed the presence of an electron leak at the node of Ranvier,[9] the physiology of which will be discussed later in this chapter. If the single fiber action potential is recorded intracellularly with an internal or crushed end reference recording, the curve is usually monophasic, rising from a negative membrane potential.

   More often recording is made from surface electrodes on single fibers or whole nerves, with biphasic potentials being recorded (Fig. 5–2A). If crushed end reference recording is used, on the other hand, the potentials are then monophasic (Fig. 5–2B). In clinical practice, the recording electrodes usually pick up potentials from many fibers and at a variably greater distance from these active fibers in the nerve, thus giving rise to compound nerve action potentials. These are at least biphasic and may be irregular in form, owing to summation of temporally dispersed responses. Such wave forms, as seen on direct measurement, can be computed from addition of individual fiber responses.[17] In recording at a distance in this fashion, from either a single fiber or a bundle of fibers (as in a peripheral nerve), the initial phase is usually negative, which in electromyography is generally recorded by an upward deflexion of the beam on the cathode ray oscilloscope. Nerve action potentials so recorded usually are bi- or triphasic.[31]

At this stage, it is useful to summarize some of the properties and character-istics of neurons. These include:

1. The all or none response, which is the ability of nerve fibers to respond completely and with a propagated impulse when the stimulus reaches thresh-old.

2. The refractory period, which is a length of time following an effective stimulus during which the nerve fiber will not respond to a further stimulus.

3. Two way conduction, which is the property of a neuron whereby a propagated action potential is transmitted in both directions from the site of the stimulus.

4. Subthreshold stimuli may sometimes summate to give a threshold stimu-lus, with a resulting response.

5. Accommodation occurs in nerves and is manifested by a decrease of excitability, with prolonged subthreshold stimulation.

6. Depolarization block may be produced by subthreshold stimuli, by ex-cessive external potassium, by anoxia and by injury. This block is counteracted by hyperpolarization.

7. Impulses are duplicated at the branching points of nerves (which always correspond to nodes of Ranvier), so that the undiminished impulse is propa-gated down each branch.

8. Interaction between adjacent fibers in a neuron by volume conduction may give rise to a change in threshold of up to 10 per cent in apparently nonactive neurons. Occasionally, current flow generated by active fibers can stimulate a previously inactive adjacent fiber to above threshold levels. This latter phenomenon is called ephaptic stimulation.

Volume Conduction

The problem of volume conduction recurs frequently in recording biologi-cal electrical potentials. Although basically it constitutes the application of Ohm's law to the electrolytic conduction around the axon, this phenomenon of volume conduction is complicated in vivo by the non-uniformity of the excit-able tissues and the nonhomogeniety of the conducting medium.

$$I_1 = K \frac{V}{r}$$

where I_1 = longitudinal current, V = axoplasmic potential, r = axoplasmic re-sistance, K = a constant, related to the units employed.

The equation is Ohm's law applied to a neuron.

Conduction Velocity

Conduction velocity varies directly with the diameter of a nerve fiber, and is greatly increased by the presence of a myelin sheath. An impulse can pass along an unmyelinated nerve fiber at the relatively slow rate of 0.4 to 1 m/sec and its speed is directly proportional to the square root of the diameter of the fiber. The more rapid transmission of the impulse along the myelinated fiber results from the insulation of the nerve segments by a myelin sheath. These

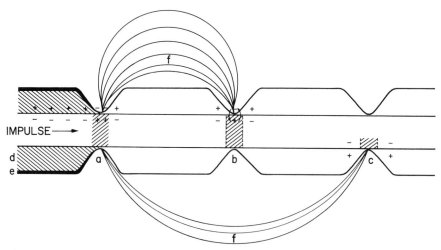

Figure 5—3 Saltatory conduction in a myelinated fiber. a = depolarized membrane at node of Ranvier; b = partially depolarized membrane at node of Ranvier (near threshold); c = beginning depolarization of membrane at node of Ranvier; d = myelin sheath; e = Schwann cell; f = electrical field.

insulated segments are separated by the myelin-free areas (1 micron) at the nodes of Ranvier. At the node of Ranvier, there is an electron leak and easy depolarization relative to the greater stability of the internode. Excitation, therefore, appears to jump from node to node as the electrical field from one node becomes sufficient to activate the next. This phenomenon is called saltatory conduction (Figure 5-3). However, there is some longitudinal current traveling at a finite rate in the internode and, therefore, it is not strictly correct to state that in saltatory conduction the nerve impulse jumps from node to node without some latency being referrable to the internode.[49] Alternatively, this more rapid conduction may be related to the low membrane capacity in the internode of the medullated fiber. Thus, two-thirds of the membrane charge is at the tiny nodal region. A safety factor is present in myelinated fibers, so that in nerve conduction the impulse can sometimes pass across one or even two nodes that have been narcotized[54] (Figure 5-3). In myelinated fibers, conduction velocity is directly proportional to diameter, and may vary from as high as 120 m/sec in some motor and sensory fibers[41] (i.e., cat) to as low as 4 m/sec in some slow myelinated fibers (A or delta). The velocity of nerve transmission also varies with the internodal distance, as there is a direct relationship between the separation of the nodes of Ranvier and the time required for the electrical field to produce appropriate depolarization in saltatory conduction.

Returning to the compound nerve action potential, if this is recorded at progressively greater distances from the stimulation point, the various spikes of the dispersed potential will become separated into distinct velocity groups[16] (Figure 5-4). This method provides one of the electrical methods of classifying nerve fibers. Three components, alpha, beta and delta, can be distinguished by the velocity rates of each group. Another electrical distinction is shown by differences in threshold for stimulation; the threshold is lower in the faster fibers and higher in the fibers with slower conduction velocity. Mixed nerves

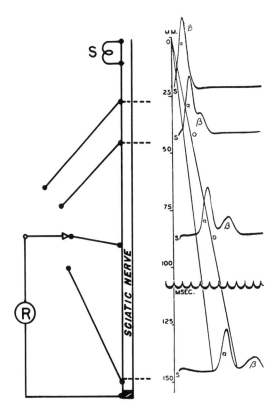

Figure 5–4 Compound action potential of frog sciatic nerve recorded at different distances from site of stimulation. Left: Diagram of recording apparatus. S = stimulus; R = recorder. Right: Only the first two elevations, α and β, are shown. As conduction increases, α and β became clearly separated in time (temporal dispersion) because they reflect activity of fibers' conduction at different rates. Diagonal straight lines are drawn through onsets of α and β deflections; slopes of these lines give conduction rates of most rapidly conducting α and β fibers. (From Ruch, T. C. and H. D. Patton: *Physiology and Biophysics.* W. B. Saunders Company, Philadelphia, 1965.)

TABLE 5–1   PROPERTIES OF MAMMALIAN NERVE FIBERS†

	A	B	sC	drC
Fiber diameter, μ	1–22	≤3	0.3–1.3	0.4–1.2
Conduction speed, m per sec	5–120	3–15	0.7–2.3	0.6–2.0
Spike duration, msec	0.4–0.5	1.2	2.0	2.0
Absolute refractory period, msec	0.4–1.0	1.2	2.0	2.0
Negative afterpotential amplitude,				
per cent of spike	3–5	none	3–5	none
Duration, msec	12–20	. . . .	50–80	. . . .
Positive afterpotential amplitude,				
per cent of spike	0.2	1.5–4.0	1.5	*
Duration, msec	40–60	100–300	300–1000	*
Order of susceptibility to asphyxia	2	1	3	3
Velocity/diameter ratio	6	?	?	1.73 average

*A postspike positivity 10 to 30 per cent of spike amplitude and decaying to half size in 50 msec is recorded from drC fibers. This afterpositivity differs from the positive afterpotential of other fibers.

†(From Ruch, T. C. and H. D. Patton: *Physiology and Biophysics.* W. B. Saunders Company, Philadelphia, 1965.)

contain components of all three velocity or threshold groups, but cutaneous nerves usually contain only alpha (faster) and delta (slower).

Nerves can also be classified functionally into groups:

Group A. These fibers are myelinated somatic, being both afferent and efferent.

Group B. These fibers are also myelinated, but are efferent and preganglionic in the autonomic system.

Group C. These fibers are unmyelinated, and are of two subgroups—sympathetic (sC), being the efferent postganglionic sympathetic axons, and dorsal root sensory (drC), being the small unmyelinated afferent axons found in peripheral nerves and dorsal roots (see Table 5–1).

Finally, fiber diameter may be used as a basis for classification:

1. Muscular nerves
   a. Myelinated
      Motor and proprioceptive afferent
      12 to 21 microns, Group I
      6 to 12 microns, Group II   } alpha
                                          } delta   } A fibers
      1 to 6 microns, Group III }   delta
   b. Unmyelinated
      0.4 to 1.2 microns, Group IV   C fibers
2. Cutaneous nerves
   a. Myelinated
      6 to 17 microns (alpha)
      1 to 6 microns (delta) }   A fibers
   b. Unmyelinated
      0.4 to 1.2 microns   C fibers

Conduction velocity is affected by physical factors such as temperature[45] and metabolic rate; a decrease of either factor reduces velocity. In disease, slow conduction velocities occur in regenerating fibers of small diameter, and also in the presence of primary or segmental demyelination of nerves.

APPLIED ASPECTS

Basic anatomical and physiological knowledge of nerve conduction can be applied in health and disease by recording the effects of nerve and muscle stimulation. The equipment consists of an amplifier-cathode ray oscilloscope (CRO) system, on which potentials may be recorded and demonstrated on the oscilloscope screen (Fig. 5–5). Preamplification is needed to visualize adequately potentials in the microvolt to millivolt range. Differential amplification enables the appropriate frequency range to be chosen, which in electromyography and nerve conduction is between 20 and 8000 cycles per second (Hz). The signal to noise ratio can be increased by the appropriate use of an input transformer. Records are usually taken from surface electrodes placed over appropriate nerves or muscles, but may also be made from needle electrodes placed in the

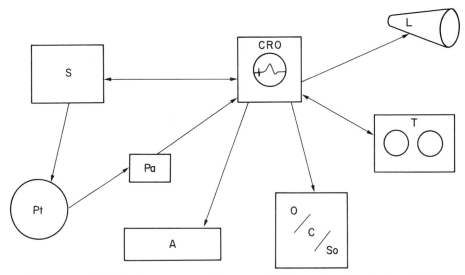

Figure 5–5   Clinical testing apparatus (diagrammatic). Pt = patient; S = stimulator; CRO = amplifier/cathode ray oscilloscope; Pa = pre-amplifier; L = loudspeaker; A = averager; T = magnetic tape; O = fiber optic recorder; C = camera; So = storage oscilloscope.

muscle or adjacent to nerves. The cathode ray oscilloscope is connected to a loudspeaker and also to a stimulator, which usually drives the sweep of the oscilloscope. The stimulator, isolated from ground, is capable of delivering a short duration pulse between 0.05 msec and 2 msec, with a maximum voltage up to 300 v. Further refinements include the use of a stimulator capable of delivering trains and multiple stimuli at given separations. A permanent recording of the tracing can be made using 35 mm film, polaroid film, fiber optic recording systems or magnetic tape. A storage oscilloscope is useful in studying the form of motor unit potentials in electromyography and the variation of potentials following repetitive stimulation in nerve stimulation studies. Electronic averaging devices are used to demonstrate low amplitude nerve action potentials which would otherwise be buried in the baseline noise level. Nerve and muscle stimulation can also be performed by a simple muscle stimulator or chronaximeter.

    Galvanic and faradic stimulations are simple tests, which formerly were in common use in clinical medicine. The muscle is stimulated at its "motor point," which is the point of lowest threshold, usually found where the nerve enters the muscle. With denervation, the threshold to faradic or rapidly alternating current rises, since the duration of the impulse is too short to excite via the damaged nerve or the muscle. The contractions at make and break of galvanic stimulation are gradually depressed in denervation, until only a sluggish response of the muscle remains. These manifestations are called "the reaction of degeneration."

    A more elegant demonstration of the effects of direct stimulation is by construction of a strength-duration curve (Fig. 5-6). Here, the voltage or current is plotted against the duration of stimulus needed to produce a mini-

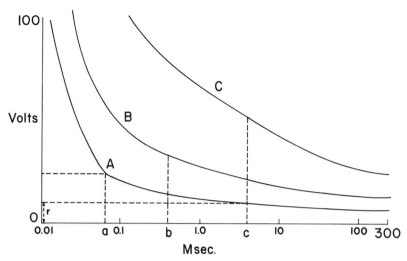

Figure 5 – 6   Strength duration curves and chronaxies. A = normal curve; B = partially denervated curve; C = fully denervated curve; a = chronaxie value of normal muscle; b = chronaxie value of partially denervated muscle; c = chronaxie value of fully denervated muscle; r = rheobase; Msec = milliseconds.

mally visible response. In denervation, a short duration pulse requires a higher stimulus (voltage or current) to obtain the minimally visible response, and the curve shifts to the right. A shorter way of detecting denervation is the chronaxy, which is the duration required to excite contraction at a voltage of twice the rheobase. The rheobase is the minimal voltage required to produce a response by a stimulus of very long duration (in practice, about 300 msec). An increase in chronaxy occurs in denervation and correlates approximately with the changes in the curve on strength-duration measurements. Chronaxy could be used to follow the progression of neuropathies, such as in the course of a facial palsy or Bell's palsy, in which repeated electromyographic or nerve conduction studies may not be desirable.

Motor Nerve Conduction

Motor conduction velocity is measured by stimulating a nerve at two points along its course and in each case recording the contraction of a peripheral muscle supplied by this nerve. In order to insure that all nerve fibers are appropriately excited, the intensity of stimulus should be supramaximal – i.e., 50 per cent above that sufficient to produce a maximum muscle response. For example (Fig. 5–7), the median nerve is stimulated at the elbow and at the wrist, and evoked potential from the thenar muscles is recorded. The time for the impulse to reach the muscle (the latency) is usually measured on a cathode ray oscilloscope from the stimulus artifact to the onset of the evoked potential. The shorter latency from the wrist stimulation is subtracted from the longer latency of the stimulation at the elbow to give the conduction time between the two points. The conduction velocity of the nerve from elbow to wrist is then calculated by dividing the difference of the latencies into the distance between

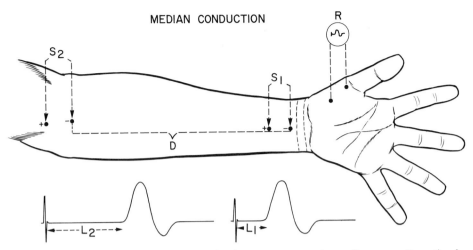

Figure 5–7 Procedure for motor conduction measurement in median nerve. S_1 = stimulus distally (wrist); S_2 = stimulus proximally (elbow); R = recording electrode over thenar muscle; L_1 = distal latency (wrist to muscle); L_2 = proximal latency (elbow to muscle); D = distance between stimulating electrodes S_1, S_2.

$$\text{Conduction velocity} = \frac{D}{L_2 - L_1}$$

stimulation points.[22] Each latency represents the time for the impulse to pass from the distal point of stimulation to the instant that the electrical reaction begins in the muscle. This, of course, also includes the time in the arborized axon and the time for neuromuscular transmission which is eliminated in the above calculation of conduction velocity. Other important parameters of the evoked muscle potential from nerve stimulation are the amplitude, duration and complexity. The voltage and duration of the stimulus required at various points is also of value, and in a few cases, the latencies from threshold as well as supramaximal stimulation should be recorded.

Sensory Nerve Conduction

This can be measured by electrical stimulation of the fingers or toes, using ring electrodes, and recording the nerve action potentials directly over the nerves more proximally (orthodromic). Alternatively, the nerve can be stimulated more proximally with the recording ring electrode over the fingers or toes (antidromic); however, the sensory potential may be obscured or misinterpreted, owing to interference by the evoked motor response. If the nerves are stimulated directly at the wrist and above, recordings from higher levels along the nerve will also include the motor fibers and should be regarded as mixed nerve potentials. When a single recording at wrist from digital stimulation is obtained, a distal sensory latency will be recorded, but the amplitude of the sensory nerve action potential should also be measured. With standard techniques, this amplitude is important as a representation of the number of active fibers within the sensory nerve. If sensory or mixed nerve action potentials are recorded at higher levels, conduction velocities can be computed. Low amplitude potentials can more easily be seen by superimposition of several traces on polaroid film or a storage oscilloscope. Averaging of low amplitude nerve action potentials, particularly those below 5 μv, which is the noise level of much commercial equipment, has improved the recording of nerve action potentials from sensory and mixed nerves in the arm, and has also made possible computation of sensory conduction velocity in the legs.[34]

Clinical Measurements and Application

Normal values of nerve conduction velocity are usually in the range of 50 to 60 m/sec in the upper limb nerves in the distal segments below the elbow, and between 60 and 80 m/sec between shoulder and elbow. In the legs, the normal values are usually between 40 to 50 m/sec (Table 5-2).

Nerve conduction in human infants at birth is about 40 per cent of the adult velocity value, owing to the small size of the fiber and to the fact that a proportion of nerve fibers are incomplete in their myelination at this age.[38] Maturation occurs mainly over the first year, and by the end of the second year[57] most myelinated peripheral nerves are conducting in the normal range. The median nerve is an exception; in this, the full velocity may not be achieved until age 5 to 7.[15] In the premature infant, there is a correlation between the postconceptional age and the nerve conduction velocity, and this correlation may prove to be the optimum way to gauge prematurity. Studies on twins, triplets, quadruplets and quintuplets in our laboratories confirm these findings[29] (Fig. 5-8).

Peripheral nerves reacting to destructive conditions, or undergoing degeneration, may be affected in three ways:

TABLE 5-2 NORMAL VALUES FOR MOTOR AND SENSORY NERVE CONDUCTION*

Nerve	Motor Conduction Velocity (m/sec)			Number of Patients
	Mean	S.D.	Lower Limit	
Median	57.2	4.2	48.8	25
Ulnar	60.0	5.8	48.4	188
Peroneal	51.0	3.26	44.5	69
Post. Tibial	48.7	3.5	41.7	12
	Sensory Distal Latency (msec)			Number of Patients
	Mean	S.D.	Upper Limit	
Median	2.8	.30	3.4	70
Ulnar	2.3	.29	2.9	28

*S.D. = Standard deviation of measurement. Lower limit is regarded as mean value − 2 S.D. measurement. (From Lovelace, R. E., and S. J. Horwitz: Peripheral neuropathy in long-term diphenylhydantoin therapy. Arch. Neurol., *18*:69–77, 1968.)

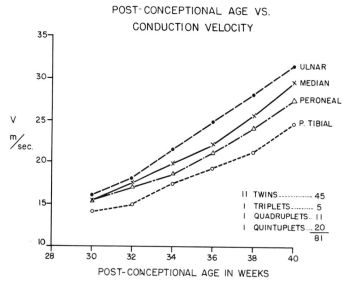

Figure 5–8 Post-conceptional age versus conduction velocity. V = velocity; m/sec = meters per second. Number of studies on multiple births is indicated. (From Koenigsberger, M. R., J. Curtin and R. E. Lovelace: Motor conduction velocities as a measure of gestational age in premature infants. A study of multiple births. Neurology, *20*:381, 1970.)

A. A temporary disturbance of function, resulting from minor injury from which the nerve usually recovers completely in a period of less than two months, is called *neuropraxia* and is not connected with any intrinsic morphological change. This produces a blockage of nerve conduction at the level of the lesion.

B. When the axon has been severely damaged, failure of conduction in the nerve distal to the lesion occurs in the condition of *axonotmesis.* Following the injury, there is secondary or Wallerian degeneration of the myelin sheath, which corresponds to the axonal disappearance. Nerve conduction returns only if a viable axon regenerates. The regenerating axon is thin at first, so that conduction velocity is slow and becomes more rapid as the fiber diameter increases and as remyelination occurs.

C. When the primary damage is to the Schwann cell—whether by toxins, compression or anoxia—*primary demyelination* or Gombault's degeneration takes place. If the axon still remains intact, conduction is possible, but at a much slower rate. With remyelination, there may be great variation in the internodal distance, which also causes slow conduction velocity. Fibrosis around a peripheral nerve, which may be associated with this segmental demyelination, increases the threshold of stimulus needed to activate the nerve and also reduces conduction velocity, relative to the degree of demyelination produced.

From the above considerations, the clinical significance of conduction velocity and nerve stimulation are apparent. The contributions of motor and sensory nerve abnormalities to the various neuropathies can be measured, and the type of nerve involvement can be determined as well; primary axonal neuropathy with failure of conduction; or segmental demyelination with slow conduction velocity. The extent of regeneration and the degree of involvement of peripheral nerves can be assessed. The involvement may be a diffuse process, such as in peripheral neuropathy; multiple individual nerve lesions, as in mononeuritis multiplex; local single nerve lesions or involvement of trunks, plexuses or spinal segments. It is possible to localize the site of a lesion on a nerve by discovering evidence of blockage of conduction at a certain level, or of localized slowing of conduction. Examples of this are the entrapment syndromes in the carpal or tarsal tunnels, or in the deep palmar branch of the ulnar nerve; here one finds prolonged distal latencies, abnormal muscle evoked potentials and impaired sensory distal conduction. The ulnar nerve may be involved similarly at the elbow, the peroneal nerve as it passes around the neck of the fibula, the median nerve passing through the pronator teres muscle and, less commonly, the femoral nerve under the inguinal ligament. A good example, which demonstrates the various stages, is a "tardy" ulnar palsy with involvement of the ulnar nerve in the groove behind the medial epicondyle of the elbow. At first, evoked potentials can be recorded from the hypothenar muscles on stimulation of the nerve below the elbow and at the wrist, but an absent or reduced amplitude response on stimulation above the elbow indicates blockage of nerve conduction at that level (neuropraxia). The next stage of development of the disorder is one of demyelination, in which the evoked muscle response to above-elbow stimulation, when present, becomes complex in shape and reduced in amplitude, with greater dispersion (axonocachexia). At this stage, there is also evidence of slow conduction velocity in the segment around the elbow. Sensory conduction is impaired, and the sensory nerve action potential at the wrist may be unrecordable, even with maximal finger stimulation. Finally, with axonotmesis, there is Wallerian degeneration over the whole distal nerve segment, with loss of response, and associated denervation noted electromyographically in relevant muscles. Concurrent re-innervation may produce further dispersion of the evoked potential. Thus, conduction velocity is useful in documenting the presence of neuropathies, in elucidating the cause for wasting or in investigating severe pain or hyperpathia, often associated with neuropathy. Nerve conduction is slowed in the neuropathies that are associated with alcoholism, diabetes and in some drug intoxications (heroin, for example) and also in uremia.

In disease of the anterior horn cell, in which severe wasting may be associated with denervation in the affected muscles, nerve conduction may be relatively unaffected, since the peripheral nerve is spared. Sensory nerve conduction is normal in anterior horn cell disease. Motor nerve conduction has occasionally been seen to be slow in patients with anterior horn cell disease, and this has been attributed to the effect of local cold on the nerve trunk, as conduction velocity is reduced about 5 per cent per degree Centigrade fall in temperature.[26]

In myopathy and myositis, conduction velocity is normal. In some familial or congenital neuropathies, particularly in the condition of peroneal muscular atrophy or Charcot-Marie-Tooth disorder, the conduction velocity may be very slow, even in nerves that do not appear to be clinically affected. Similar involvement occurs in the allied Roussy-Lévy syndrome, familial hypertrophic polyneuritis (Dejerine-Sottas disease) and Refsum's disease. Less marked impairment of conduction velocity is seen in Friedreich's ataxia and ataxia telangiectasia. A-beta-lipoproteinemia (the Bassen-Kornzweig syndrome) and Tangier disease (serum alpha-lipoprotein deficiency[2]) are also associated with neuropathy having slow conduction times. Conduction studies may be particularly useful in diagnosing metachromatic leukodystrophy in children. Conduction velocity is likely to be slow in the metabolic, deficiency, hereditary and allergic neuropathies. From such observations, these have been called demyelinating neuropathies.

The differentiation between demyelinating neuropathies and axonal neuropathies is no more clear-cut than is the anatomical distinction into sensory and motor neuropathies.[18] In diabetes, both demyelination and axonal degeneration occur, with demyelination predominating.[58] In porphyria, both also occur, with axonal degeneration greater.[60] In general, the acute toxic neuropathies tend to be axonal,[30] such as those seen with organophosphate poisoning, or those resulting from drugs, such as thalidomide or vincristine, but an exception is the now rare diphtheritic neuropathy, which is demyelinating.

Sensory conduction may be lost in any lesion of the sensory pathway distal to the dorsal root ganglion, and is valuable in distinguishing a brachial plexus disorder from involvement of the anterior horn cell in the spinal cord.[3] Normal sensory nerve action potentials may be recorded at the wrist from digital stimulation when anesthesia or analgesia is present as the result of a spinal cord lesion such as syringomyelia. Distal latencies may be increased or sensory nerve action potentials may be lost in a variety of neuropathies, often in diabetic neuropathy and Friedreich's ataxia[46] and invariably in Charcot-Marie-Tooth disorder[8] and the hypertrophic neuropathy of Dejerine-Sottas. When the total clinical condition is one of a mild, chronic, purely sensory neuropathy (frequently seen in diabetes or in hereditary sensory neuropathy), especially if it is confined to the legs, the peroneal and posterior tibial nerve action potentials obtained with averaging techniques may be helpful.[34] In children—and with difficulty in adults—it has been possible to record sural sensory nerve action potentials directly, without the aid of computerization.[6] In subliminal nerve lesions associated with subclinical neuropathy, threshold conduction velocity may be more valuable, as shown by Preswick in the carpal tunnel syndrome.[47] Provocative ischemia may give rise to nerve conduction failure or slowing at an earlier point in time than would be normally expected in such lesions.[14] Subclinical diabetic and uremic neuropathies may also be revealed by nerve conduction studies.

H-Reflex

This is the reflex produced by low threshold stimulation of a muscle nerve so that the large myelinated sensory fibers from the muscle spindles are activated, but the stimulus is subthreshold to the direct motor fibers. The response in the muscle occurs, therefore, via a reflex pathway through the spinal cord, thence to activation of the motor fibers. The spindle afferent conduction velocity may thus be estimated by the H-reflex measurement. As an example, this delayed or H-reflex may be produced in the gastrocnemius muscle at a latency of approximately 30 msec by stimulation of the posterior tibial nerve behind the knee; this is thought to represent the time of a single synapse reflex arc. In the normal adult, this is practically the only convenient site for H-reflex recording, but in the first few years of life, H-reflexes can be recorded from other nerves, including the ulnar.[36] In adults, abnormal H-reflexes can be recorded in the presence of spinal cord disease at the appropriate level.[37]

F-waves are of shorter latency, and probably involve only the motor axon and no synapse: The impulse presumably is rebounded at the anterior horn cell and passes back down the motor neuron to the muscle.[42] Unlike the H-reflex, they are not obliterated when the direct motor response appears, and are more consistently present, although they are of more variable latency. They may prove useful in measuring abnormal neuroconditions in the root zone, as in the early stage of postinfectious polyneuritis or the Guillain-Barré syndrome, at a time when motor conduction velocity of the fastest fibers may be quite unimpaired on distal conduction studies.[20]

Because conduction of fastest fibers does not always give information as to the extent of change in the neurons, it is useful to analyze more fully the compound nerve action potential. Even with averaging techniques, this is not easy to perform with recording in situ, but if nerves are stimulated after appropriate excision at biopsy in a constant temperature mammalian chamber, the velocities of the individual nerve fibers (i.e., alpha, delta, and C fibers) can be demonstrated. Lambert[7] has shown that whereas alpha fibers are very slow and delta fibers are lost in hypertrophic interstitial neuropathy, and both lost in hereditary sensory neuropathy, the C fibers in the sural nerve are still intact in both.

The future of nerve conduction studies may largely evolve around the more detailed development of reflex measurements, with the resultant information that these will give about the proximal motor and sensory neuron and the state of the spinal cord.

NEUROMUSCULAR TRANSMISSION

Motor End Plate Anatomy and Chemistry

Neuromuscular transmission is the means by which the nerve impulse activates the muscle fiber and results in contraction of the muscle fiber. The usual response in mammalian muscle fibers is a propagated action potential and twitch. The morphological means by which this is effected is the end plate and its component structures.

The size and morphology of end plates vary with species, but generally, the end plate is circular or oval and usually of a diameter less than 70 microns. There is usually one motor end plate for each muscle fiber, situated centrally and supplied by one terminal twig from a neuron.[12] Histologically, the end plate consists of three portions:
1. The terminal apparatus of the nerve

2. The specialized region of muscle fiber surface in contact with this terminal apparatus
3. The area of teloglia surrounding it

The area of teloglia contains the "sole nuclei" and appears to be continuous with the Schwann cell envelope of the myelinated fiber. The end plate of the muscle is separated from the terminal apparatus of the nerve by a space of less than 1 micron, called the synaptic cleft. Electron microscopic studies (Fig. 5-9) indicate that in mammalian (including human) tissue, the end bulb of the nerve has a curved surface which is cupped into a partially concave foot plate on the muscle, thereby forming a primary cleft. The foot plate of the muscle is further subdivided into numerous secondary clefts. In disease, the primary cleft may become distorted and the secondary clefts abnormal in shape and number. The developing end plate in the fetus is similar to the abnormal end plates in diseases of neuromuscular transmission.[11] With maturity, organization of the end plate involves the development of the primary and secondary clefts.

The function of the end plate region has been studied by chemical and electrical means. Following the response of repetitive stimulation on the nerve, the muscle contracts in forms that vary from single twitches to a completely fused tetanus. The end plate can transmit frequencies up to 40 per sec before significant fatigue occurs. Microelectrode studies have indicated that, in the resting state, small electrical disturbances occur on the cleft side of the postsynaptic membrane.[13] These discrete changes are of the order of 0.5 mv amplitude and occur at a frequency of about 1 per sec. In nerve excitation[43] these electrical disturbances become large enough to produce an end plate potential which, when it reaches threshold level on the foot plate of the muscle, will discharge the postjunctional membrane and produce a propagated action potential in the muscle, spreading in both directions from the end plate. Histochemical studies have demonstrated vesicles containing acetylcholine in the end

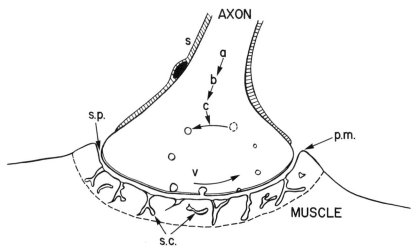

Figure 5–9 Motor end plate (diagrammatic). s = Schwann cell; s.p. = synaptic space: primary cleft; s.c. = secondary clefts; p.m. = post-junctional membrane; a = synthesis of acetylcholine; b = store (reserve) of acetylcholine; c = readily available acetylcholine; v = discharge and re-charge cycle of synaptic vesicles.

bulb of the neuron[1] (Fig. 5–9). These vesicles are continually discharging and being regenerated; the contents of acetylcholine are released in packets into the short synaptic cleft and are responsible for the production of the small electrical disturbances at the postsynaptic membrane, referred to previously, called miniature end plate potentials. After discharge of the vesicle, a recharging process occurs in the same vesicle, causing accumulation of further supplies of acetylcholine, which appear to be stored in immediately proximal regions of the neuron.[39] The acetylcholine acts on a receptor site in the postjunctional membrane, and is then immediately destroyed by acetylcholinesterase present either in the synaptic cleft or possibly at a second receptor site. Anticholinesterase preparations will compete with the acetylcholine for the cholinesterase and so will preserve acetylcholine for a longer period. Curare preparations, on the other hand, compete with acetylcholine for the primary receptor sites on the postjunctional membrane and prevent depolarization.

When depolarization of the postjunctional membrane has occurred, a propagated action potential is produced. The action potential triggers the mechanical contraction of the muscle by an excitation-contraction-coupling reaction.[12] To account for the speed of this change, there is a mechanism for rapid transmission of the information from the surface to the center of the fiber that involves the transverse tubular system of the sarcoplasmic reticulum (see Chapter 4).

The end plate mechanism appears to be acutely dependent on the concentrations of divalent cations. If we consider an end plate potential as being produced as a result of the discharge of 100 to 200 quanta (each equivalent to a miniature end plate potential) of acetylcholine from the nerve terminals, the magnitude of the action potential will depend on the ability of the terminal ending of the nerve to produce an adequate quantity of acetylcholine.[43] Sufficient acetylcholine is usually produced only when the action potential arriving at the terminal nerve ending increases the quantal release of acetylcholine and when the depolarization produced by the nerve impulse is of sufficient magnitude. Reducing the external calcium and raising the external magnesium concentrations may cause a reduction in the number of quanta produced per impulse; thus, the action of calcium appears to be to increase the release of these quanta caused by the action potential in the nerve terminal.[32] This corresponds to raising the frequency of the miniature end plate potentials. Further studies, however, with curarized mammalian preparations have indicated that at the start of repetitive stimulation using low calcium–high magnesium treated preparations, a potentiation under normal physiological conditions is masked. Such masking could be attributed to reduced available store of acetylcholine in the nerve terminal and would certainly fit in with the fall of end plate amplitude occurring on repetitive stimulation in a curarized preparation. Following a train of nerve impulses to a normal physiological end plate, a potentiation in neuromuscular transmission occurs.[44] Studies with preparations blocked by magnesium and d-tubocurarine have indicated that this post-tetanic potentiation results from an increase in the store of available acetylcholine and that it reaches a peak in about 100 msec. Secondary potentiation, reaching a peak in 4 to 7 sec, may result from increased mobilization of the acetylcholine, so building up the available store.[24]

Clinical Application

The simplest test for neuromuscular transmission is to observe the muscular fatigue on repetitive stimulation of the appropriate nerve. This is called the "Jolly" reaction.[27]

One of the simplest methods of demonstrating the efficiency of the neuromuscular junction is the observation of single firing motor unit potentials. The motor unit potential is composed of the many single fiber potentials making up one motor unit, which is a group of muscle fibers and its single neuron. If every muscle fiber in the motor unit fires consistently with each neuronal impulse, the shape of the motor unit potential recorded from the same position on each occasion should be exactly comparable. In practice, there is a small variation of up to 5 per cent in amplitude and duration. When, however, individual end plates with their muscle fibers show excessive fatigue, the motor unit potential becomes lower in amplitude or fragmented as individual muscle fiber potentials disappear. Thus, a significant variation in amplitude of the same motor unit potential, repetitively firing, will appear in defects of neuromuscular transmission, as in myasthenia gravis. This may take the form of a simple progressive decrement of the motor unit potential as more fibers become fatigued, or it may present with variation in amplitude of the same motor unit potential. In a similar fashion, the amplitude and numbers of potentials firing in a maximal interference pattern of motor unit potentials produced by a strong contraction decrease in the presence of a defect of neuromuscular transmission. When such a fall-off in the interference pattern is observed during needle electromyography of a patient with myasthenia gravis, intramuscular or intravenous administration of an anticholinesterase drug preserves acetylcholine in the synaptic cleft and corrects the defect of neuromuscular transmission for as long as the drug acts.

Miniature end plate potentials can be recorded from excised muscle in a suitable constant-temperature nutrient bath medium. In excised myasthenic muscle, one microelectrode study showed that the miniature end plate potentials are not consistently abnormal in amplitude[5] but are reduced in frequency, whereas several other studies indicated that their amplitude was reduced, thus suggesting that the packets contained smaller amounts of acetylcholine.[10, 56] These latter studies failed to confirm a change in frequency. More recently, in our laboratory[35] and in the Mayo Clinic,[59] experiments have been performed with small macroelectrodes on mammalian and human muscle in situ. When inserted at the motor point, miniature end plate potentials (of 30 to 60 μv) can be recorded extracellularly. Two recent reports[21, 35] using this technique in patients with myasthenia gravis have indicated, in fact, that the miniature end plate potentials may not be abnormal in amplitude, but are very significantly reduced in frequency in this disorder. This conflict between the data from some of the microelectrode recordings in excised muscle on the one hand, and from small macroelectrode recordings from muscle in situ on the other hand, may occur because the disorder of neuromuscular transmission as seen in myasthenia gravis is partly a result of a morphological change in the end plate in which the contact of the nerve terminal with the postjunctional membrane on the muscle is drastically reduced. This is confirmed by electron microscopic studies showing a change in the size of the end bulb of the neuron and by alterations in the shape and dimensions of the primary and secondary clefts of the synaptic space[11] (Fig. 5–9).

The remainder of electrodiagnostic studies associated with neuromuscular transmission can be considered as an extension of the original Jolly test. If the evoked potential from muscle produced by supramaximal stimulation is recorded with surface electrodes in such a fashion that consistent results can be produced by repetitive stimulation, the effects of repetitive stimulation can be interpreted to describe the function of the neuromuscular junction. At stimulation rates between 1 and 5 per sec, no significant variation is noted in the amplitude of this supramaximally evoked potential. At more rapid stimulation in normal patients, post-tetanic potentiation results in a rise of between 5 and 20 per cent in amplitude. This becomes more apparent at stimulation rates up to 40 per sec and, usually, repetitive stimulation up to 50 per sec is not associated with significant decrement. In disorders of neuromuscular transmission, decrement usually appears at the slow rates of stimulation, best seen at 2 and 5 per sec; with prolonged stimulation, further decrement usually occurs. The commonest disorder of neuromuscular transmission in which this type of decrement occurs is myasthenia gravis, in which decrements greater than 20 per cent are usually noted, especially when testing a weakened muscle. Anticholinesterase therapy tends to correct this decrement and may invalidate results of tests on a patient under such therapy. At high rates of stimulation in patients with myasthenia gravis, potentiating effects may be noted following an initial decrement, but prolonged stimulation usually produces further decrement. Thus, post-tetanic facilitation is usually not lost in disorders of neuromuscular transmission, such as myasthenia gravis. Lesser decrements with repetitive stimulation are also noticed in neuronal muscle wasting diseases, such as amyotrophic lateral sclerosis, syringomyelia and carcinomatous neuromyopathy. In patients with myasthenia gravis with mild defects, potentiating measures such as prolonged exercise and ischemia may be needed to bring out the decrement on repetitive stimulation.

Occasionally, a paradoxical myasthenic reaction is seen in some patients, principally those with small cell carcinoma of the bronchus. This has sometimes been called the myasthenic syndrome or the Lambert-Eaton syndrome. It consists of a fatiguing type of muscular weakness, but without the specific exercise fatigue so characteristic of myasthenia gravis. These patients may also have evidence of peripheral neuropathy. Characteristically, the patient exhibits a slow onset to the hand grip. Electrical studies show a marked potentiation of the supramaximal muscle evoked potential on repetitive stimulation, even at very low rates. The initial amplitude of the supramaximally evoked potential in the previously rested nerve-muscle system is reduced from normal, but even at stimulation rates as low as 1 per sec, there may be a rapid potentiation of as much as 200 per cent. Repetitive stimulation at 2, 5, 10, and 25 per sec produces similar potentiation. Electromyographic recordings may also show variation in the amplitude of single motor unit potentials, perhaps because of the presence of many end plate potentials of just subthreshold level. Intracellular investigation on excised muscle shows that the miniature end plate potentials are normal in amplitude, but that there is reduced number of quanta released by the impulse. Thus, many end plate potentials at subthreshold level are produced, but these rapidly advance to threshold levels with repetitive stimulation. Administration of guanidine improves the condition and increases the amplitude of the end plate potentials, perhaps by increasing the number of quanta of acetylcholine released from the nerve ending. In some ways, the defect in neuromuscular transmission of the myasthenic syndrome is similar to that produced experimentally by excess circulating magnesium (Mg^{++}).

Another manifestation of abnormal neuromuscular transmission is seen in the response to curare. Patients with myasthenia gravis are markedly sensitive to curare. Although part of the defect in this disorder has been thought to be connected with the nerve terminal and acetylcholine concentration in the vesicles, there may also be some disturbance in the postjunctional membrane. Blockage of the primary receptor sites for acetylcholine by the curare may further reduce drastically the safety factor in the myasthenic motor end plate and give rise to the excessive paralysis easily produced by low dosages of this substance. This is the basis of the curare test performed in myasthenia gravis.

Finally, various chemicals and toxins may act on the end plate region. In particular, some of the mycin antibiotics, such as neomycin and kanamycin, may produce disorder of neuromuscular transmission resembling myasthenia gravis or may seriously exacerbate myasthenia gravis. Botulinum toxin probably produces its effects by presynaptic action or by disturbance in the synthesis or storage of acetylcholine.

REFERENCES

1. Barrnett, R. J.: Ultrastructure histochemistry of normal neuromuscular junction. Ann. N. Y. Acad. Sci., *135*:27-34, 1966.
2. Beranek, R.: Intracellular stimulation myography in man. Electroenceph. Clin. Neurophysiol., *16*:301-304, 1964.
3. Bonney, G., and Gilliatt, R. W.: Sensory nerve conduction after traction lesions of the brachial plexus. Proc. Roy. Soc. Med., *51*:365-367, 1958.
4. Cole, K. S.: *Membranes, Ions and Impulses.* Los Angeles, University of California Press, 1968.
5. Dahlback, O., Elmqvist, D., Johns, T. R., Radner, S., and Thesleff, S.: An electrophysiological study of the neuromuscular junction in myasthenia gravis. J. Physiol. (London), *156*:336-343, 1961.
6. DiBenedetto, M.: Sensory nerve conduction in the lower extremity. Arch. Phys. Med. Rehabil., *51*:253-258, 1970.
7. Dyck, P. J., and Lambert, E. H.: Numbers and diameters of nerve fibers and compound nerve action potentials of sural nerves: Controls and hereditary neuromuscular disorders. Transactions of American Neurological Association, *91*:214-217, 1966.
8. Dyck, P. J., Lambert, E. H., and Mulder, D. W.: Charcot-Marie-Tooth disease: nerve conduction and clinical studies of a large kinship. Neurology, *13*:1-11, 1963.
9. Eliasson, S. G.: Properties of isolated nerve fibers from alloxanized rats. J. Neurol. Neurosurg. Psychiat., *32*:525-529, 1969.
10. Elmqvist, D., Hofmann, W. W., Kugelberg, J., and Quastel, D. M. J.: An electrophysiological investigation of neuromuscular transmission in myasthenia gravis. J. Physiol. (London), *174*:417-434, 1964.
11. Engel, A. G.: Ultrastructure of the neuromuscular junction—Myasthenia gravis and the Myasthenic Syndrome. Fourth International Conference on Myasthenia Gravis., Ann. N. Y. Acad. Sci., Dec., 1970.
12. Fatt, P.: Skeletal neuromuscular transmission. In: *Handbook of Physiology*, Vol. 1, pp. 199-213. American Physiol. Soc., Washington, D.C., 1959.

13. Fatt, P., and Katz, B.: Spontaneous subthreshold activity at motor nerve endings. J. Physiol., *117*:109-128, 1952.
14. Fullerton, P. M.: The effect of ischemia on nerve conduction in carpal tunnel syndrome. J. Neurol. Neurosurg. Psychiat., *26*:385-397, 1963.
15. Gamstorp, I.: Normal conduction velocity of ulnar, median and peroneal nerves in infancy, childhood and adolescence. Acta Paediat. (Stockholm), suppl. *146*:68-76, 1963.
16. Gasser, H. S., and Erlanger, J.: *Electrical Signs of Nervous Action.* Philadelphia, University of Pennsylvania Press, 1937.
17. Gasser, H. S., and Grundfest, M.: Axon diameters in relation to spike dimensions and conduction velocity in mammalian fibers. Am. J. Physiol., *127*:393-414, 1939.
18. Gilliatt, R. W.: Nerve conduction in human and experimental neuropathies. Proc. Roy. Soc. Med., *59*:989-993, 1966.
19. Goodgold, J., and Eberstein, A. F.: Transmembrane potentials of human muscle cells in vivo. Exp. Neurol., *15*:338-346, 1966.
20. Graham, J.: Studies on the F wave in the Guillain-Barré Syndrome. Personal communication, Cardiff, U.K., 1970.
21. Grob, D., Rosenfalck, A., and Buchtal, F.: Spontaneous end-plate activity in normal subjects and in patients with myasthenia gravis. Fourth International Conference on Myasthenia Gravis, New York. Ann. N. Y. Acad. Sci., Dec., 1970.
22. Hoder, R., Larrabee, M. G., and German, W.: The human electromyogram in response to nerve stimulation and the conduction velocity of motor axons. Arch. Neurol. Psychiat., *60*:340-365, 1948.
23. Hodgkin, A. L., and Keynes, R. O.: Active transport of cations in giant axons Sepia and Loligo. J. Physiol. (London), *128*:28-60, 1955.
24. Hubbard, J.: Repetitive stimulation at the mammalian neuromuscular junction and the mobilization of transmitter. J. Physiol., *169*:641-662, 1963.
25. Johns, R. J.: Microelectrode studies of muscle membrane potentials in man. Res. Publ. Assoc. Nerv. Ment. Dis., *38*:704-713, 1958.
26. Johnson, E. W., Guyton, J. D., and Olsen, K. J.: Motor nerve conduction velocity studies in poliomyelitis. Arch. Phys. Med. Rehabil., *41*:185-190, 1960.
27. Jolly, F.: Über Myasthenia Gravis Pseudoparalytica. Klin. Wschr., *33*:4, 1895.
28. Katz, B.: *Nerve, Muscle and Synapse.* New York, McGraw-Hill Book Co., Inc., 1966.
29. Koenigsberger, M. R., Curtin, J., and Lovelace, R. E.: Motor conduction velocities as a measure of gestational age in premature infants. A study of multiple births. Neurology, *20*:381, 1970.
30. Kremer, M.: Clinical aspects of toxic neuropathies. In: *Biochemical Aspects of Neurological Disorders,* Oxford, 2nd. series, pp. 89-100. Blackwell, 1965.
31. Lenman, J. A. R., and Ritchie, A. E.: *Clinical Electromyography.* Philadelphia, J. B. Lippincott Co., 1970.
32. Liley, A. W.: The effects of presynaptic polarization on the spontaneous activity at the mammalian neuromuscular junction. J. Physiol., *134*:427-443, 1956.
33. Ling, G. and Gerard, R. W.: The normal membrane potential of frog sartorius fibers. J. Cell. Comp. Physiol., *34*:383-396, 1949.
34. Lovelace, R. E., Myers, S. J., and Zablow, L.: Sensory conduction in peroneal, posterior tibial and sural nerves using averaging techniques. Electroenceph. Clin. Neurophysiol., *27*:726, 1969.
35. Lovelace, R. E., Stone, R., and Zablow, L.: A new test for myasthenia gravis: Recording of miniature end-plate potentials in situ. Neurology, *20*:385, 1970.
36. Magladery, J. W., Porter, W. E., Park, A. M., and Teasdall, R. D.: Electrophysiological studies of nerve and reflex activity in normal man. Bull. Johns Hopkins Hosp., *88*:499-519, 1951.
37. Magladery, J. W., Teasdall, R. D., Park, A. M., and Languth, H. W.: Electrophysiological studies of reflex activity in patients with lesions in the central nervous system. Bull. Johns Hopkins Hosp., *91*:219-275, 1952.
38. Marinacci, A. A.: *Applied Electromyography,* Philadelphia, pp. 1-22. Lea and Febiger, 1968.
39. Martin, A. R.: Mechanisms of transmitter release from nerve terminals. Fourth International Conference on Myasthenia Gravis. Ann. N. Y. Acad. Sci., Dec., 1970.
40. McComas, A. and Johns, R. T.: Potential changes in the normal and diseased muscle cell. In: *Disorders of Voluntary Muscle,* pp. 877-907. (J. Walton, ed.). Boston, Little, Brown, 1969.
41. McDonald, W. I.: Nerve conduction muscle afferent fibers during experimental demyelination in cat nerve. Acta Neuropathologica, *1*:425-432, 1962.
42. McLeod, J. G., and Wray, S. H.: An experimental study of the F wave in the baboon. J. Neurol. Neurosurg. Psychiat., *29*:196-200, 1966.
43. Nastuk, W. L.: Fundamental aspects of neuromuscular transmission. Ann. N. Y. Acad. Sci., *135*:110-135, 1966.

44. Otsuka, M., Endo, M., and Nonomura, Y.: Presynaptic nature of neuromuscular depression. Jap. J. Physiol., *12*:573-584, 1962.
45. Petajan, J. H., and Daube, J. R.: Effects of cooling the arm and hand (on neuromuscular function). J. Applied Physiol., *20*:1271-1274, 1965.
46. Preswick, G.: The peripheral neuropathy of Friedreich's Ataxia. Paper presented at International Meeting on Electromyography, Glasgow, Scotland, 1967.
47. Preswick, G.: The effect of stimulus intensity in the carpal tunnel syndrome. J. Neurol. Neurosurg. Psychiat., *26*:398-401, 1963.
48. Riecker, C., and Bolte, H. D.: Membranpotentiale einzelner Skeletmuskelzellen bei hypokaliämischer periodischer Muskelparalyse. Klin. Wschr., *44*:804-807, 1966.
49. Stampfli, R.: Saltatory conduction in nerve. Physiol. Rev., *34*:101-112, 1954.
50. Tasaki, I., Carnay, L., and Watanabe, A.: Transient changes in extrinsic fluorescence of nerve produced by electric stimulation. Proc. Nat. Acad. Sci., *64*:1362-1368, 1969.
51. Tasaki, I.: *Nerve Excitation.* Springfield, Ill., Charles C Thomas, 1968.
52. Tasaki, I., Barry, W., and Carnay, L.: Optical and electrophysiological evidence for conformational changes in membrane macromolecules during nerve excitation. Physical Principles of Biological Membranes (Coral Gables Conference), pp. 17-34. Gordon and Breach, 1968.
53. Tasaki, I.: Conduction of the nerve impulse. In: *Handbook of Physiology*, pp. 75-121. Am. Physiol. Soc., Washington, D.C., 1959.
54. Tasaki, I.: *Nervous Transmission.* Springfield, Ill., Charles C Thomas, 1953.
55. Tasaki, I., and Mizuguchi, K.: The changes in the electric impedance during activity and the effect of alkaloids and polarization upon the bioelectric processes in the myelinated nerve fiber. Acta Biochem. Biophys., *3*:484-493, 1949.
56. Thesleff, S.: Acetylcholine utilization in myasthenia gravis. Ann. N.Y. Acad. Sci., *135*:195–206, 1966.
57. Thomas, J. E., and Lambert, E.: Ulnar nerve conduction velocity and H-reflex in infants and children. J. Applied Physiol., *15*:1-9, 1960.
58. Thomas, P. K., and Lascelles, R. C.: The pathology of diabetic neuropathy. Quart. J. Med., *35*:489-509, 1966.
59. Weiderholt, W. C.: End-plate noise. Neurology, *20*:214–224, 1970.
60. Zimmerman, E. A., and Lovelace, R. E.: The etiology of neuropathy in acute intermittent porphyria. Transactions of American Neurological Association, *93*:294-296, 1968.

Chapter 6

THE MOTOR UNIT AND MUSCLE ACTION POTENTIALS

by Stanley J. Myers, M.D., and Robert E. Lovelace,
M.B. (Lond.), M.R.C.P. (Lond.)

Brief History

Electromyography plays a significant role in the clinical laboratory for diagnostic and prognostic purposes as well as in physiological and kinesiological research. That electricity is generated from muscle was postulated by Redi in 1666, but this was first demonstrated by Matteucci, using an improved galvanometer, in 1838. DuBois-Reymond confirmed this work and in 1851 performed the first human electromyography (he used jars of liquid as electrodes) by recording action currents from the contracting arm of a man. The development of more sophisticated apparatus, especially Einthoven's string galvanometer, made further investigations of muscle action potentials possible and allowed correlation of laboratory findings with normal human muscle potentials. The first extensive clinical EMG study was made in Germany by Piper, who published the first book on electromyography in 1912. In 1929, Adrian and Bronk introduced the coaxial (concentric) needle electrode which made it possible to pick up potentials from a single muscle fiber. They also amplified the muscle action potentials through a loudspeaker as an additional aid in interpreting results. The introduction of the cathode ray oscilloscope by Erlanger and Gasser (1937) freed workers from the limitations of mechanical galvanometers.

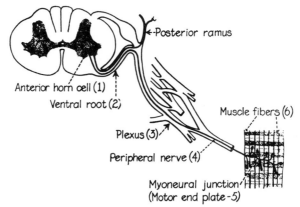

Figure 6–1   The motor unit. Terminal and subterminal branching of the nerve fiber occurs between (4) and (5). (From Rodriquez and Oester: Fundamentals of Electromyography. *In* Licht, S. (ed.): *Electrodiagnosis and Electromyography.* New Haven, E. Licht, 1971.)

MOTOR UNIT

Definition

The motor unit as the anatomical unit of muscle function was defined by Liddell and Sherrington in 1925. The motor unit consists of a single anterior horn cell (motoneuron), its axon cylinder (including the terminal and subterminal branching within the muscle body), the motor end plates and all the muscle fibers innervated by that neuron (Fig. 6–1).

Anatomical and Physiological Make-Up

The motor axon branches many times to provide end plates for its multiple muscle fibers. Most of the divisions occur within the terminal intramuscular nerve bundles at the points of branching of the nerve bundles proper at a node of Ranvier.[19] Normally the division is into two groups of fibers of approximately equal caliber containing 10 to 50 nerve fibers each, which, after emerging from the bundle as subterminal nerve fibers, run in isolation across the muscle fibers to terminate in the end plates. In man only 1.5 to 10 per cent of nerve fibers branch after they leave as subterminal nerve fibers.

The number of muscle fibers per motor unit is estimated in humans by counting the total number of muscle fibers in a muscle and dividing this by the total number of motor nerve fibers.[17, 23] Some representative values of the number of muscle fibers per motor unit are as follows: opponens pollicis, 13; superior rectus, 23; platysma, 25; biceps brachii, 163; sartorius, 300; rectus femoris, 305; first dorsal interosseous, 340; gracilis, 527; anterior tibial, 610; gastrocnemius, 2037. These estimations assume that 60 per cent of the nerve fibers in muscles are motor fibers, as determined from measurements on the nerves to the anterior tibial and gastrocnemius muscles in the cat. No correction is made for motor nerve fibers supplying the intrafusal muscle fibers. Furthermore it is unlikely that the proportion of motor nerve fibers will be equal for functionally different muscles. Thus, the estimate given for the number of muscle fibers per motor unit is imprecise and is likely to be on the low side. In general, however, the size of the motor unit varies according to its function, with those muscles responsible for precision movements having the least number of muscle fibers per motor unit.

Multi-innervation

It is not known definitely whether multiple innervation of muscle fibers occurs. There is evidence that it may be present in the cat, dog and the frog,[32, 47] but no reliable evidence exists that it plays any significant role in man. The evidence of its existence in the animals mentioned above is mostly indirect, obtained from the measurement of tensions produced by stimulation of single motor nerve fibers compared with the tension produced by stimulation of two or more fibers together.[9, 47] Most muscle fibers do not seem to have more than two motor end plates, and it is not possible to determine if these doubly innervated fibers received their nerve from branches of the same neuron, from separate axons or from nerve fibers supplied by different cord segments.

Double and multiple innervation has been reported in human gracilis and soleus muscles, based on histochemical staining of muscle fibers for motor end plates. However further studies utilizing the muscles of stillborn infants do not support these conclusions.[17] In most muscles motor end plates are found in the middle of the muscle fibers. The gracilis and sartorius are exceptions since two end plate bands are noted in the gracilis, and in the sartorius the end plates are disseminated. In the sartorius these end plates correspond to the numerous short muscle bundles seen in serial longitudinal sections and are developed from a chain of myoblasts in series, each supplied with only one end plate. In adult muscles these longitudinal fiber chains fuse together and create the impression that one is dealing with multiple innervation and multiple end plates in a single muscle fiber.

The location of the end plates in the middle portion of the muscle belly provides for the fastest activation of all its contractile material, and multiple nerve endings may increase the rate at which tension is developed by the muscle fiber. If nerve impulses reach terminations synchronously at several points along the muscle fiber, impulses will be initiated and spread over the length of the fiber in less time than if activity began at only one locus.

The biceps brachii and opponens pollicis muscles of man have been demonstrated to have 1.3 to 1.5 motor end plates per muscle fiber,[17] and this too has been interpreted as indicating a multiple innervation of some fibers. The end plate zone in these muscles is centrally located, as it is in most other muscles. Therefore, if present, the two end plates are only a short distance from each other and multiple innervation can play only a limited role in reducing the activation time.

Motor Unit Territory

Individual muscle fibers extend throughout the length of most muscles and are arranged in parallel. The gracilis and sartorius muscles are exceptions, where the fibers are arranged in series. The topographical arrangement of the muscle fibers of a motor unit as seen in cross section is not firmly established, but most workers agree that in animals there is an intermingling and wide scattering of fibers from different motor units.

If single ventral root fibers innervating the rat anterior tibial muscle are isolated and stimulated repetitively, the glycogen in the muscle fibers responding to the stimulation of the single axon becomes exhausted. Immediately after stimulation the whole muscle is excised, frozen, and cross sections are cut and stained by PAS technique for glycogen so that the muscle fibers of the stimulated motor units can be seen. Such preparations show that there is moderate variation in the total number of muscle fibers and motor unit territory and that there is a diffuse scattering of the muscle fibers throughout the territory of that motor unit.[6] The vast majority of fibers, approximately 70 per cent of the motor unit, have no contact with other fibers of the same unit. A motor unit occasionally contains groups of muscle fibers, with each group usually consisting of two fibers but rarely more than three.

In man indirect methods of analysis have been made by Buchthal, Guld and Rosenfalck using the multilead electrode (Fig. 6-2). Different multielectrode types of up to 14 leads were constructed. One type having twelve 50 to 100μ leads, arranged in a row of 2.5 mm total length, was used for the study of the volume conduction of the spike of motor unit potentials.[15] Other types having greater leading-off areas and larger interelectrode distances (14 leads, 1.5 mm each, with a distance of 2.5 mm between the centers of adjacent leads) were used to scan total muscle cross section and to study the territory of the motor unit.[16] The spatial spread of action potentials from a given motor unit so

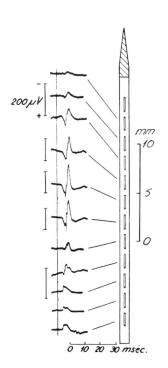

Figure 6–2 Diagram of and examples of recording from a multilead electrode. Action potentials from a motor unit in the human biceps brachii. The lead nearest the tip is the indifferent electrode. (From Buchthal, Guld and Rosenfalck: Multielectrode study of the territory of a motor unit. Acta Physiol. Scand., 39:89, 1957.)

obtained indicates the territory occupied by the fibers of a motor unit. A spike component in the motor unit potential is taken to signal the presence of active muscle fibers closer than 0.5 mm from the recording electrode, since there is a reduction in the amplitude of a potential to less than one-tenth of its maximum at a distance of 0.3 to 0.65 mm from a spike source. The spike potentials with a voltage of 50 μv or more recorded on the outer leads of a multielectrode that passes through the center of a motor unit indicate the limits of its territory. With two multielectrodes perpendicular to each other and transverse to the fiber direction and another electrode situated at the periphery of the motor unit field it is found that the territory of a motor unit is roughly circular, or oval-shaped in some muscles, with an average diameter of 5 mm (range 2 to 22 mm). Within the same muscle the territory of different motor units varies by a factor of four. The area of territory of a single motor unit may enclose fibers of up to 30 motor units. For example, in the biceps brachii, with an average territory of 4 to 6 mm, there is theoretically space for the fibers of 10 overlapping motor units. In fact, up to six different motor units were identified in the same lead owing to different rates of discharge.[16] These findings agree with the histological evidence of overlap between fibers of different motor units.

The Subunit

The area mapped by the occurrence and propagation of individual spike sources has been called a subunit by Buchthal et al.[11] and is considered to be innervated by a single neuron. The average radius of 0.085 to 0.15 mm could contain 10 to 30 muscle fibers of 56μ diameter. When two spike sources are found within the area scanned by the multielectrodes, the mean distance between the center of each pair of spike sources is 0.7 mm. If the motor unit is assumed to contain 1000 muscle fibers and the territory to be 5 mm, then each spike source would contain 19 muscle fibers, which falls in the range of 10 to 30 fibers mentioned earlier.[16] The space between the subunits of a single motor unit but within its total territory is considered to be occupied by subunits of other motor units. The subunit gives rise to a smooth motor unit potential of high voltage and short duration.

The concept of the subunit is not accepted by all. Analysis of the volume conduction of fibrillation potentials, which are assumed to arise from single muscle fibers, has at times disclosed maximum voltages of the same order as found for motor unit potentials and also a voltage-distance relationship identical with that of the motor unit spike. This implies that the motor unit spike could originate from single muscle fibers. Buchthal feels that this may be the case in some instances but that under most circumstances several muscle fibers give rise to the motor unit spike. As an alternate explanation, the smooth course of the subunit spikes (in spite of being generated by 10 to 30 fibers of different diameters and with different sites of innervation) could result from a mutual interaction of the potentials from adjacent fibers, thus equalizing the propagation of the individual fiber action potentials. This phenomenon has been thought to occur in human muscle in which the action potentials of two electrically activated muscle fibers could be brought to synchronize as a single spike potential; but the work cited below casts doubt on this.

Using a multilead electrode, Ekstedt[21] has measured extracellular single muscle fiber action potentials in voluntary activated human skeletal muscle. Single muscle fibers were activated in situ by injection of sodium citrate into the muscle. Muscle fibers chemically activated in this way are independently discharged and all consecutive discharges are of identical shape. However, in the voluntary activated muscle the fibers do not discharge independently, and yet two or more adjacent fibers do not generate composite potentials that simulate those from a single fiber. The difference in arrival time to the electrode of two fiber action potentials from the same motor unit was not constant from discharge to discharge and so led to variations in the waveform, the "jitter phenomenon" on the order of 10 to 30 μsec in the mutual time interval between the spike components of the composite potentials. The absence of jitter is the most important criterion for single muscle fiber recordings.

Ekstedt's results in humans, as well as Brandstater's[6] and others' in animals, are not consistent with the concept of a subunit arrangement of fibers of the motor unit with clean, smooth spikes resulting from contraction of up to 30 perfectly synchronized, tightly packed fibers. Non-simultaneous action potentials from closely adjacent fibers belonging to the same motor unit and intermingling of fibers belonging to different motor units have been demonstrated.

Excitation and Depolarization

In many ways muscle fibers and nerve fibers resemble one another in the behavior of their surface membranes to excitatory stimuli. The physiology of the membrane potential will be dealt with in more detail in other chapters and will be summarized here.

The differences in potential between the inside and outside of single muscle cells have been measured by microelectrodes. The resting potential difference between the interior of the muscle cell and the extracellular space is approximately 100 mv in the mouse and somewhat lower (60 to 80 mv) in human muscle.[8] The resting membrane has a high impedance (10 megohms) and a low permeability for most ions. The extracellular concentration of sodium ions is high and of potassium ions low, the opposite being found intracellularly. Potassium ions are 32 to 50 times more permeable than sodium ions. However, there is a continuous flux of sodium ions across the membrane by action of a metabolic sodium pump in the cell membrane, which keeps the ionic distribution constant. Because of the higher intracellular concentration, potassium ions diffuse through and accumulate at the outer surface of the membrane to be held there by the negatively charged impermeable anions at the inner surface. This equilibrium is responsible for the positive polarization of the membrane; its magnitude can be predicted correctly from theoretical laws (Nernst equation).

Initiation of the excitatory state occurs at the myoneural junction. Small disturbances are rapidly attenuated, but when a stimulus of critical current density is applied to a critical membrane area, a propagating electrical potential will result. This "action potential" follows an "all or none law"; it travels the length of the muscle fiber with constant velocity and undiminished amplitude. The action potential is due to a specific increase in the permeability of the membrane to sodium ions (the reverse of the resting situation), as shown by the fact that the absence of sodium in the surrounding fluid makes the muscle non-excitable, and the action potential can be made smaller or larger by varying the extracellular sodium concentration.[38] At the height of excitation there are more positive sodium ions entering than there are potassium ions leaving, so that the membrane potential changes from the potassium equilibrium potential (−100 mv inside), through zero when the membrane is depolarized, to an overshoot — the sodium equilibrium potential (+30 mv). Repolarization occurs with the passive outward flux of potassium ions and the restoration of sodium ions by active pumping. The action potential of the muscle fiber differs from that of the nerve fiber in that the repolarization curve for muscle fiber takes longer because of events occurring in the submembrane tubular structure.

RECORDING OF MUSCLE ACTION POTENTIALS

Muscle is a source of electrical activity and is surrounded by a low resistance conducting medium (the interstitial fluid, blood and other tissue), usually referred to as a volume conductor. This in turn is surrounded by skin, the surface of which consists of a layer of horny dead and dying cells which have a high electrical resistance. Electromyography is the recording of electrical changes occurring in muscle by electrodes either in contact with the skin over the muscle area or inserted into the muscle.

Surface Electrodes

Surface electrodes consist of paired metal (often silver) plates or pads placed on the skin with one electrode over the motor end plate area of the muscle to be studied. Although summated electrical potentials are recorded, rapid, low amplitude potentials are attenuated and fine detail of individual motor units cannot be routinely obtained because of alteration in electrode position, varying degrees of skin and subcutaneous tissue thickness and the large areas encompassed. Surface electrodes have been used to give a broad survey of action potentials from a whole group of fibers and can be of value in studying kinesiological patterns such as time relationships and correlation with muscle tension.

Needle Electrodes

Three principal types of recording needle electrodes are utilized: (1) *concentric (coaxial) needle electrodes* (Fig. 6–3B), (2) *bipolar needle electrodes* (Fig. 6–3C) and (3) *monopolar (unipolar) needle electrodes* (Fig. 6–3A).

The concentric (coaxial) needle electrode introduced by Adrian and Bronk in 1929[1] is still used today. It consists of a steel hypodermic injection type needle with a centrally mounted insulated wire of stainless steel, silver or platinum. The tip of the central exploring electrode is exposed flush with the bevel of the cannula. Voltage differences are measured between the center core (average diameter 100μ) and the outer needle (diameter 0.35 to 0.65 mm).

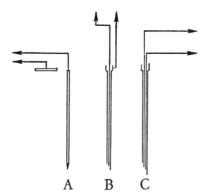

A B C

Figure 6 – 3   Schematic representation of EMG needle electrodes. (A) Unipolar needle, insulated except at its tip. Separate reference and ground electrodes are necessary. (B) Coaxial (concentric) needle. The recording electrode is exposed at the tip while the barrel acts as the indifferent lead. A separate ground is used. (C) Bipolar needle electrode. The two recording leads are bare at their tips and the barrel is grounded. (From Rodriquez and Oester: Fundamentals of Electromyography. *In* Licht, S. (ed.): *Electrodiagnosis and Electromyography.* New Haven, E. Licht, 1971.)

The coaxial needle can selectively record potentials close to the needle and in the direction determined by the bevel.

The bipolar needle electrode consists of two insulated central cores, often of copper or platinum, cemented side by side in a grounded steel cannula. The tips of the electrodes are flush with the bevel of the cannula and can be parallel in the bevel or in tandem. The diameters of the core electrodes are usually 100μ with an interelectrode distance of 500μ or more. The angle of the bevel determines the recording surface of the core as well as ease of muscle penetration.

The monopolar (unipolar) needle electrode consists of a thin wire, usually stainless steel, insulated with lacquer, plastic or, more recently, teflon, except at its tip. The outer diameter is normally 0.3 to 0.5 mm and the bare tip has a diameter of 25 to 50μ. Voltage differences between the needle tip, acting as the exploring electrode in the muscle, and a more distant reference electrode, usually a metal plate on the skin surface, are recorded.

Recording Characteristics

Lundervold,[35] utilizing a single needle that could be used for monopolar, concentric or bipolar recording, observed that the amplitude of a motor unit or fibrillation potential as recorded by monopolar leads was only slightly larger than that recorded with concentric needles but usually considerably larger than that measured with a bipolar electrode. The duration of the negative spike of the action potential was shortest with bipolar and longest with monopolar leads and concentric needle recordings. The electrode records a mean value of the potential which is spread over the sampling area.[13] The smaller the sampling area, the less the amplitude variation and the higher the amplitude. The amplitude of the recorded potential is also a function of the distance of the surface of the electrode to the current source.

With unipolar electrodes the shape and duration of the muscle action potential (MAP) is determined by the fact that the muscle acts as a volume conductor, picking up more distant fibers and units. With bipolar electrodes the duration of potential is shorter, with less distance between the cores. There is a partial canceling of the initial and terminal portions of the potentials recorded by each of the inner cores.

To obtain maximum amplitude and to avoid directional properties, monopolar needles are most desirable. For analysis of motor action potential form (including polyphasicity) in maximal interference patterns bipolar needles are best. Standardization of the recording devices as well as the needles is necessary in order to compare results of investigators.

Several other needle electrodes may be used for special purposes. For example, in kinesiological recordings an electrode consisting of two fine nylon-insulated wires is introduced into the muscle by an injection needle that is subsequently withdrawn.[2] These fine wires cause little discomfort, but their position can only be altered by withdrawing them through the insertion channel created by the needle.

MUSCLE ACTION POTENTIALS – EMG FINDINGS

The electrode registers the average potential existing over its leading-off area, the recording surface of which is in direct contact with approximately eight muscle fibers, only one or two of which belong to the same motor unit. The sharp spike of the potential recorded is primarily the result of the excitation of a single muscle fiber.[21] This reflects the potential of the motor unit of which it is a part but is not the whole motor unit potential.

The amplitude of the action potential is dependent on several variables, particularly the distance between the recording electrode and the contracting muscle fibers. There is some correlation between the number of muscle fibers per unit and the amplitude of the potential, because summated spikes of contracting fibers near the electrode contribute to the spike component. The relationship between the leading-off surface area of the electrode and the amplitude recorded has been demonstrated by Buchthal.[15] It is estimated that eight muscle fibers can be in contact with the surface of a concentric needle electrode of dimensions 0.1×0.4 mm, but at the most three out of the eight fibers belong to the same unit and contribute to the potential, which totals 4.0 mv. With electrodes of smaller surface, such as a multilead electrode, the higher proportion of contracting fiber to surface area produces a larger potential, i.e., 10 mv. Also, muscles having a larger fiber diameter produce potentials of greater amplitude.

The duration of the muscle action potential is dependent on, but not proportional to, the mean size of the motor unit.[53] For example, eye muscles, which have small units, produce potentials with a duration of only 1.6 to 1.8 msec, while the platysma, with larger units (25 fibers per unit), have a mean duration of 4.9 msec. Potentials from the medial head of the gastrocnemius (1600 to 2000 fibers per unit) have a duration of 9.6 msec.

Nerve impulses have been demonstrated to arrive synchronously at all the end plates of the motor unit; transmission of the muscle action potentials from

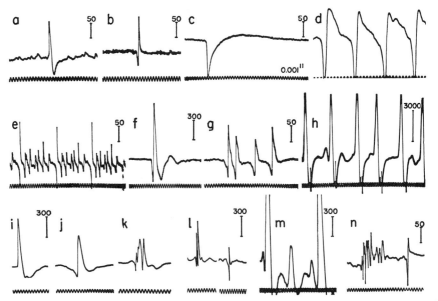

Figure 6-4 Muscle action potentials (MAP) in electromyography: (a) end plate potential; (b) fibrillation potential and (c) positive wave from denervated muscle; (d) myotonic discharge; (e) bizarre high frequency discharge; (f) fasciculation potential, single discharge; (g) fasciculation potential repetitive or grouped discharge; (h) synchronized repetitive discharge in muscle cramp; (i) diphasic, (j) triphasic and (k) polyphasic MAPs from normal muscle; (l) short duration MAPs in progressive muscular dystrophy; (m) large potentials in anterior horn cell disease; (n) reinnervation "nascent" units. Calibration scales are in microvolts; time scales are in milliseconds. An upward deflection indicates a change of potential in the negative direction at the needle electrode. (From Mayo Clinic: *Clinical Examinations in Neurology.* Sections of Neurology and Physiology, 3rd Edition. Philadelphia, W. B. Saunders Company, 1971.)

different fibers at varying distances from the recording electrode lead to a broadening of the resultant potential curve. Variation in synaptic delay also plays a role in modifying the duration of the action potential. There is little difference in conduction velocity for the individual muscle fibers of one motor unit (4 to 5.5 m per sec at 36.5°C) for the human biceps brachii.[21] This constant velocity has been explained in part on the basis of the low external resistance of the extracellular fluid around the muscle fibers, which facilitates mutual interaction between fibers of different diameters.

The shape of the muscle action potential is influenced by factors similar to those affecting amplitude and duration, i.e., the number, distance and distribution of fibers of the same unit in relation to the recording electrode. A slight temporal dispersion of the component spikes can cause potentials with several phases or humps. The position of the electrode relative to the innervation zone is important because if an electrode is situated near the end plates, the potential starts with a steep negative deflection.* Muscle acts as a volume conductor, so the gradual onset and tail of the muscle action potential may be distorted by potentials picked up from more distant motor units.

---

*By convention in EMG recording the negative deflection is upward.

With monopolar or concentric needle electrodes di- and triphasic potentials (Fig. 6–4i, j) will comprise about 80 per cent of all potentials recorded in normal adult subjects[13]; these have a voltage range of 100 to 3000 μv and a duration of from 2 to 10 msec. The duration of the sharp negative spike is approximately 2 msec. The action potential parameters vary from one muscle to another, since the innervation ratio is not the same. Monophasic and polyphasic potentials are seen in 1 to 12 per cent of all potentials recorded. Polyphasic potentials by definition contain more than four phases and occur with increased frequency in neuropathic and myopathic disorders, although they comprise 1 to 3 per cent of normal potentials (Fig. 6–4k-n).

Interference Patterns and Recruitment

Electromyographic examination of a normal relaxed skeletal muscle at rest reveals an isoelectric base line, i.e., electrical silence (Fig. 6-5). With minimal voluntary contraction one or several motor units are activated and these are usually of low amplitude (500 μv). As tension increases, the firing frequency of the individual potential increases. If the amplitude increases at the same time, it is assumed that the number of muscle fibers activated within the same motor unit has increased, presumably because all the end plates of a unit are not in an

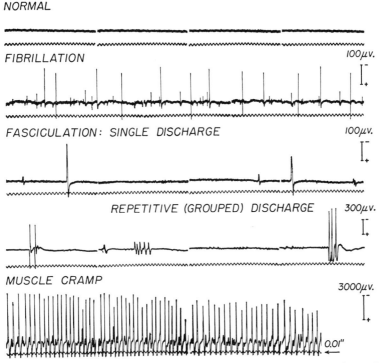

Figure 6–5 Records of spontaneous electric activity in voluntarily relaxed muscle. There is no electrical activity from a normal muscle; the slight irregularity of the baseline is "noise" inherent in high amplification. Lower tracings show spontaneous electrical activity in various conditions. (From Mayo Clinic: *Clinical Examinations in Neurology.* Sections of Neurology and Physiology, 3rd Edition. Philadelphia, W. B. Saunders Company, 1971.)

identical state of physiochemical readiness. Other evidence comes from studies with protected microelectrodes of the human rectus femoris and gastrocnemius muscles; in these it was noted that motor unit potentials tended to increase in amplitude with heightened tension during isometric contraction.[41] This increase is attributed to an increase in the number of active muscle fibers involved in successive discharges of a single motor unit.

With increasing tension additional motor units are recruited, some of higher amplitude. Buchthal et al.[14] found the amplitude of the second and third recruited units to be larger than the first and felt that this was due to decreasing distance between the recording electrode and the active unit as the strength of contraction increased. With further rises in tension even more units are recruited, and there is temporal and spatial summation of potentials, producing a characteristic interference pattern, so that with monopolar and concentric needle electrodes muscle action potentials from individual units can no longer be clearly distinguished. There is an order of recruitment of motor units. At low strength of contraction only a few motor units are active and these have a slow discharge rate and a relatively low amplitude. With increasing tension there is an increase in frequency of discharge by the active motor units and a recruitment of previously inactive units.

It appears that recruitment has a more important role in grading of activity than does changing of frequency, except at very low and very high contraction strengths. With bipolar electrodes it is possible to identify separate motor units during most voluntary contractions.[5] Frequencies above 50 per sec were never observed, and frequencies between 40 and 50 per sec only occurred when the tension was above 75 per cent of the maximum voluntary contraction (MVC) strength. Under most conditions (25 to 75 per cent MVC) the fastest units responded at frequencies between 25 and 35 per sec. Over the tension range of 5 to 60 per cent MVC the firing starts and stops abruptly, and the frequency increases but not in proportion to strength. For example, in one unit observed the firing commenced at 20 per sec when the tension was 15 per cent of maximum and increased with tension rise but only to 30 per sec. Units that are active at lower tensions, below 5 per cent MVC, usually have a lower starting frequency and a greater frequency range with irregular discharge rates. In the human biceps brachii the slower firing, low threshold units tend to be located deep in the muscle, while the rapid firing, higher threshold units are more superficial.[18]

Synchronization

In anterior horn cell diseases such as polio, amyotrophic lateral sclerosis (ALS) and syringomyelia "synchronization" is demonstrated when simultaneous action potentials are recorded from two or more widely separated electrodes. The cause of this phenomenon is not clear. One speculation is that there is an intraspinal mechanism for synchronization of rhythm of discharge in a number of different motor units supplied by the same spinal segment.[40] Another possibility is that in the same muscle single units of very large area (as noted in anterior horn cell disorders) are responsible.

The occurrence of occasional, true synchronization of motor units in a number of muscles in human subjects and animals has not received valid confirmation. An electronic model and statistical analysis of EMG records made under a variety of conditions seem to bear out the absence of true synchronization of motor neuron activity in voluntary contractions,[46] although grouping of discharges may be seen in the single action potential of the tendon jerk and partial synchronization and grouping in clonus and various tremors.[20]

Effect of Age, Temperature, Fatigue and Disuse

The mean duration of the muscle action potential increases with age so that at age 70 to 80 years the average duration is up to 75 per cent longer than in children under four years.[14] This is explained as a decrease in the propagation velocity of the impulse over the muscle fiber. Peterson and Kugelberg[42] noted that normal values in young individuals are obtained from the first recruited, low threshold muscle action potentials, whereas aging selectively destroys muscle fibers with the largest calibers and lowest thresholds.

The total number of muscle fibers of the rat soleus muscle decrease with age, but no difference has been found in the number of α motor nerve fibers to the muscle.[28] Thus, it can be assumed that there is no loss of motor nerve cells in the spinal cord because of aging, and the decrease in the size of the motor unit is due to peripheral loss of muscle fibers. This is substantiated by evidence of random degeneration of the end plates and some terminal end plate regeneration. These factors may explain the increased duration of action potentials and greater number of polyphasic potentials noted with aging.

As the intramuscular temperature is lowered, the mean duration of the muscle action potential increases by 10 to 30 per cent and the mean amplitude decreases by 2 to 5 per cent for each degree centigrade reduction. The number of polyphasic potentials can increase as much as tenfold with a 10°C fall in temperature.[14] This prolongation of duration is due to the temperature coefficient of the propagation velocity. The slower propagation velocity of the impulse over the muscle fiber and the terminal nerve fibers can cause a temporal dispersion of fibers within the motor unit.

In the absence of fatigue the sum of electrical activity recorded by surface electrodes of a muscle bears a simple linear relation to the force developed.[45] The increase in force is due to the activation of more motor units and, to a lesser degree, to their greater frequency of discharge. In fatiguing muscle the relative force developed and the sum of electrical activity also remains linearly related until the level of mechanical activity cannot be maintained. However, in the fatigued muscle each increment of physical force requires a larger electrical activity, presumably because of a deficiency in the contractile process rather than changes in electrical propagation. Transmission across the neuromuscular junction may also be modified. The EMG recorded with surface electrodes reveals an increased amplitude of the summated potentials and a decrease in their frequency with fatigue[37] as a result of synchronization. Needle EMG study shows that discharges of fibers from different motor units tend to group during fatiguing muscular work; there is also an increase in the total number of active motor units. The individual action potentials are decreased in amplitude with little change in frequency or duration of the potentials. The number of polyphasic potentials is increased with fatigue,[45] presumably owing to incomplete synchronization between fibers of different motor units[14] or to end plate alterations with more irregular firing of individual fibers of the motor unit occurring in the vicinity of the needle electrode tip.

In muscles with disuse atrophy, polyphasic potentials of more than four phases occurred in 25 per cent of all action potentials compared with 1 to 3 per cent in normal muscle.[43] A reduction or increase in duration of the action potentials is occasionally noted. This may be due to alteration in fiber conduction velocity. No significant changes of muscle fiber membrane characteristics have been demonstrated in animals up to one month after disuse was induced by section of the spinal cord at a higher level than the muscle supply and after sectioning of the dorsal roots.[7] In these animals, in whom a total flaccid paraplegia without lower motor neuron denervation was produced, a reversible fall of 10 mv in the resting membrane potential was noted in the first week only.

Spontaneous Activity

THE FIBRILLATION POTENTIAL.   Fibrillations are muscle action potentials of short duration and are caused by firing of single muscle fibers spontaneously (Fig. 6–5), or they may be the result of mechanical irritation such as needle insertion. They are not visible at the skin surface but may be seen in an exposed muscle or on the tongue. They are not exclusively indicative of lower motor neuron disease, as 10 to 15 per cent of apparently normal subjects have demonstrated a single region of fibrillation potentials,[10] and fibrillation potentials are noted in 15 to 30 per cent of primary myopathic diseases such as primary muscular dystrophy and polymyositis. Not all patients with lower motor neuron disease show fibrillation potentials. They are less in evidence after prolonged denervation because of atrophy and replacement fibrosis of the muscle fibers. Fibrillations are most pronounced in patients with peripheral nerve injuries, less in those with most anterior horn cell diseases and least in patients with higher nervous system lesions.

When recorded with standard monopolar or concentric needle electrodes, fibrillation potentials are usually diphasic discharges with an initial positive deflection (Fig. 6-4b). The usual amplitude is from 50 to 150 μv, but potentials of up to 3 mv have been recorded, and duration is usually 0.5 to 2.0 msecs. They occur rhythmically or arrhythmically with a frequency of from 2 to 30 per sec. Hypoxia or cooling will decrease the frequency. Neostigmine increases the frequency.

Fibrillation potentials are to be distinguished from potentials recorded in the area of the neuromuscular junction.[27, 51] The so-called "nerve potential" manifests as spontaneous spikes of low amplitude (but greater than 100 μv) (Fig. 6–6), usually diphasic with a sharp initial negative deflection (Fig. 6-4a) and are considered to be due to firing of single muscle fibers in the end plate area. Another response in the end plate area, the miniature end plate potentials, are localized non-propagated potentials of less than 100 μv amplitude

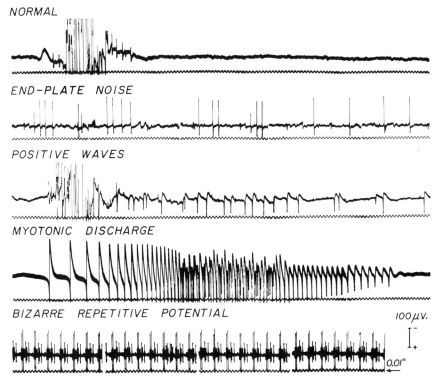

NORMAL

END-PLATE NOISE

POSITIVE WAVES

MYOTONIC DISCHARGE

BIZARRE REPETITIVE POTENTIAL

100 μv.

0.01″

Figure 6–6   Insertion potentials, evoked by insertion of a needle electrode into muscle. In a normal this consists of a brief discharge of electric activity lasting little longer than the movement of the needle. (From Mayo Clinic: *Clinical Examinations in Neurology.* Sections of Neurology and Physiology, 3rd Edition. Philadelphia, W. B. Saunders Company, 1971.)

which, when recorded with standard extracellular needle electrodes, appear as a thickening of the baseline (the end plate noise). When microelectrodes are used, voltages of approximately 1 mv are obtained. These potentials are irregular in rhythm and are characteristically monophasic and negative with a slow return to baseline.

Studies employing intracellular microelectrode techniques on living white mice have shown that the resting potential remains near the normal level of 100 mv following denervation until the muscle begins to fibrillate, at which time the potential falls rapidly, ultimately reaching a value of 77 mv.[49] It is postulated that denervation causes an absolute or relative alteration of the sodium pump mechanism, wherein the increased extrusion of sodium caused by the active fibrillatory process results in a lowering of the membrane resting potential.[49]

If the end plate zone is excised from actively fibrillating muscle, the fibrillation continues in the strip bearing the end plate but ceases in the other sections as soon as they are cut off.[30] Intracellular recording at or close to a denervated muscle shows fibrillation potentials that are preceded by a slowly rising depolarization ("prepotential"). In other areas of the muscle the potentials take off abruptly from the baseline and exhibit the characteristics of conducted spikes.[3] The membrane at the denervated end plate zone seems to have properties different from the rest of the muscle fiber membrane. Cathodal currents applied to the denervated end plate area increase fibrillatory frequency, while anodal currents decrease frequency. However, currents of a similar magnitude do not change fibrillation frequency when applied to other areas of the muscle fiber. Acetylcholine and norepinephrine in certain concentrations also increase the frequency of fibrillation when applied to the muscle at the denervated end plate zone, while larger doses of acetylcholine depress fibrillation frequency. In spite of the fact that these two agents induce membrane potential changes (depolarization) wherever they are applied, fibrillation frequency was only affected when these agents act on the end plate area. Thus, the denervated end plate region acts as a pacemaker site for fibrillation potentials and has chemical and electrical properties different from the rest of the denervated muscle fiber membrane.[3] There has been recent speculation that sensitivity to circulating catecholamine is more important than increased susceptibility to acetylcholine in the production of fibrillation.

Muscles studies in premature infants prior to innervation and in patients with meningomyelocoele where complete innervation has been prevented showed fibrillations.[36] Muscle fibers of a fetus apparently fibrillate until innervated. This preinnervation activity differs from denervation fibrillations only in its low amplitude (usually less than 15 μv) and slow frequency (less than 10 per sec). Fibrillatory activity decreases as the time of normal gestation approaches and innervation is accomplished.

POSITIVE SHARP WAVES.   Positive sharp waves are spontaneous potentials often seen in association with fibrillations, usually after denervation, and may appear days or weeks before the onset of fibrillation. They may also be seen in myopathies.

Positive sharp waves are initiated by needle insertion (Fig. 6–6) and have an initial rapid positive (downward) sharp deflection that is followed by an exponential negative change, which can continue into a prolonged low voltage negative phase (Fig. 6–4c). The duration usually exceeds 10 msec and may be as long as 30 to 100 msec. The voltage is variable and the frequency ranges from 2 to 100 per sec.

Little is known about the etiology of positive waves. One theory is that they represent the synchronous discharge of a number of denervated muscle fibers, but it seems unlikely that they would produce such a continuously characteristic shape. Buchthal[10] observed that there is a radial distribution of the electrical field corresponding to the positive wave and suggested that they arise from single muscle fibers and that they are probably due to the placement of the recording electrode near a blocked or damaged region of the fiber.

FASCICULATION.   Fasciculations are involuntary muscle twitchings that can often be seen on the surface of the skin. They are irregular in rhythm, form, voltage and duration. Rarely individual potentials recorded may have the same characteristic appearance as in repetitive myokymic discharges (Fig. 6–4f–h; Fig. 6–5). Fasciculations are noted in many conditions, including benign myokymia, anterior horn cell disease, nerve root compression, ischemia and various forms of muscle cramps. Although frequently seen in diseases of anterior horn cells, fasciculations are thought to arise from a peripheral phenomenon in the region of the myoneural junction. Section of the motor nerve in cases of advanced disease of anterior horn cells (ALS) is followed by the same degree of fasciculation for several days before Wallerian degeneration begins,[25] and spontaneous muscular fasciculations are not affected by spinal anesthesia or peripheral nerve block. Neostigmine will produce or increase fasciculations, even during spinal anesthesia. Curare abolishes spontaneous fasciculations and prevents the induction of fasciculations by neostigmine in normal subjects. The impulse is presumed to start in the area of the end plate and to spread antidromically to involve other axon branches, thus accounting for the frequently observed polyphasicity and prolonged duration of the potentials. The location of the myoneural junction originating the impulse within the motor unit may vary, explaining the presence of changing polyphasic waveforms.[44]

After nerve section, fasciculations disappear with the development of Wallerian degeneration. Immature terminal collateral sprouts of motor neurons were found in biopsies from fasciculating muscle regions in patients with ALS.[53] These immature neuromuscular junctions may be more sensitive to humoral agents, and thus fasciculation twitchings may be initiated by normal levels of neurohumoral transmitters (e.g., acetylcholine). Fine, beaded nerve fibers are seen in the intramuscular nerve bundles of patients with motor neuron diseases. These fibers are unmyelinated and many do not have Schwann-cell cover. It is possible that ephaptic transmission across these fibers could produce fasciculatory movements.

Idiopathic benign fasciculations and muscle cramps (Fig. 6-4h) often occur in the calf muscles; they can be associated with salt depletion and are often facilitated by ischemia. The twitches are irregular and of varying polyphasicity; they can be stopped by voluntary activity. Their polyphasic form would seem to indicate that they arise in the terminal branches of the lower motor neuron and have a changing focus of origin. It is unlikely that the focus is at the myoneural junction because they are not influenced by neostigmine.

The fasciculations that occur after root compression are often of simple diphasic form (Fig. 6-4g) and usually are associated with other signs of denervation such as positive waves and fibrillations.

Fasciculations may be caused by a central mechanism as well as by a peripheral one.[40] Giant bizarre spontaneous potentials are seen in ALS and related diseases, and these, unlike other fasciculations, may be eliminated by nerve block. The anatomical basis for these abnormal potentials may in part be intramuscular axonal budding or collateral regeneration from normal to denervated elements. However, EMG studies of motor unit territory in ALS indicate that the motor units are larger than can be accounted for by intramuscular sprouting. In some instances several neural elements at the same spinal level interact to produce synchronous fasciculation in different muscles, which seems to originate from a spinal locus of hyperexcitability. Intraspinal axonal sprouting occurs in ALS patients; there is uncertainty whether this sprouting is analogous to the intramuscular collateral regeneration of partially denervated muscle.

CLINICAL APPLICATIONS

Diseases of the motor unit pathway at any point from the anterior horn cell to the muscle fiber itself can produce an abnormal pattern in the EMG (Fig. 6-1). In addition, the higher nervous centers influence the motor neuron apparatus so that upper motor neuron lesions may alter electromyographic findings. This section is not intended to be a clinical manual, and while specific disease entities may produce characteristic EMG findings, these will not be discussed in detail except to illustrate pathophysiological changes which apply to a group of disorders as a whole.

Unipolar or concentric needle electrodes are used in clinical electromyography. The electrical activity produced by insertion of the needle, the spontaneous activity in the relaxed resting muscle, the interference pattern in full forceful contraction against resistance and the character of the individual muscle action potentials during weak or submaximal contraction are all recorded. The muscle is usually examined in several locations, and it is often helpful to amplify the sound equivalent of the potentials, as the ear is quite sensitive to variations.

Lower Motor Neuron Disease

The electromyogram in lower motor neuron disease has certain general characteristics which include: fibrillation potentials and positive sharp waves (Fig. 6-4b,c), fasciculation potentials (Fig. 6-4f), increase in amplitude (Fig. 6-4m) and decrease in the number of muscle action potentials observed during full effort (Fig. 6-10), increase in average duration of muscle action potentials and increased incidence of polyphasic potentials (Fig. 6-4m). Some of these changes also occur in myopathy, so a single criterion is insufficient to characterize the level of involvement along the motor unit pathway.

A brief word should be mentioned about collateral and terminal regeneration (Figs. 6-7, 6-8, 6-9). Collateral regeneration consists of the ingrowth of

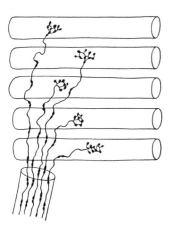

Figure 6–7 Normal arrangement of terminal innervation. Note one-to-one-to-one relationship, i.e., one nerve fiber, one end plate, one muscle fiber. (From Coërs and Woolf: *The Innervation of Muscle.* Springfield, Ill., Charles C Thomas, 1959.)

Figure 6–8 Collateral sprouting and reinnervation. Degeneration has taken place in all but one nerve fiber (see normal arrangement in Figure 6–7). A sprout has arisen from the intact axon at a node of Ranvier and invaded the Schwann column of a degenerated fiber. One nerve fiber now innervates five muscle fibers and there is variation in the form of the end plates. (From Coërs and Woolf: *The Innervation of Muscle.* Springfield, Ill., Charles C Thomas, 1959.)

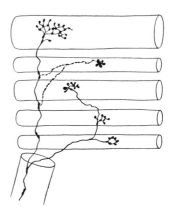

Figure 6–9 Probable mechanism of development of changes in terminal innervation in distal neuropathies and also in cases with primary degeneration of muscle fibers. Note tendency for nerve fibers to form several end plates with more than one of the latter on most muscle fibers. (From Coërs and Woolf: *The Innervation of Muscle.* Springfield, Ill., Charles C Thomas, 1959.)

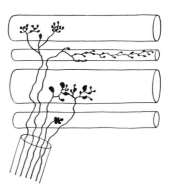

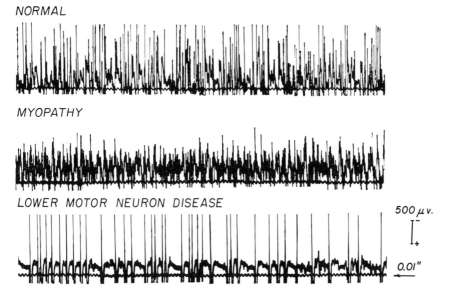

NORMAL

MYOPATHY

LOWER MOTOR NEURON DISEASE

500 μv.

0.01"

Figure 6–10 MAPs during maximal voluntary contraction (biceps brachii). (From Mayo Clinic: *Clinical Examinations in Neurology.* Sections of Neurology and Physiology, 3rd Edition. Philadelphia, W. B. Saunders Company, 1971.)

branches from *intact* nerve fibers to adjacent denervated fibers (Fig. 6-8).[53] This axonal sprouting has been demonstrated in man for both sensory and motor neuron fibers. Terminal regeneration occurs in interrupted nerve fibers whereby new end plate connections are established by the peripherally regenerating terminal axonal branches within the muscle fibers (Fig. 6-9).

ANTERIOR HORN CELL DISORDERS.   The anterior horn cell is involved in disorders such as poliomyelitis, ALS, the progressive spinal muscular atrophies (e.g., Werdnig-Hoffman disease) and in hereditary degenerative conditions such as Charcot-Marie-Tooth disease. The characteristic features and clinical course vary according to the particular entity, but in general fibrillations and fasciculations are common. There is a decrease in total number of motor units but an increase in the number of fibers making up each individual unit (Fig. 6–11D). Most muscle action potentials have a prolonged duration and increased amplitude that is more pronounced than is seen in muscles with impairment of peripheral nerves or roots (Fig. 6–4m). The motor unit territory may be increased by 80 to 140 per cent and the maximum voltage five to eight times the normal value in severely involved muscles.[22] There is extensive collateral regeneration, since

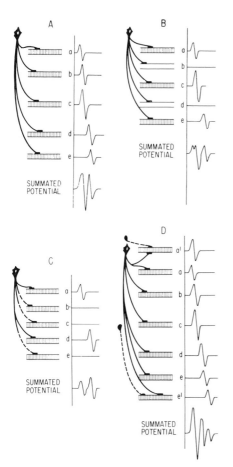

Figure 6–11 Simple diagrams to illustrate possible mechanisms for normal and abnormal motor unit potentials. (A) Normal situation with muscle fiber (c) closest to the electrode. Excitation arrives first in fiber (a) and last in fiber (e). The summated potential differs from any component action potential. (B) Myopathy with loss of fibers (b) and (d) causing bizarre alteration of summated potential. (C) Early terminal regeneration after a nerve lesion. The regenerated axon branches (a) and (d) excite muscle fibers (a) and (d) after increased latency; regeneration is incomplete in the other axon branches (dashed), and the corresponding muscle fibers are not activated. (D) Motor neuron degeneration with collateral growth from healthy axon branches to innervate muscle fibers (a') and (e'). Fiber (a') is closer to the electrode than (a), thus increasing the amplitude of the summated potential. Fiber (e') is excited later than (e) and increases the duration of the summated potential. This summated potential is a giant potential. (From Norris: *The EMG*. New York, Grune and Stratton, 1963.)

the degenerating nerve fibers are scattered over wide areas and intact and degenerating nerve fibers often lie close together, giving rise to tremendous collateral branching from the surviving fibers. In ALS polyphasic fasciculations of increased duration may be observed in atrophic muscles and also in certain muscles that do not show weakness or wasting. EMG findings suggest that this is caused by the firing of a single motor unit rather than the synchronous firing of two or more units, and the fact that the twitching muscle region is larger than that normally corresponding to a single unit may be explained by the collateral branching that results in a pathologically enlarged motor unit. The action potentials are often polyphasic and of increased duration, again because of temporal dispersion of the enlarged unit.

NERVE ROOT AND PLEXUS INJURY.   A nerve root or plexus lesion causes denervation corresponding to the segments involved, manifested by fibrillation potentials, occasional fasciculations, reduced numbers of muscle action potentials and complex polyphasic units often of increased duration. In the acute phase there may be electrical silence with spontaneous activity appearing only as Wallerian degeneration occurs. The peripheral nerve supply to individual muscles is composed of fibers from several spinal cord segments; as a result, normal and diseased motor units may be observed together. When atrophic changes occur in the muscle fibers, spontaneous activity disappears and evidence of chronic denervation is noted in the muscles supplied by the affected cord segments. Plexus lesions can be differentiated from nerve root lesions by examination of the paraspinal muscles, which are supplied by the posterior primary division of the ventral nerve root proximal to the plexus. In root lesions the paraspinal muscles innervated by the involved root manifest signs of denervation. On the other hand, the paraspinal muscles will be normal in the more distal plexus lesions.

PERIPHERAL NERVE LESIONS.   A peripheral nerve damaged by disease or trauma may exhibit temporary loss of conductivity or varying degrees of degeneration.

In physiological block (neuropraxia) continuity of the nerve sheath is maintained without Wallerian degeneration, and the condition is characterized by electrical silence at rest. There will be no voluntary action potentials if the block is complete and a reduced number of normal potentials if it is partial.

Immediately following severance of the nerve trunk, no voluntary muscle action potentials are seen. The axon cylinder begins to fragment at about the third day, and at this time nerve conduction velocity distal to the site of injury rapidly decreases. The motor end plate retains its excitability for another 5 to 10 days. It is not until the end plate is reduced to the same degree of excitability as the muscle fiber that fibrillation potentials begin to appear (Fig. 6-5). Denervation potentials at rest begin approximately 10 days after the injury and occur in all areas of the muscle receiving their supply distal to the site of injury. Fibrillations last until the regenerating axon arrives at the surface of the muscle fiber and penetrates the end plate, or until the muscle fibers atrophy. Fibrillations can last for periods as long as 18 years[50] even after many normal units have recovered.

The voluntary motor potentials first seen on return of function are called nascent units and are of low amplitude, short duration and are often polyphasic (Fig. 6–4n; Fig. 6–11C). They are due to early terminal reinnervation of a reduced unit as well as to varying rates of distal conduction. As reinnervation progresses, the motor unit increases in area and number of fibers, so that three months after injury the motor unit territory is within normal limits and the maximum voltage ranges from normal to 1.8 times normal. Eight months or longer after nerve injury the maximum voltage is 2.5 to 3.5 times normal and the motor unit territory is increased by an average of 15 to 40 per cent.[22] The changes in motor unit territory and maximum voltage do not correlate with the degree of paresis as measured by muscle testing. The presence of normal-appearing action potentials is usually indicative of the return of near synchronous discharging of the fibers of the unit. Giant or large-spike potentials of up to 15 mv may be seen three to five years after regeneration,[55] owing to collateral innervation from surviving axons in incomplete lesions and to regenerating nerve fibers escaping normal channels and innervating several end plates in series.

In peripheral neuropathies there is axonal degeneration, and denervation potentials proportional to the severity and extent of the lesion are seen at rest. If progressive degeneration occurs distally before the onset of (or in the absence of) nerve regeneration, there is a gradual loss of muscle fibers in the unit, which causes a decrease in amplitude and fragmentation of the action potentials. As the degeneration spreads, there is a reduction of low voltage initial and terminal deflections of the action potential. This rare electromyographic picture of distal neuronitis is indistinguishable from that seen with the myopathies (Fig. 6–11B). In peripheral neuropathies with primary axonal degeneration, spontaneous recovery is possible if there is anatomical continuity of the myelin sheaths. The recovery time depends upon removal of the pathological agent, site of the lesion and the distance through which regeneration must take place.

In polyneuritis, recovery occurs by collateral and terminal regeneration. During and following reinnervation the potentials are complex and of prolonged duration because of temporal dispersion of the motor unit as well as alterations of conduction velocity along the regenerating distal nerve branches and across the immature end plates.

Upper Motor Neuron Lesions

Physiologically the higher nervous centers influence the lower motor neuron in normal motor activity. It has generally been denied that disease of the upper motor neurons affects the motor unit proper. This concept has been challenged by one study that shows a 57 per cent incidence of fibrillations and a 70 per cent incidence of positive waves.[26] Another study has recorded a 73.5 per cent incidence of spontaneous activity in involved hemiplegic limbs, but a 9 per cent incidence of fibrillations on the unaffected side.[4] Nerve conduction times were normal. In patients with spinal injuries fibrillations have been observed in muscles innervated by nerve root segments quite distal to the level of injury. It is possible that trans-synaptic neuronal degeneration occurs; this is supported by experimental work on animals.

In a classic study of action potentials in spastic conditions by Hoefer and Putnam in 1940[31] it was noted that voluntary contraction produced a pattern of decreased frequency and amplitude, but these parameters were proportional to the strength of the contraction. In this study there was no evidence of lower motor neuron disease and accordingly the results of examination of individual discharges were essentially normal. In spastic muscles studied during clonus there was a strong tendency to synchronization with alternating activity between protagonist and antagonist groups.

Motor End Plate Disturbances

A defect in transmission across the neuromuscular junction, as in myasthenia gravis, is characterized by a decrease in amplitude of the successively evoked potentials on repetitive stimulation. The amplitude of single motor units with voluntary contractions varies widely[34] until, because of fatigue, the unit may fail to respond. A normal pattern may be restored by an injection of neostigmine or edrophonium chloride. The changing amplitude is explained by a blocking of excitation at the end plate to a variable number of muscle fibers supplied by the neuron, with fibers recovering at different rates. This may also account for the "myopathic picture," which is sometimes seen, of complex polyphasic potentials of normal to decreased amplitude and normal to decreased duration. Defects in neuromuscular transmissions have been noted in other conditions such as ALS and disseminated carcinomatosis.

"MYASTHENIC" SYNDROME. In patients with malignant intrathoracic tumors (and at times in non-malignancies) signs suggestive of a neuromuscular transmission defect have been noted. Clinically the weak resting patient becomes weaker with continuing muscle contraction or stimulation after an initial period of enhanced strength. Unlike myasthenia gravis, the initial response to a supramaximal stimulus is only a fraction of normal amplitude, and as contraction continues there is a period of facilitation characterized by increasing responses, but these are often short of normal expected amplitude. The etiology of this disorder is not explainable at this time.

Myopathy

Myopathies may exhibit one or more of the following electromyographic findings: (1) the presence of spontaneous activity at rest with potentials resembling or identical to fibrillation potentials; (2) myotonic discharges induced by voluntary contractile activity, insertion of the needle or by tapping the muscle near the needle (Fig. 6-6); (3) a relatively normal interference pattern of muscle action potentials (in spite of muscle weakness and wasting) (Fig. 6-10); (4) a decrease in amplitude and average duration of individual motor unit potentials (Fig. 6-4l); (5) an increase in the number of polyphasic potentials; and (6) diminished territory of the motor units with decreased fiber density within the motor unit.[10] Fibrillatory activity is most common in myositis and myotonic discharges in myotonia dystrophica, but these phenomena can be seen in other conditions.

Fibrillations have been noted in most myopathies. The mechanisms of the abnormal spontaneous muscle potentials are not clear. In progressive muscular dystrophy and hyperkalemic periodic paralysis the spontaneous discharges may be related to the increase in excitability resulting from low levels of intracellular potassium.[10] It is also possible that the degenerating muscle fibers in the dystrophies may initially lose their terminal innervation. In the myositic disorders inflammatory involvement of the subterminal intramuscular nerve endings and end plate areas has been demonstrated[19] and could cause in-increased irritability. There is evidence of collateral reinnervation, and prolonged action potentials are noted; but since the sprouting is entirely peripheral, very large motor units and enlargement of motor unit territory are not found. This myositic picture is similar to that found in a distal neuronitis.

Bizarre, high frequency potentials are often noted in myositis. These are high frequency runs of identical-appearing potentials, usually polyphasic, that start and stop abruptly (Fig. 6-6).

In the myopathies most of the EMG changes are due to a reduction of the number of muscle fibers in the individual unit; however, the total number of motor unit potentials remains unchanged until the very late stages, so that muscle force and summated voltage is decreased, but the number of potentials with increased frequency of discharge is maintained.[33] More electrical activity of action potential spikes is necessary to achieve the same amount of force as was attained prior to illness. Because of the random degeneration of muscle fibers, the smooth summated effect of the normal muscle action potential is lost and complex potentials of low amplitude are noted (Fig. 6–11B). The fibers furthest from the recording electrode are likewise decreased, so there is a shortening of the duration of the recorded potentials. It is difficult to explain the decrease in motor unit territory noted with multilead electrodes purely on the basis of muscle degeneration, as almost every muscle fiber would have to be destroyed. If there is associated distal denervation, this decrease in territory can be more readily accounted for.

Myotonia

Myotonia is an abnormally sustained contraction with difficulty in relaxation. The electromyogram shows runs of repetitive high frequency waxing and waning discharges, usually of positive waves or biphasic potentials, the initial deflection being positive (Fig. 6-6; Fig. 6-4d).

In humans myotonia may be seen as a dominantly inherited form of muscular dystrophy (myotonia dystrophica), myotonia congenita, associated with periodic paralysis (principally the hyperkalemic type) or with Pompé's disease (a glycogenosis accompanied by acid maltase deficiency of muscle). Myotonic phenomena may also be seen in inflammatory disease of muscle (dermatomyositis), although the discharges are not as pronounced and manifest less waxing and waning; they tend to begin abruptly and then to gradually taper off. This has been called pseudomyotonia, and in patients with pseudomyotonia clinical myotonia is absent.

Myotonic discharges persist after procaine block of the nerve or after curarization, which suggests that they originate in muscle. During intracellular recording of human myotonic muscle, Norris[39] found spontaneous slow depolarization of the muscle membrane leading to repetitive spikes or an abortive spike followed by further slow depolarization. Procaine amide is often used in the treatment of myotonic dystrophy, and since this drug is thought to reduce membrane permeability to ions, its stabilizing effect on the myotonic membrane may indicate a membrane permeability disorder. The slow depolarization of the membrane, leading to repetitive spikes, and the lower resting membrane potential are similar to those conditions found in denervated striated muscle. The electromyogram on voluntary contraction resembles more closely a neuropathy than a myopathy and shows high voltage polyphasic potentials of prolonged duration,[54] suggesting primary involvement of the neuron as well as the membrane. The subterminal nerve fibers grow and ramify to form large, multiple end plates. They also extend parallel with the muscle fibers, giving off short collateral sprouts that terminate in diminutive expansions upon the muscle fiber. This, together with the central position of the nuclei in the extrafusal fibers in myotonic dystrophy, suggests a conversion of normal extrafusal muscle fiber innervation into the multiple motor innervation characteristic of the intrafusal muscle fibers of the spindles. Thus, the conversion of the innervation of the muscle fibers from an extrafusal to an intrafusal form can lead to hyperexcitable "pseudo-muscle spindles" that are spread throughout the involved muscles and accompanied by resultant depolarization and membrane changes as noted earlier.

AUTOMATIC ANALYSIS OF THE ELECTROMYOGRAM

The electromyogram does not lend itself to automatic analysis because it is a constantly and often randomly appearing signal. The main benefit of automatic analysis is to replace qualitative information with precise quantitation to reduce the sources of human error in interpretation and to provide rapid on-line read-outs.[29] The main features used in recognition of an abnormal electromyogram are (1) reduction in number of active units, (2) changes in mean amplitude of individual spikes and (3) changes in form of the individual spike potentials.

Integration of the electromyographic signal provides an automatic measurement of the summated potentials. The total activity of the signal for the time period desired is measured and includes both frequency and amplitude. The signal may be rectified before being integrated so that the positive and negative summated potentials do not cancel out. This gross measure of the electrical activity of the muscle is often used in conjunction with other methods of analysis.

The terms *power density spectrum* and *frequency analysis* are commonly used in analytical procedures but are not specifically defined. It is possible to count the number of spikes per unit time automatically by setting limits to the amplitudes of direction changes of potential that can be recorded. Thus, an output pulse can be recorded for each directional change of 100 μv, giving both total amplitude in units of 100 μv or more and the number of changes of direction of the input voltage exceeding 100 μv.[52] For example, the number of counts is increased in myopathy. Neuropathies may show high or low counts, depending upon the number of units destroyed and the complexity of potentials. Other techniques utilize the distance between potentials or the duration of a single measured potential to extrapolate overall frequencies.

More sophisticated procedures of applying mathematical computation to biological data make use of Fourier analysis, autocorrelation and cross-correlation techniques. In these methods the electromyographic signal is treated as a stationary value, and when the signal for a specific period of time is broken down into component harmonic sine and cosine waves, a reasonable approximation of the frequency spectrum can be given.

Audiospectral analysis of the electromyogram has also been done.[48] A shift to higher frequencies was found in myopathies as compared to a control peak audiofrequency characteristic of 100 to 200 Hz in normal subjects. Another technique using band-pass filters to measure the frequency spectrum of the surface electromyogram of muscle contracting to fatigue showed that low frequency components of 10 to 30 Hz are most prevalent and that the percentage of these components compared to the total spectrum increases as fatigue occurs.[37] The raw electromyographic data show an increase in amplitude and a decrease in overall frequency (decreased interference pattern). This would be expected since the frequency of the individual component motor units is approximately 10 to 70 Hz (mean 30), and with fatigue the number of units firing increases, but synchronization takes place, giving a reduced interference pattern. The technique of band-pass filtration is cumbersome and requires corrections to reduce inaccuracies in the filters. Digital filter programs are being devised which may speed up the analysis. The development of small, online, hybrid analogue-to-digital computers has been a significant advance. Raw data or data already treated in another fashion can be fed into properly programmed computers that give almost instantaneous analysis and complicated statistical calculations. This is obviously an area that holds high potential for future development.

REFERENCES

1. Adrian, E. D. and Bronk, D. W.: The discharge of impulses in motor nerve fibres. Part II. The frequency of discharge in reflex and voluntary contractions. J. Physiol., 67:119-151, 1929.
2. Basmajian, J. V.: *Muscles Alive*, 2nd edition. Baltimore, Williams and Wilkins Company, 1967.
3. Belmar, J. and Eyzaguirre, C.: Pacemaker site of fibrillation potentials in denervated mammalian muscle. J. Neurophysiol., 29:425-441, 1966.
4. Bhala, R. P.: Electromyographic evidence of lower motor neuron involvement in hemiplegia. Arch. Phys. Med. Rehabil., 50:632-637, 1969.
5. Bigland, B. and Lippold, O. C. J.: Motor unit activity in the voluntary contraction of human muscle. J. Physiol., 125:322-335, 1954.
6. Brandstater, M. E. and Lambert, E. H.: A histological study of the spatial arrangement of muscle fibres in single motor units within rat tibialis anterior muscle. Bull. Amer. Assoc. Electromyog. Electrodiag., Aug., 1968.
7. Brooks, J. E.: Disuse atrophy of muscle. Arch. Neurol., 22:27-30, 1970.
8. Brooks, J. E. and Hongdalarom, T.: Intracellular electromyography. Resting and action potentials in normal human muscle. Arch. Neurol., 18:291-300, 1968.
9. Brown, M. C. and Matthews, P. B. C.: An investigation into the possible existence of polyneu-

ronal innervation of individual skeletal muscle fibres in certain hind-limb muscles of the cat. J. Physiol., *151*:436-457, 1960.

10. Buchthal, F.: Spontaneous and voluntary electrical activity in neuromuscular disorders. Bull. N.Y. Acad. Med., *42*:521-550, July, 1966.
11. Buchthal, F., Ermino, F. and Rosenfalck, P.: Motor unit territory in different human muscles. Acta Physiol. Scand., *45*:72-87, 1959.
12. Buchthal, F., Guld, C. and Rosenfalck, P.: The origin of the motor unit potential. Acta Physiol. Scand., *31*(suppl. 114):7-8, 1954.
13. Buchthal, F., Guld, C. and Rosenfalck, P.: Action potential parameters in normal human muscle and their dependence on physical variables. Acta Physiol. Scand., *32*:200-218, 1954.
14. Buchthal, F., Pinelli, P. and Rosenfalck, P.: Action potential parameters in normal human muscle and their physiological determinants. Acta Physiol. Scand., *32*:219-229, 1954.
15. Buchthal, F., Guld, C. and Rosenfalck, P.: Volume conduction of the spike of the motor unit potential investigated with a new type of multielectrode. Acta Physiol. Scand., *38*:331-354, 1957.
16. Buchthal, F., Guld, C. and Rosenfalck, P.: Multielectrode study of the territory of a motor unit. Acta Physiol. Scand., *39*:83-105, 1957.
17. Christensen, E.: Topography of terminal motor innervation in striated muscles from stillborn infants. Am. J. Phys. Med., *38*:65-77, 1959.
18. Clamann, H. P.: Activity of single motor units during isometric tension. Neurology, *20*:254-260, 1970.
19. Coërs, C., and Woolf, A. L.:*The Innervation of Muscle.* Oxford, Blackwell, 1959.
20. Denny-Brown, D.: Interpretation of the electromyogram. Arch. Neurol. Psychiat., *61*:99-128, February, 1949.
21. Ekstedt, J.: Human single muscle fibre action potentials. Acta Physiol. Scand., *51*(suppl. 226):1-96, 1964.
22. Ermino, F., Buchthal, F. and Rosenfalck, P.: Motor unit territory and muscle fibre concentration in paresis due to peripheral nerve injury and anterior horn cell involvement. Neurology, *9*:657-671, 1959.
23. Feinstein, B., Lindegård, B., Nyman, E. and Wohlfart, G.: Morphologic studies of motor units in normal human muscles. Acta Anat., *23*:127-142, 1955.
24. Fleck, H.: Action potentials from single motor units in human muscle. Arch. Phys. Med. Rehabil., *43*:99-107, 1962.
25. Forster, F. M. and Alpers, B. J.: The site of origin of fasciculations in voluntary muscle. Arch. Neurol. Psychiat., *51*:264-267, 1944.
26. Goldkamp, O.: Electromyography and nerve conduction studies in 116 patients with hemiplegia. Arch. Phys. Med. Rehabil., *48*:59-63, 1967.
27. Goodgold, J. and Eberstein, A.: The physiological significance of fibrillation action potentials. Bull. N.Y. Acad. Med., *43*:811-818, 1967.
28. Gutmann, E. and Hanzliková, V.: Motor unit in old age. Nature, *209*:921-922, 1966.
29. Halliday, A. M.: Computing techniques in neurological diagnosis. Brit. Med. Bull., *24*:253-259, 1968.
30. Hayes, G. J. and Woolsey, C. N.: The unit of fibrillary activity and the site of origin of fibrillary contractions in denervated striated muscle. Fed. Proc., *1*:38, 1942.
31. Hoefer, P. F. A. and Putnam, T. J.: Action potentials of muscles in spastic conditions. Arch. Neurol. Psychiat., *43*:1-22. 1940.
32. Hunt, C. C. and Kuffler, S. W.: Motor innervation of skeletal muscle: Multiple innervation of individual muscle fibres and motor unit function. J. Physiol., *126*:293–303, 1954.
33. Kugelberg, E.: Electromyography in muscular dystrophies. J. Neurol. Neurosurg. Psychiat., *12*:129-136, 1949.
34. Lindsley, D. B.: Myographic and electromyographic studies of myasthenia gravis. Brain, *58*:470-480, 1935.
35. Lundervold, A., and Li, C.: Motor units and fibrillation potentials as recorded with different kinds of needle electrodes. Acta Psychiat. Neurolog. Scand., *28*:201-212, 1953.
36. Marinacci, A. A.: *Applied Electromyography.* Philadelphia, Lea & Febiger, 1968.
37. Myers, S. J. and Sullivan, W. P.: Effect of circulatory occlusion on time to muscular fatigue. J. Appl. Physiol., *24*:54, 1968.
38. Nastuk, W. L. and Hodgkin, A. L.: The electrical activity of single muscle fibers. J. Cell. and Comp. Physiol., *35*:39-73, 1950.
39. Norris, F. H., Jr.: Unstable membrane potential in human myotonic muscle. Electroenceph. Clin. Neurophysiol., *14*:197-201, 1962.
40. Norris, F. H., Jr.: Synchronous fasciculation in motor neuron disease. Arch. Neurol., *13*:495-500, 1965.

41. Norris, F. H., Jr. and Gasteiger, E. L.: Action potentials of single motor units in normal muscle. Electroenceph. Clin. Neurophysiol., 7:115-126, 1955.

42. Petersen, I. and Kugelberg, E.: Duration and form of action potential in the normal human muscle. J. Neurol. Neurosurg. Psychiat., 12:124-128, 1949.

43. Pinelli, P. and Buchthal, F.: Muscle action potentials in myopathies with special regard to progressive muscular dystrophy. Neurology, 3:347-359, 1953.

44. Richardson, A. T.: Muscle fasciculation. Arch. Phys. Med. Rehabil., 35:281-285, 1954.

45. Scherrer, J. and Bourguignon, A.: Changes in the electromyogram produced by fatigue in man. Am. J. Phys. Med., 38:148-158, 1959.

46. Taylor, A.: The significance of grouping of motor unit activity. J. Physiol., 162:259-269, 1962.

47. Walker, L. B., Jr.: Multiple motor innervation of individual muscle fibres in the m. tibialis anterior of the dog. Anat. Rec., 139:1-11, 1961.

48. Walton, J. H. The electromyogram in myopathy: Analysis with the audiofrequency spectrometer. J. Neurol. Neurosurg. Psychiat., 15:219-226, 1952.

49. Ware, F., Jr., Bennett, A. L. and McIntyre, A. R.: Membrane resting potential of denervated skeletal muscle measured in vivo. Am. J. Physiol., 177:115-118, 1954.

50. Weddell, G., Feinstein, B., and Pattle, R. E.: The electrical activity of voluntary muscle in man under normal and pathological conditions. Brain, 67:178-257, 1944.

51. Wiederholt, W. C.: End-plate noise in electromyography. Neurology, 20:214-224, 1970.

52. Willison, R. G.: Some problems in the diagnosis of primary muscle disease. Proc. Roy. Soc. Med. (England), 59:998-1000, 1966.

53. Wohlfart, G.: Clinical considerations on innervation of skeletal muscle. Am. J. Phys. Med., 38:223-230, 1959.

54. Woolf, A. L.: The theoretical basis of clinical electromyography. Part II. Ann. Phys. Med., 6:241-266, 1962.

55. Yahr, M. D., Herz, E., Moldaver, J. and Grundfest, H.: Electromyographic patterns in reinnervated muscle. Arch. Neurol. Psychiat., 63:728-738, 1950.

Energy Expenditure and Transfer

Chapter 7

PHYSIOLOGY OF TEMPERATURE REGULATION IN MAN

by John A. Downey, M.D., D.Phil. (*Oxon*)

INTRODUCTION

"La fixité du milieu intérieur est la condition de la vie libre." Thus Claude Bernard recognized the biological significance of a regulated body temperature in man.[3] Fever had been recognized since Biblical times, but it was not until the development of the thermometer in the eighteenth century that accurate temperature measurements could be made, leading to the knowledge of the constancy of body temperature in health. It is now clear that in man and warm blooded animals temperature is closely regulated most of the time despite exposure to wide extremes of environmental temperature. The effect of a changing environmental exposure to all or part of the body causes the skin temperatures over the body to vary widely and without a systematic pattern. Some workers have attributed all or most of body temperature regulation to responses from the skin, but both physiological evidence and logic indicate that a less variable temperature must be the regulated temperature. The best evidence is obtained when internal temperature is measured and compared with some reference temperature; when significant deviation occurs, appropriate corrective responses are initiated to reduce the difference. In this Chapter I will discuss the several temperatures of the body and their contribution to the sensing of total body heat content. In addition, the means of adjusting heat loss and production for man at rest and during exercise and fever will be discussed.

137

TEMPERATURE MEASUREMENT

Skin

The temperature of the skin varies over the body because of exposure to the environment and changes in the circulation to the skin, due in part to thermoregulatory responses. The temperature of the fingers and toes vary most widely (up to 15°C); the proximal part of the limbs and the trunk vary the least (3 to 4°C).

Central or Deep Body Temperature

There is evidence, which will be developed later, that the hypothalamus is the site of temperature receptors that regulate body temperature. It is not possible to measure temperature there in man, but it is important to measure temperature at a site that reflects and parallels the temperature changes occurring in the brain. Traditionally temperature measured rectally has been the most reliable and constant. This is true when the body is in thermal balance, whether at rest, during exercise or with a fever. Rectal temperature does not, however, accurately reflect rapid changes in body heat. When, for example, hot saline is injected into a vein to cause a rise in oral temperature and a compensatory vasomotor reaction in the skin, the rectal temperature shows little or no response. The rectal temperature is the highest of the several deep body temperatures that can be measured and is usually about 0.3°C higher than the temperature of aortic blood.[7]

The temperature in the mouth under the tongue is a more sensitive and rapid indicator of the blood temperature and, presumably, of the tissues of the brain. Figure 7-1 compares the oral, subclavian arterial and rectal tempera-

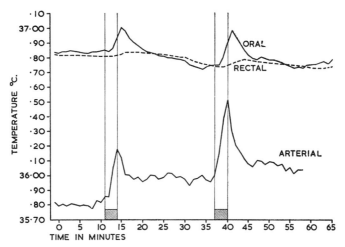

Figure 7—1   Temperature measured in the mouth, rectum and subclavian artery in a normal subject during immersion of one forearm in a bath of warm water (shaded areas indicate duration of immersion.) (From Cranston: Temperature regulation. Brit. Med. J., 2:69, 1966.)

tures during the introduction of heat into the body. The oral temperature more closely follows the temperature of the blood, while the rectal temperature does not vary.[8] If the measurement of relatively small heat loads is desired, the oral temperature is clearly much more accurate than the rectal temperature. However, oral temperature can be affected by local conditions. A high reading will be found after the patient has consumed a hot drink. Breathing through the mouth will cause a false low reading.

In special circumstances, particularly in the laboratory, other temperatures may be measured. The temperature of the lower one-third of the esophagus reflects oral temperature accurately in both resting and exercise states. The temperature of the ear drum or of the external auditory canal has been introduced as even more closely reflecting blood and brain temperatures and can be useful, although it is uncomfortable when taken over long periods.

Normal Body Temperature

There is a remarkable constancy of body temperature in man when measurements are taken under standard circumstances. Ivy[21] measured the oral temperatures of 276 students in class between 8 and 9 A.M. and found a mean temperature of 36.7 ± 0.2°C. However, small but significant changes in body temperature are related to factors such as time of day, age and sex. Studies of these factors have increased understanding of the general subject of temperature regulation.

Diurnal Changes

Body temperature varies throughout the day with a minimum of about 36.1°C in the early morning (4 to 6 A.M.) to a maximum of about 37.4°C in the late afternoon.[28] This variation seems to be one manifestation of the circadian rhythm seen in other areas of physiology and is affected by sleeping, eating, light and time.[5] The cycle changes with travel; for example, when a person flies east or west for 8 to 10 hours, the cycle readjusts slowly over three to four days to the new time.[20] Similarly, when workmen change shifts from day to night, an adjustment takes place. Fasting reduces the extent of the variation.

Age

Regulation of body temperature in the premature and newborn child is different from that found in adults owing to immaturity of the infant's nervous system and also to special mechanisms of heat production; these differences will not be covered here. During the first year of life, temperature changes due to emotion, crying or activity are greater than in the adult.

Elderly patients regulate body temperature at about the same level as the younger adult,[26] but they are less able to withstand exposure to cold or extreme heat, resulting in hypo- or hyperthermia. This fragility does not seem to be caused by any single factor but rather to overall changes in nutrition, health and exposure.

Sex

Preovulatory women have the same oral temperature as men. At ovulation body temperature tends to rise 0.2 to 0.5°C and remains higher throughout the remainder of the cycle. The cause for this rise in temperature is not known. Some hormones, including pregnenolone and pregnanediol, cause fever when injected in man, and this may be a partial explanation.

Men and women do not respond the same to thermal stresses. Women begin sweating in the heat at a higher skin temperature and sweat at a lower rate than do men. In the cold, women have a lower skin temperature than men and a heat loss of about 10 per cent less. This is in part due to a more effective vasoconstriction in women, but also to greater thickness of the subcutaneous tissues.[18] Some of the differences in temperature regulation between men and women, especially in the heat, may be due to the greater acclimatization or training of men.[14]

Race

Certain primitive non-Caucasians respond differently to thermal stress than do Caucasians. With whole body exposure to moderate cold the metabolic rate of an urban Caucasian rises markedly as his deep body temperature falls. The metabolic rate of a central Australian aborigine starts near basal but decreases as the rectal and skin temperatures fall to levels below that of the urban Caucasian. On the other hand, Alacaluf Indians of southern Chile have a higher resting metabolism that declines slightly, as does the rectal temperature on cold exposure, but the rectal temperature goes no lower than that of Caucasians. Other groups have responses intermediate to these.

Urbanized men of different races respond in the same way to cold.[16] This would indicate that at least some of the reactions are not racial in origin but manifestations of acclimatization.

Influence of Pharmacological Agents

Anesthetic agents, even in doses less than required to cause sleep, may impair temperature regulation,[13] as do other medications, particularly the psychotropic drugs (e.g., chlorpromazine). The modes of action are not clear, but it is important to realize that physiological studies on man or animals under medication must be interpreted with caution.

REGULATION OF BODY TEMPERATURE

Body temperature is maintained by a precise balance between heat production and heat loss. The afferent or sensory side of this balance includes temperature sensitive structures both in the superficial and in the deep or central regions of the body.

Skin Receptors

Temperature sensations of warmth and cold are important in the regulation of body temperature. There are thermal receptors in the skin that appear to be undifferentiated free nerve endings. However, even though the nerve endings do not appear to be different morphologically, they do differ significantly in physiological function. Neurophysiological studies[17] indicate that there are three types of receptors:

1.   One type of receptor responds to heating with a burst of electrical activity and an increase in the static neural discharge.

2.   Another type responds to cooling with a burst of activity and an increase in static discharge.

3.   A third type responds to several stimuli, including warming, with a continuous barrage of activity.

It is not possible to extrapolate directly from receptor discharge to thermal sensation and regulation, but it would appear that nervous activity from the skin is able to signal to the central nervous system the absolute temperature of the skin as well as changes and the direction of change of skin temperature. The number of temperature receptors in various parts of the skin is different, but acting together they provide a form of early-warning system to the central receptors, initiating appropriate corrective thermoregulatory reactions to minimize changes in central temperature.

Central Receptors

Extensive research on animals, employing ablation techniques or warming and cooling of the brain, has clearly shown that there are temperature sensitive receptors in the anterior preoptic region of the hypothalamus and that in that region temperature changes of as little as 0.2 to 0.3°C can initiate peripheral thermoregulatory responses. Furthermore, recent studies in which electrical activity from single nerve cells in the hypothalamus was recorded have shown the existence of cells that increase firing activity with cooling, others that increase firing activity with heating and others, perhaps reference cells, that do not change their rate of firing with changing temperature. These may be the actual cells that sense temperature changes.[19]

In man direct neurophysiological studies are not possible, but there is increasing evidence that central temperature sensitive structures are present.

Pickering[29] first showed that the return of warm or cool blood from an extremity to the central regions of the body caused peripheral vasomotor responses. Snell[32] infused measured amounts of hot or cold saline intravenously. He found a linear response between heat introduced and the vasomotor responses in the hand and calculated that the threshold of the central receptors would respond to temperature changes of as little as 0.1 to 0.2°C. Downey et al.[10, 12] cooled the insensitive lower body of spinal patients to cause a decrease in central body temperature. When the central temperature fell to approximately 35.6°C, shivering occurred in the innervated muscles even when the sentient skin was not allowed to cool (Fig. 7-2). If the sentient skin was allowed to cool, simultaneous central cooling produced an earlier and perhaps

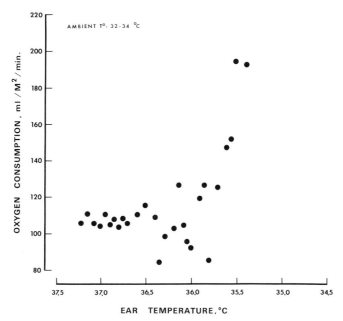

Figure 7–2   A demonstration of the oxygen consumption of seven spinal patients when the insentient part of their bodies was cooled in a surgical cooling blanket. Each point is the average of the oxygen consumption at that temperature. The ambient temperature was maintained at 32 to 34° C to keep the sentient skin warm. Increased oxygen consumption and shivering occurred when the ear temperature fell to approximately 35.6 to 35.8° C. (From Downey, Miller and Darling: Thermoregulatory responses to deep and superficial cooling in spinal man. J. Appl. Physiol., *27*: 209, 1969.)

more vigorous response (Fig. 7-3). These results indicate that deep temperature receptors are present in man which can act independently of receptors in the skin, but that there are synergistic reactions with the skin.

There is little direct evidence as to the site of the temperature receptors in man, although they are presumed to be at least in part in the hypothalamus. Head injury can cause disorders of temperature regulation, but this may only indicate that the integrity of the central nervous system and reflex pathways are involved in the thermoregulatory response. Cranston[8] infused hot saline into arteries in several areas of the body. Infusions into the carotid artery caused the greatest increase in hand blood flow. This suggests that temperature sensitive structures are within the distribution of the carotid circulation that responded to the warmth by increasing heat loss in the periphery, results which would be in line with the results of animal studies.

Extracranial Receptors

In addition to temperature receptors in the skin and brain of animals and man, investigators have searched for receptors elsewhere in the body. In man temperature receptors have been postulated to be in the proximal great veins, thus explaining the rapid temperature responses during exercise, but positive evidence of these or other receptors is currently unavailable.

In animals there is some evidence that receptors may be present in the heart (rabbits),[13] pulmonary vessels (sheep)[4] and particularly in the spinal cord

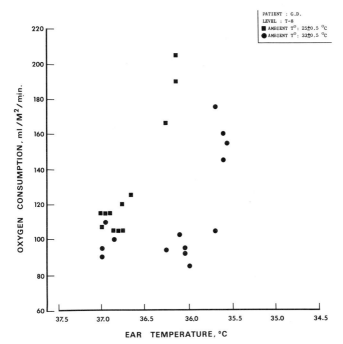

Figure 7–3 A demonstration of the oxygen consumption of a spinal patient (level T8) when the insensitive part of his body was cooled, while the sentient body is in a warm ambient (33 ± 0.5° C) and in a cool ambient (25 ± 0.5° C). When the sentient skin was warm, increased oxygen consumption and shivering occurred when the ear temperature fell to 35.6° C. When the skin was cool, simultaneous central cooling caused shivering to start at 36.4° C. (From Downey, Miller and Darling: Thermoregulatory responses to deep and superficial cooling in spinal man. J. Appl. Physiol., 27:209, 1969.)

(dogs).[31] Cooling the spinal cord of unanesthetized dogs to about 34°C caused vigorous shivering in the legs. The importance of this response in normal thermoregulation is not known.

THERMOREGULATORY RESPONSES

Behavioral and Environmental Selection

The most primitive response of an animal to heating or cooling is to change its habitat. This response is seen in all vertebrates, even in animals such as lizards, which control their body temperatures by moving in or out of the warmth. Modern man attempts to avoid extremes of temperature by either modifying his dress or his environment, the environment being modified by such means as central heating or air conditioning. These reactions are so effective that even people living in extremely cold climates may experience only short-term and limited cold stress.

Vasomotor Responses

Control of the blood flow to the skin regulates the flow of heat from the central or core regions of the body to the periphery. Increased skin circulation reduces the gradient of heat from central to peripheral and increases heat loss if the body temperature is greater than the ambient temperature. Conversely, decreased skin circulation reduces heat loss to the periphery. The peripheral circulation is controlled through the autonomic nervous system, and there are considerable regional differences in the control. The circulation in the skin of the fingers and toes, for example, is much more vasoactive than that of the trunk. Only the skin circulation takes part in thermal reflexes, the muscle blood flow remaining constant unless locally heated. The circulation through the skin effects the fine adjustment of body temperature; the coarse adjustment is effected by changes in evaporative heat loss or increases in heat production. In an ambient temperature of approximately 24 to 32°C most, if not all, of the heat balance of a naked man at rest is achieved through skin circulatory changes.

Evaporative Heat Loss

The high heat of evaporation of water (approximately 0.5 Kcal per gm) affords a potent method of eliminating heat from the body when regulation demands a large heat loss. The two avenues for evaporative heat loss are via the lungs and respiratory passages and from sweating onto the general skin surface.

The expired air of the lungs is saturated with water vapor, the moisture being taken up by evaporation from the respiratory passages. In animals, panting provides an effective mode of heat loss, but in man this is of relatively little importance even though respiratory rate and volume are increased with both fever and heating.

In man heat loss by evaporation occurs mostly through sweat secreted on the skin. There are two types of sweat glands in man: (1) The eccrine sweat glands, which secrete a dilute solution containing NaCl, urea, lactic acid and several trace elements, are distributed over the whole body and are under the control of sympathetic cholinergic nerves. Eccrine sweating is abolished with atropine; (2) Apocrine glands are found in association with hair follicles, particularly in the axilla, nipples and pubic region, and secrete a creamy substance rich in organic matter. The apocrine glands respond to adrenergic transmitters, and atropine does not abolish the secretion. It is the eccrine glands that sweat with heating, except on the palms and soles. The amount of secretion may be up to a maximum of 15 Kg a day, and by varying the sweat rate the amount of heat the body can lose is great.[25]

Thermogenesis

Increased heat production is an early response to cold exposure in man and warm blooded animals. Shivering, the involuntary contraction of muscle, is the most evident form of response. Initially the muscle contractions may be invisible, in the form of muscle tensing; but with increasing stimulus they become visible, often starting in the face and shoulders, but ultimately extending to all the muscles of the body. Shivering is a potent source of increased heat production through which oxygen consumption can be increased up to 500 per cent for short periods and by 200 to 300 per cent for the longer periods. It is mediated by the somatic nerves and requires an intact spinal cord and posterior hypothalamus. No shivering, for example, occurs below the level of spinal cord transection or in muscles paralyzed with poliomyelitis.

Other ways of increasing heat production include specific dynamic action of food, exercise and hormonal secretion. In acclimatized and newborn animals there is evidence for non-shivering thermogenesis particularly associated with increased secretion of norepinephrine and thyroid hormones. There is no definite evidence for non-shivering heat production in adult man, and in totally paralyzed man there is no increased heat production, at least during short-term cold exposures.[22]

Activation of Thermoregulatory Responses

Thermoregulatory reflexes can be activated by heating or cooling the skin alone before any change in central or deep body temperatures takes place. Warming[23] or cooling[29] the skin in one part of the body causes vasomotor reaction elsewhere in such a short time that these reactions can be mediated only by a nervous reflex. However, unless there is a subsequent change in central temperature, the reaction will not persist for more than a few minutes.[29] Sudden severe cooling of the whole body can precipitate shivering, and often there will be a rise in central temperature owing to the concomitant vasoconstriction (conserving heat) and the shivering (producing heat). However, the shivering will last only a few minutes and will not start again until the central temperature falls below resting levels. With a further fall in central temperature shivering will increase progressively. Heating an area of the skin can cause sweating to begin before a rise in central temperature occurs.[30]

A rise in central temperature can cause vasodilation and sweating in the periphery, but a cool skin will reduce the response.[2] Central cooling can produce vasoconstriction and shivering even when the skin is warm, provided the central temperature falls to approximately 35.6°C.[10, 12]

In day-to-day life the exposure to heating or cooling is not usually limited, except temporarily, to either the peripheral or central region of the body, that is, the whole thermoregulatory system reacts together. There is good evidence that there is a synergistic relationship between the superficial and deep sensors working to enhance the effectiveness of the regulation. For example, when there is skin cooling as well as central cooling, shivering occurs at a higher central temperature. Sweating rate is greater when both the skin and central temperatures are raised together rather than separately.

Full understanding of all the interrelationships involved in thermoregulation has not been achieved, and even the relative influences of peripheral and central receptors cannot be determined at this time.

In summary, it would appear that there is a high degree of control of central body temperature, whereas the skin temperature varies greatly. Thus the central receptors probably play a dominant role in thermoregulation, with the responses of the skin important mainly in short-term regulation and probably in modifying the form and sensitivity of the central receptors.

Regulation of Body Temperature in Exercise

Exercise causes a rise in body temperature, even in a cold environment. Nielsen[27] found that the elevation of body temperature during exercise is proportional to the metabolic work performed and independent of the ambient temperature (between wide extremes). The constancy of the elevation of central temperature, whether the exercise was performed in a hot (35°C) or a cool (5°C) room, implies a re-regulation of the temperature center in the body by the work and not simply an overload of the body's heat loss mechanism. The mechanism of this re-regulation is not known. It does not appear to be similar to the fever of infection, as the temperature rise due to exercise is not affected by salicylates.[11]

Regulation of Body Temperature in Fever

The most commonly recognized abnormality of temperature regulation in man is fever of infections, or inflammation. Rather than being a breakdown of regulation, it has recently been demonstrated that this fever too is a re-regulation of body temperature at a higher level.

At the onset of fever, as occurs after an injection of pyrogen, the body acts as if it were hypothermic, and there is a sharp vasoconstriction to conserve heat, often followed by shivering ("the chill") until a new higher level of temperature is reached. When the temperature is constant at the higher level, the body will respond to heating or cooling quantitatively in the same manner as before the fever. This indicates that the sensitivity of the regulation of body temperature during fever is as precise as at normal levels.[6] When the cause of the fever is removed or the fever is abolished by anti-pyretics, the body invokes heat loss mechanisms—i.e., vasodilation and sweating—until the temperature is reduced to the normal regulated levels.

Much study has been done in the last 20 years on the mode of production of fever in infections. When bacteria are incubated with granulocytes, a fever producing substance is formed called endogenous pyrogen. This pyrogen can also be elicited by incubating granulocytes with endotoxin[9] and can be extracted from the blood of animals having bacterial infections,[24] viral infections[1] and even from those with hypersensitivity states.[15] It appears to be the final common pathway for most, if not all, fevers of infection and probably exerts its action directly on the central nervous system.[8]

The integrity of the control system for maintaining a constant internal body temperature can be broken, allowing hypo- or hyperthermia to occur. The most common cause of such a breakdown is exposure to heat or cold after the ingestion of some chemical agent or drug, which interferes with either the effectiveness of the central nervous system, such as barbiturates or alcohol, or agents that may more selectively block some of the effects or mechanisms, such as the effect of chlorpromazine in reducing shivering. Extremes of environmental exposure can overwhelm the body despite the integrity of the control mechanism. Men exposed to cold water, such as after a shipwreck, cannot maintain body temperature despite vigorous shivering and intense vasoconstriction. In extreme heat, as on a desert, hyperthermia can occur. There is a loss of a large volume of body water and electrolytes by sweating; if not replaced, this can lead to circulatory collapse, and a failure of sweating and hyperthermia can occur if the exposure is continued. If heat loss is blocked, as when a person is immersed in a tub of hot water, temperature will rise. In illness, especially when there is damage to the central nervous system, the mechanism for either heat loss or heat production may be impaired, and temperature regulation may be abnormal.

SUMMARY

Body temperature is a closely regulated physiological function that is essential to health. It is effected by achieving a neat balance between heat production and heat loss, a balance that is brought about by an intricate system of thermal sensors in the skin, the brain and possibly other regions of the body. The responses of a man to activity, environment, stress and illness can be understood and predicted by a knowledge of the basic system of physiological controls.

REFERENCES

1. Atkins, E. and Huang, W. C.: Studies on the pathogenesis of fever with influenzal viruses. I. The appearance of an endogenous pyrogen in the blood following intravenous injection of virus. J. Exp. Med., *107*:383–401, 1958.
2. Benzinger, T. H.: Heat regulation: homeostasis of central temperature in man. Physiol. Rev., *49*:671–759, 1969.
3. Bernard, C.: *Leçons sur les Phénomènes de la Vie. Communs aux Animaux et aux Végétaux.* Paris, Ballière et Fils, 1878.
4. Bligh, J.: The receptors concerned in the respiratory response to humidity in sheep at high ambient temperature. J. Physiol. (London), *168*:747–763, 1963.
5. Bünning, E.: *The Physiological Clock: Endogenous Diurnal Rhythms and Biological Chronometry,* 2nd ed. New York, Academic Press, Inc., 1964.
6. Cooper, K. E., Cranston, W. I. and Snell, E. S.: Temperature regulation during fever in man. Clin. Sci., *27*:345–356, 1964.
7. Cooper, K. E. and Kenyon, J. R.: A comparison of temperature measured in the rectum, oesophagus, and on the surface of the aorta during hypothermia in man. Brit. J. Surg., *44*:616-619, 1957.
8. Cranston, W. I.: Temperature regulation. Brit. Med. J., *2*:69-75, 1966.
9. Cranston, W. I., Goodale, F., Jr., Snell, E. S. and Wendt, F.: The role of leucocytes in the initial action of bacterial pyrogens in man. Clin. Sci., *15*:219-226, 1956.
10. Downey, J. A., Chiodi, H. P. and Darling, R. C.: Central temperature regulation in the spinal man. J. Appl. Physiol., *22*:91-94, 1967.
11. Downey, J. A., and Darling, R. C.: Effect of salicylates on elevation of body temperature during exercise. J. Appl. Physiol., *17*:323-325, 1962.
12. Downey, J. A., Miller, J. M. and Darling, R. C.: Thermoregulatory responses to deep and superficial cooling in spinal man. J. Appl. Physiol., *27*:209-212, 1969.
13. Downey, J. A., Mottram, R. F. and Pickering, G. W.: The location by regional cooling of central temperature receptors in the conscious rabbit. J. Physiol. (London), *170*:415-441, 1964.
14. Fox, R. H., Löfstedt, B. E., Woodward, P. M., Eriksson, E. and Werkstrom, B.: Comparison of thermoregulatory function in men and women. J. Appl. Physiol., *26*:444-453, 1969.
15. Hall, C. H., Jr. and Atkins, E.: Studies on tuberculin fever. I. The mechanism of fever in tuberculin hypersensitivity. J. Exp. Med., *109*:339-359, 1959.
16. Hammel, H. T.: Terrestrial animals in cold: Recent studies of primitive man. *In*: Field, J. (ed.): *Handbook of Physiology.* Washington, American Physiological Society, 1964, Sect. *4,* pp. 413-434.

17. Hardy, J. D.: Physiology of temperature regulation. Physiol. Rev., *41*:521-606, 1961.
18. Hardy, J. D. and Du Bois, E. F.: Differences between men and women in their response to heat and cold. Proc. Nat. Acad. Sci. U.S., *26*:389-398, 1940.
19. Hardy, J. D., Hellon, R. F. and Sutherland, K.: Temperature-sensitive neurones in the dog's hypothalamus. J. Physiol. (London), *175*:242-253, 1964.
20. Hauty, G. T. and Adams, T.: Phase shifts of the human circadian system and performance deficit during the periods of transition: I. East-west flight. Aerospace Med., *37*:668-674, 1966.
21. Ivy, A. C.: What is normal or normality? Quart. Bull. Northwestern Univ. Med. School, *18*:22-32, 1944.
22. Johnson, R. H., Smith, A. C. and Spalding, J. M. K.: Oxygen consumption of paralysed men exposed to cold. J. Physiol. (London), *169*:584-591, 1963.
23. Kerslake, D. McK. and Cooper, K. E.: Vasodilation in the hand in response to heating the skin elsewhere. Clin. Sci., *9*:31-47, 1950.
24. King, M. K. and Wood, W. B., Jr.: Studies on the pathogenesis of fever. IV. The site of action of leucocytic and circulating endogenous pyrogen. J. Exp. Med., *107*:291-303, 1958.
25. Kuno, Y.: *Human Perspiration.* Springfield, Ill., Charles C Thomas, 1956.
26. MacPherson, R. K. and Ofner, F.: Temperature regulation in elderly men in bed. Med. J. Aust. *1*:889-893, 1967.
27. Nielsen, M.: Die Regulation der Körpertemperatur bei Muskelarbeit. Skand. Arch. Physiol., *79*:193-230, 1938.
28. Pembrey, M. S.: Animal heat. *In*: Schäfer, E. A. (ed.): *Textbook of Physiology.* Edinburgh, Pentland, 1898, Vol. 1, p. 785-867.
29. Pickering, G. W.: The vasomotor regulation of heat loss from the human skin in relation to external temperature. Heart, *16*:115-135, 1932.
30. Randall, W. C., Rawson, R. O., McCook, R. D. and Peiss, C. N.: Central and peripheral factors in dynamic thermoregulation. J. Appl. Physiol., *18*:61-64, 1963.
31. Simon, E., Rautenberg, W. and Jessen, C.: Initiation of shivering in unanaesthetized dogs by local cooling within the vertebral canal. Experientia, *21*:476-477, 1965.
32. Snell, E. S.: The relationship between the vasomotor response in the hand and heat changes in the body induced by intravenous infusions of hot or cold saline. J. Physiol. (London), *125*:361-362, 1954.

Chapter 8

CONTROL OF THE CIRCULATION IN THE LIMBS

by John A. Downey, M.D., D.Phil. *(Oxon.)*

INTRODUCTION

The major factor influencing the resistance to flow within a vascular bed is the tone of the smooth muscle in the wall of the arterioles. There is an intrinsic and automatic tone of the arteriolar smooth muscle, but this intrinsic tone can be modified or even dominated by nervous, chemical and physical agents.

In this chapter factors influencing the control of the blood vessels of the arms and legs will be discussed as well as the responses of this portion of the peripheral circulation to changes in posture, temperature and activity.

Measurement of Peripheral Circulation

The circulation to the limbs has been extensively studied over many years with the aid of several techniques. Most commonly the flow to a segment of a limb (the hand or foot, the calf or forearm) has been measured by venous occlusion plethysmography. For years it was assumed that the circulation to the hand and foot occurred predominantly through the skin, while the forearm or calf flow reflected largely muscle flow and that the skin contribution to that total flow could be ignored. It has since been found that this is not true and that a change in muscle flow could be masked or negated by a shift in skin flow of the opposite direction and vice versa. Thus, attempts have been made to separate the relative contribution of each to the total flow. The circulation of the skin has been followed by measuring skin temperature, heat flow, calorim-

149

etry or clearance of radioactive substances. Estimation of muscle flow is difficult and has best been achieved by clearance of radioisotopes or the measurement of the oxygen content of venous blood draining predominantly from muscle or skin. More studies have been made of the hand and forearm than of the leg, but in general the comparable segments of the upper and lower limbs seem to respond in a similar fashion.

The effects of drugs on the circulation can be studied in several ways. Drugs can be injected into a peripheral vein so that they diffuse through the whole circulation. Measurements can then be made of the blood flow in the extremities. When given in this way, however, the drug's effect on the circulation to be studied may be modified by the systemic reactions to the drug, such as the effect on other vascular beds, the heart, cardiac output and blood pressure, and by the rate of metabolism and excretion of the drug. If the direct effect of a substance on a portion of the circulation is desired, the drug can be injected into the artery just proximal to the vascular bed to be studied. The dose of the intra-arterial infusion can be given at a high enough concentration so as to cause a direct local reaction, but when the drug circulates back to the rest of the body it is so dilute that the systemic effects will be minimal or absent.

NERVOUS CONTROL OF THE BLOOD VESSELS

One of the dominant influences on the blood vessels of the skin and muscle of the extremities is the sympathetic division of the autonomic nervous system. The sympathetic nerves originate in nerve cells in the intermediolateral columns of the thoracolumbar spinal cord, and the axons emerge with the ventral spinal nerve roots at the same level. The neurons pass via the white rami to paraspinal sympathetic ganglia and either: (a) synapse within the ganglia with postganglionic fibers or (b) pass through the ganglia and communicate with more remote ganglia or with other segments of the sympathetic chain before synapsing. The postganglionic fibers pass to innervate the blood vessels in the same bundle as the peripheral nerves. These are called the *sympathetic adrenergic vasoconstrictor* fibers, and the transmitter substance released from the postganglionic endings is norepinephrine. In addition there are certain postganglionic fibers following the sympathetic nerve pathways that liberate acetylcholine at the nerve endings. These cholinergic fibers cause vasodilatation. Acetylcholine does not appear to have a role in the regulation of the peripheral circulation other than acting as a transmitter at the ganglia and from these *sympathetic cholinergic vasodilator* fibers.

The nerve supply to the blood vessels of the arm and leg is not the same in all areas. The blood vessels of the hand and foot have only sympathetic adrenergic constrictor nerves. In contrast the vessels of the skin and muscles of the forearm or calf have both adrenergic constrictor nerves and cholinergic vasodilator nerves. This means that in the hand increased blood flow can occur only by a release of the vasoconstrictor tone, but in the arm or leg there can be an added active vasodilatation when cholinergic nerves are activated. Sympathectomy will abolish both adrenergic and sympathetic cholinergic nerve activity. The adrenergic nerves can be blocked by selective chemical blocking agents (e.g., phentolamine). The cholinergic effects are abolished with atropine or hyoscine (hyoscine is the more effective).

HUMORAL CONTROL OF BLOOD VESSELS

Catecholamines

There are two catecholamines which occur naturally in the body and are of great importance in the control of the circulation:

1. Norepinephrine is the main transmitter at the postganglionic adrenergic nerve endings but is also present in the adrenal medulla, although in lesser quantities than epinephrine.

2. Epinephrine is the main hormone of the adrenal medulla.

The actions of these substances on the circulation are complex. It has been postulated that there are at least two types of "receptors" in the smooth muscle of the blood vessels in vascular beds and these have been called the α and β adrenotropic receptors. When activiated, the α site or receptor causes constriction of the vascular smooth muscle. Stimulation of the β site causes smooth muscle relaxation and vasodilatation. More recently chemical substances have been found which selectively block each site, thereby allowing separation of the various actions of drugs. Epinephrine has both α and β effects on vascular smooth muscle, the dominant effect on any given occasion being dependent on dosage. For example, epinephrine usually dilates muscle blood vessels (β effect), but in large doses its vasoconstrictor (α effect) overrides this.

Effects on the Circulation to the Limbs

Norepinephrine, whether given intravenously or intra-arterially, causes a fall in skin blood flow of the hand or forearm, and the constriction continues for as long as the infusion persists[30] (Fig. 8-1).

The circulation to muscles is always reduced with intra-arterial infusion of norepinephrine, but when the constrictor effect of norepinephrine is blocked by an α adrenergic blockade (phentolamine), a small vasodilatory effect on muscle due to the stimulation of β receptors[12] becomes apparent.

Epinephrine causes a decrease in skin circulation[22] when administered intravenously, intra-arterially or by iontophoresis. However, when an intravenous infusion is continued for a long time (over an hour), the effect on the skin diminishes and the flow may rise to levels greater than resting. The cause of this response is not known.

The initial effect of intravenous epinephrine on forearm blood flow is a marked vasodilatation, which is followed by a return of flow to about double the resting levels for the remainder of the infusion. Intra-arterial epinephrine at low doses causes forearm blood flow to increase transiently and then to return to resting levels or below. Information from simultaneous forearm blood flow measurements and venous oxygen saturations suggests that muscle blood flow is increased throughout the infusion (Fig. 8-2). With large doses of epinephrine both muscle and skin flow are reduced.[40]

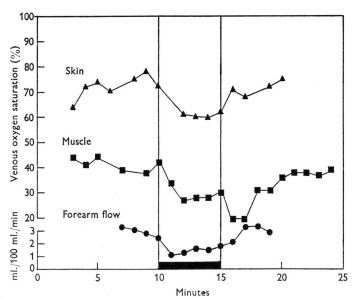

Figure 8–1   The effect of an intra-arterial infusion of norepinephrine (0.1 μg per min. during black rectangle) on the forearm blood flow and on forearm skin and muscle venous oxygen saturation. (From Cooper, Fewings, Hodge, Scroop and Whelan: The role of skin and muscle vessels in the response of forearm blood flow to noradrenaline. J. Physiol., *173*:67, 1964.)

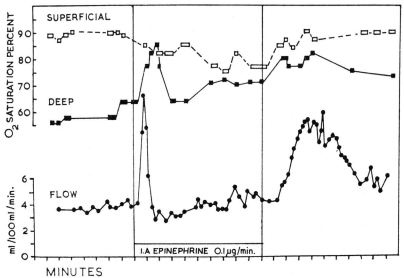

Figure 8–2   The effect of intra-arterial infusion of epinephrine (0.1 μg per min.) on forearm blood flow and on the oxygen saturation of blood from veins draining predominantly muscle and skin. (From Skinner and Whelan: The circulation in forearm skin and muscle during adrenaline infusions. Aust. J. Exp. Biol. Med. Sci., *40*:163, 1962.)

In summary, norepinephrine mainly stimulates the α sites on blood vessels and causes constriction. There is a lesser β stimulating effect that is only seen when the α site is blocked. Epinephrine has a more evenly balanced α and β effect, with the net effect varying with dose and route of infusion.

There are several other vasoactive agents normally found in the body; two of these, angiotensin and serotonin, will be mentioned briefly.

Angiotensin

Angiotensin is a polypeptide formed by the action of the enzyme renin on a substrate in plasma. It is thought to be important in the regulation of the circulation and maintenance of blood pressure in normal and diseased states.

Intra-arterial infusion of angiotensin causes a constriction in hand and forearm blood flow owing to a direct effect on the smooth muscle of the blood vessels. Intravenous infusion of angiotensin also causes a vasoconstriction in the hand and foot and a rise in blood pressure. The hand vasoconstriction caused by intravenous angiotensin is blocked by an α adrenergic blockade (phentolamine), but the rise in blood pressure is not. This suggests that angiotensin has a dual effect: (1) a direct constrictor effect on vascular smooth muscle and (2) a central (preganglionic) stimulating effect on the sympathetic nervous system.[39]

Serotonin

Serotonin (5-hydroxytryptamine) has been demonstrated in many body tissues and fluids, including the brain, serum and platelets. The role of serotonin in normal vascular tone is not clear, but circulating levels are high in patients with carcinoid tumor.

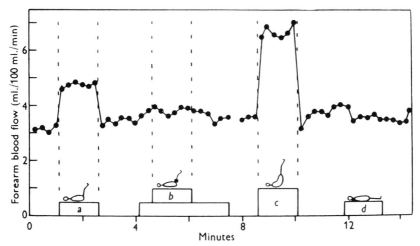

Figure 8–3   The effect of raising the legs and lower trunk on forearm blood flow: (*a*) legs raised alone; (*b*) legs raised but venous return prevented by cuffs inflated around the upper thighs; (*c*) legs and lower trunk raised; (*d*) cuff inflated to 30 mm Hg around neck. (From Roddie, Shepherd and Whelan: Reflex changes in vasoconstrictor tone in response to stimulation of receptors in a low pressure area of the intra-thoracic vascular bed. J. Physiol. (London), *139*:372, 1957.)

The direct effects of serotonin by arterial infusion include: (1) reduction of flow to the skin due to arteriolar constriction, but dilatation of the capillaries, causing redness of the skin; (2) dilatation of muscle vessels; and (3) constriction of veins. The systemic effect of intravenous infusions is variable.

POSTURAL REFLEXES

The marked changes in the hydrodynamics within the circulation in man that occur between the lying and standing positions makes the nervous control of the circulation most important in maintaining a nearly constant blood pressure. When a subject is passively tilted from a lying to a standing position, there is a transient constriction in the skin circulation in the arms and a sustained constriction in the muscle blood vessels. Conversely, when the legs and lower trunk are raised, there is a vasodilatation in the forearm muscle vessels. These responses seem to be mediated by low pressure baroreceptors in the thorax, since the responses to leg raising can be abolished if the blood is prevented from returning to the chest by cuffs inflated around the upper thighs (Fig. 8–3).[34] If the pressure within the chest is raised, as with the Valsalva maneuver or resisted breathing, vasoconstriction occurs in the arms. In summary, a rise in intrathoracic pressure causes peripheral vasoconstriction, while a fall in intrathoracic pressure causes vasodilatation.[10] The efferent pathway of this reflex is through the adrenergic sympathetic nerves.

These reflexes from the great veins are important in preventing a fall in arterial blood pressure on standing. When the venous return to the heart is decreased, as with standing, the cardiac output, and hence the blood pressure, would fall unless there is a compensatory increase in peripheral arterial resistance. On the other hand, in circumstances when the venous return is increased and the cardiac output is raised, a decrease in peripheral arterial resistance prevents an undue rise in blood pressure.

The high pressure arterial baroreceptors do not affect the vascular tone of the muscle directly,[33] but they do participate in maintaining vascular homeostasis by modifying heart rate and cardiac contractility. The veins also participate in the reflexes associated with posture and will be dealt with later.

EXERCISE

During exercise the distribution of the circulation is considerably readjusted (1) to meet the increased metabolic needs of the exercising muscle, (2) to accomplish the re-regulation of body temperature to a new higher level and (3) to accommodate any changes in posture that occur during the exercise.

Circulatory Changes in Exercising Muscle

There is an increase in blood flow through skeletal muscle during and after exercise[5] (Fig. 8–4); this occurs even after a brief contraction. The increased flow then returns to resting level over several minutes (Fig. 8–5).[21] The mechanism of this response is not fully understood. The hyperemia after muscle contraction is proportional to the strength of the contraction, which

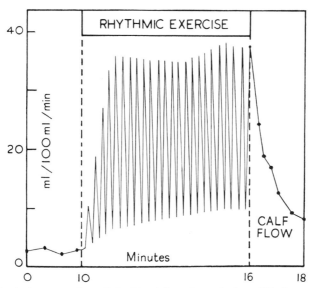

Figure 8—4 A demonstration of the blood flow through the calf before, during and after rhythmic, mild exercise. (From Barcroft and Donhorst: The blood flow through the human calf during rhythmic exercise. J. Physiol. (London), *109*:402, 1943.)

suggests that it is a result of metabolites from muscle acting directly on the blood vessels. Several metabolic or chemical factors have been investigated. Hypoxia, absolute or relative, is a likely cause, but intense investigation has not been able to demonstrate a direct relationship between the hyperemia and tissue oxygen needs.[4] Metabolites of muscle contraction, including lactic acid, adenosine diphosphate, adenosine triphosphate and ions such as potassium, can cause vasodilatation but do not appear to be quantitatively correlated with the hyperemia. Patients who lack muscle phosphorylase, and therefore cannot

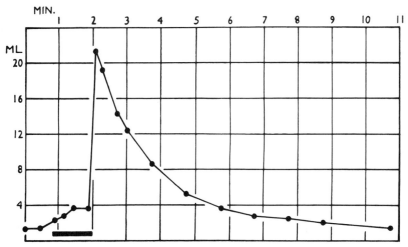

Figure 8—5 A demonstration of the forearm blood flow before, during and after a contraction of the forearm muscle for 90 seconds. (From Grant: Observation on the blood circulation in voluntary muscle in man. Clin. Sci., *3*:157, 1938.)

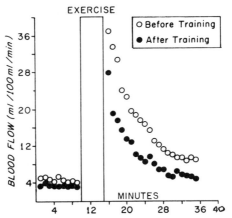

Figure 8—6   A demonstration of blood flow in the calf before and after exercise in subjects before training and after training. (From Elsner and Carlson: Postexercise hyperemia in trained and untrained subjects. J. Appl. Physiol., *17*:436, 1962.)

make lactic acid, a commonly postulated factor, do have hyperemia after exercise or ischemia.[27] Baroreceptors within muscle vessels that could be stimulated by muscle contractions have been postulated but not demonstrated conclusively.

Vasomotor nerves of the sympathetic system do not appear to be involved in the vasodilator response to exercise, as the response occurs in sympathectomized limbs, and patients with sympathectomy can perform strenuous activity without apparent detriment.

Postexercise hyperemia is increased by heating the exercising muscles; cooling tends to reduce hyperemia. However, if the limb is markedly cooled before rapid rhythmic exercise, the hyperemia is increased. This phenomenon has been attributed to changes in tissue viscosity by the cooling, which increases the internal work of the exercise.[13]

Physical training results in a lessening of the hyperemia during and after the performance of a standard exercise, even though the oxygen consumption for trained and untrained patients remains the same (Fig. 8-6).[18] The effect of training could be due to a reduction in the local tissue metabolites produced by the exercise or to a more efficient removal of metabolites by the circulation.

Vascular Responses in Non-exercising Limbs

At the onset of exercise of one part of the body there is a prompt vasoconstriction in the skin of non-exercising parts. The skin over the exercising muscles becomes warmed and vasodilated as the exercise continues, and depending on the heat load on the body, the vasodilatation may extend over the whole body. This would occur, for example, with heavy exercise in a hot room. During leg exercise there may be a temporary increase in the muscle blood flow in the arm at the beginning of exercise, which is a result of a transient rise of blood pressure. In severe exhausting exercise peripheral vascular resistance of the non-exercising parts is increased to maintain blood pressure in the face of marked vasodilatation in the exercising muscles. When the exercise is stopped there is a prompt and widespread vasodilatation in the skin due to release of the vasoconstrictor tone. This vasodilatation facilitates loss of heat and thus reduces the increased heat content of the body and returns the body temperature to its resting level.

REACTIVE HYPEREMIA

If the arterial blood supply to an extremity is occluded, there is a reactive hyperemia of the extremity after the occlusion is released.

The increased flow occurs in both muscle and skin[19] and is present in sympathectomized or completely denervated arms.[17] The maximum flow occurs immediately after the occlusion is released; the longer the occlusion, the greater the hyperemia that follows. Possible mechanisms of the increased flow include the following.

1. During the arrest of the circulation the arterial pressure, and thus the transmural pressure, in the vessels distal to the occlusion is reduced and the vascular tone is decreased. Maintenance of this decreased tone after release of the circulation permits increased circulation into the unoccluded part.[8]

2. The release of histamine by the tissues, as antihistamine infused intra-arterially reduces the hyperemia of prolonged periods of arrest.[16]

3. The accumulation of metabolites or anoxia is also considered a factor in increased blood flow, but, as in postexercise hyperemia, the relative contribution of each has not been established.

Severe arterial insufficiency prolongs the time for the circulation to return to resting levels after either exercise or arterial occlusion.

EFFECTS OF HEAT AND COLD

Reflex Effects of Heating or Cooling on the Circulation

Normal man maintains a constant temperature by balancing heat loss and heat gain. The effects of heating or cooling can best be understood as part of this balance. When exposed to an ambient temperature of 26 to 30°C, a naked man, lying quietly, regulates his temperature by finely adjusting heat loss or conservation from the surface of the skin by periods of vasodilatation and vasoconstriction. When the ambient temperature is lowered, the blood flow to the skin is progressively reduced to conserve heat; if the ambient temperature is raised, the blood flow to the skin is increased to enhance loss of heat. The responses of the skin circulation to temperature change are brought about by two mechanisms. Heating[29] or cooling[32] one part of the body will produce vasodilatation or vasoconstriction, respectively, in other parts of the body in three to five seconds, a response mediated by a nervous reflex through the sympathetic system. These reflexes, however, are transient, and it is only when enough heating or cooling occurs to change the temperature of the blood returning to the deep or central regions of the body that the response becomes sustained, continuing for as long as the perturbation of the central temperature is present.

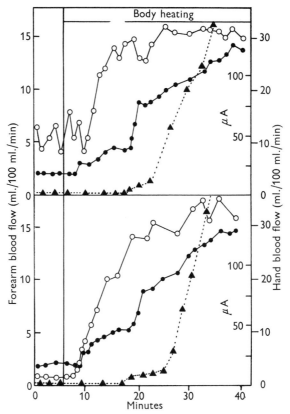

Figure 8—7 Forearm and hand blood flow before and during indirect body heating in two subjects. (●) forearm; (○) hand. The current (M.A.) flowing through the forearm skin (▲) is taken as an index of sweat gland activity. (From Roddie, Shepherd and Whelan: The contribution of constrictor and dilator nerves to the skin vasodilation during body heating. J. Physiol. (London), *136*:489, 1957.)

The reflex response to indirect heating or cooling occurs only in the skin. The muscle blood vessels do not participate.[36] The mechanism of the vasodilatation in the skin differs, depending on the nerve supply to the part. In the hand and foot vasodilatation occurs as a result of release of vasoconstrictor tone, since there are no vasodilator nerves in these areas.[35] In the forearm skin blood flow increases in three steps. The first is due to the reduction in vasoconstrictor tone; this is followed by an active vasodilatation that is mediated by the sympathetic cholinergic nerves and that can be blocked with atropine. Finally, when sweating begins there is a further rise in flow probably because of the release of the vasoactive polypeptide bradykinin with the sweat (Fig. 8-7).[37]

Direct Effects of Heating and Cooling

Direct heating of the skin causes vasodilatation.[1] The blood flow through the hand is lowest at about 15°C and heating in water up to 45°C causes an increase in flow,[23] although the general thermoregulatory state of the patient influences the responses. If the patient is cool, the flow in the hands will be less

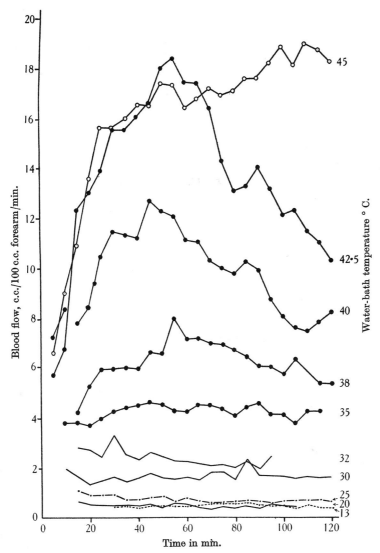

Figure 8–8 A demonstration of the effect on forearm blood flow of immersing the arm in water at different temperatures. (From Barcroft and Edholm: The effect of temperature on blood flow and deep temperature in the human forearm. J. Physiol. (London), *102*:5, 1943.)

with heating than if the patient were warm. The responses in the foot are similar to those in the hand, but the foot tends to have lower blood flow and responds more slowly to warming.[3]

Heating the arm in water at temperatures from 37 to 42°C causes an increased blood flow, but this increase is not sustained, even when the heating is continued[6] (Fig. 8–8), until the water is warmed to 45°C. Forearm flow is decreased when the arm is cooled in water down to 18°C. When the arm is placed in colder water, the flow increases to several times the resting level despite the continued cooling.[6] The mechanism of these special responses to

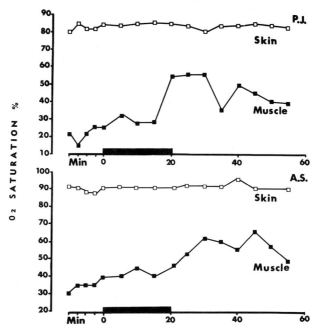

Figure 8–9 A demonstration in two subjects of the effect of short wave diathermy heating on the superficial and deep venous blood of the forearm. The black rectangle on the horizontal scale indicates the duration of heating. The venous oxygen saturation, and therefore blood flow, of muscle increased during and after heating. Skin venous oxygen was not changed. (From Downey, Frewin and Whelan: Vascular responses of the forearm to heating by shortwave diathermy. Arch. Phys. Med. Rehabil. *51*:354, 1970.)

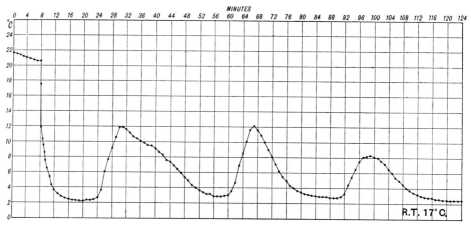

Figure 8–10 Skin temperature of the index finger cooled in crushed ice. The periodic increases in skin temperature were termed "hunting reaction." (From Lewis: Observations upon the reactions of the vessels of the human skin to cold. Heart, *15*:177, 1930.)

heating and cooling is not clear, although the cooling responses may be of a similar nature to those responses to be described later for the skin of the fingers.

The relative contribution of the muscle and the skin circulation to total forearm flow has not been separated, so the effects of heating or cooling on muscle circulation are not fully known. However, muscle flow does increase with heating by diathermy (Fig. 8–9),[15] and thus muscle flow may have contributed to the changes in forearm flow recorded in some studies.

The skin circulation of certain areas of the body responds to marked cooling in a special fashion. Cooling the hand in water from 18 to 10°C does not further reduce the blood flow.[20] Below 10°C there are periods of vasodilatation followed by vasoconstriction (Fig. 8-10). This phenomenon of vasodilatation in the cold was first reported by Sir Thomas Lewis in 1930[31] and occurs in the fingers, the toes, the ears and possibly the nose. It appears to be due to a local vascular reaction as it is still present in chronically denervated fingers, although of a lesser magnitude than in normal fingers, or in the same fingers after nerve regeneration.[24] Recent studies of Keatinge[28] may indicate a mechanism of cold vasodilatation; he demonstrated that cooling blood vessels to 5°C caused vasoconstrictor chemicals to become inactive in producing their effects and even allowing relaxation. It is possible that the subsequent dilatation and warming of the vessels by the inflowing blood could make the vessels reactive again to the vasoconstrictor stimulus. In the skin regions showing cold vasodila-

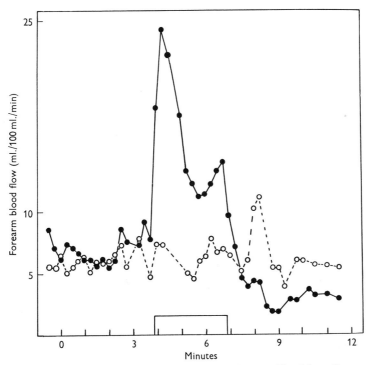

Figure 8–11   A demonstration of the effect of stress on forearm blood flow of a normal (●) and sympathectomized (○) arm. Mental arithmetic was performed during minutes 4 to 6. (From Blair, Glover, Greenfield and Roddie: Excitation of cholinergic vasodilator nerves to human skeletal muscles during emotional stress. J. Physiol. (London), *148*:633, 1959.)

tation there are a large number of arteriovenous anastomoses, and much of the flow during cold vasodilatation may be through them. Again the general thermal state of the patient affects the peripheral response; when cooled, a person develops cold vasodilatation less readily than when warm.

EMOTION

Sir Thomas Lewis first showed that the fall in blood pressure in a faint is not due to the slow heart rate.[14] It has since been shown that anxiety, mental concentration and emotional fainting all cause a widespread muscle vasodilatation (Fig. 8–11.[7, 43] This vasodilatation is limited to muscle and is mediated by the sympathetic cholinergic nerves.[11] Skin circulation may be reduced by emotional tension or in fright owing to the effect of both the vasoconstrictor nerves and circulating epinephrine released from the adrenal medulla. The epinephrine may also contribute to the muscle dilatation.

AGE

Hand blood flow does not change with age, but forearm flow is significantly greater in older men.[26] It is not known whether this increased flow is in muscle or skin, nor is the cause apparent. Reactive hyperemia in the calf after

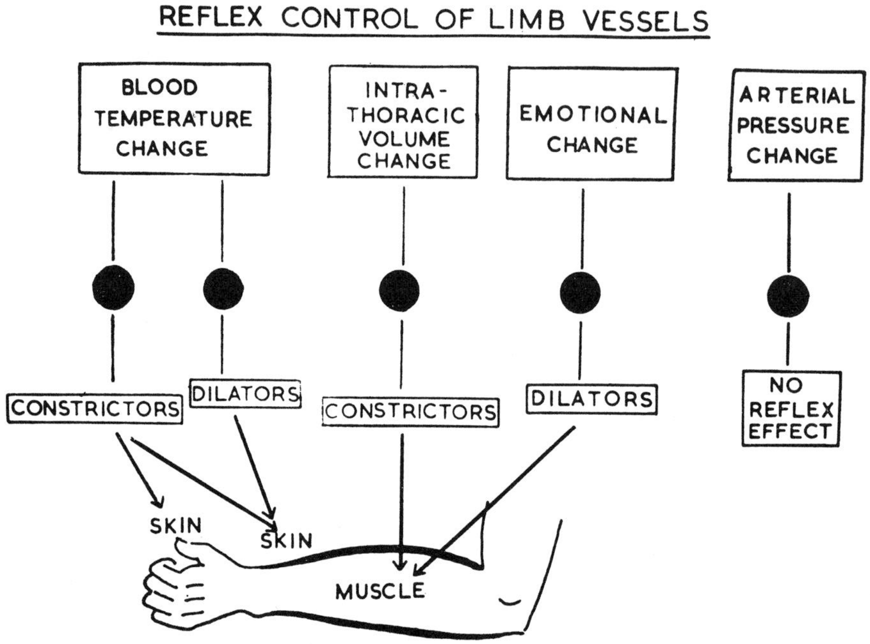

Figure 8–12 A schematic presentation of the neural reflexes involved in the control of the circulation of the arm. (From Whelan: *Control of the Peripheral Circulation in Man.* (Courtesy of Charles C Thomas, Publisher, Springfield, Ill., 1967.)

arterial occlusion is less in elderly men than in youths. It is not clear why this should be so, but it is possible that vascular changes or disease were present, although not detected by usual clinical methods.[2]

The nervous control of the skin and muscle of the forearm and hand is summarized in Figure 8-12.

VEINS

Veins are not passive conduits of blood; they are actively influenced by neural and humoral factors, and their responses complement the changes of the arterial system. General cooling, as when a person sits in a room in which the ambient temperature is falling, causes an increase in the venous tone. Local cooling of an arm causes a local venoconstriction but the responses are not as marked, as rapid or as constant as those of the arterioles. Local or general heating causes a decrease in the tone of veins.[42]

Exercise results in an increase in the tone of veins in all parts of the body, the increase being proportional to the work performed.[9] The increase in tone is minimized by local heating or when exercise is performed in a hot environment, and sympathectomy or sympatholytic drugs abolish it.

Changes in central venous pressure also modify venous tone. Increased intrathoracic pressure causes peripheral venoconstriction; decreased intrathoracic pressure causes venodilatation. These reflexes act in concert with those of the arterial circuit to help maintain a more constant cardiac output and blood pressure during exercise and postural change. Changes in posture, perhaps

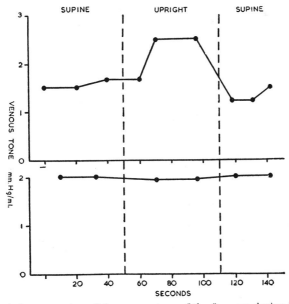

Figure 8–13   A demonstration of the venous tone of the forearm during lying and standing. The upper graph is from a normal subject, the lower graph from a patient with tabes dorsalis. (From Sharpey-Schafer: Venous tone. Brit. Med. J., 2:1589, 1961.)

also through changes in the pressure in the large veins in the thorax, cause reflex venomotor responses. These reflexes may be absent in patients with nervous diseases such as polyneuropathy or tabes (Fig. 8–13).[38]

Veins respond to humoral agents. Epinephrine and norepinephrine cause constriction and an increase in venous pressure. Angiotensin has a minor constrictor effect, while bradykinin has not been shown to influence venomotor tone.

LYMPH SYSTEM

The functions of the lymphatic system include the following:

1. The prevention of excessive change in the composition of the interstitial fluid.

2. The return to the plasma of substances that have passed from the capillaries but that cannot return directly.

There are several factors that influence the rate of lymph flow along the lymph channels. Lymph vessels are rhythmically pulsatile, generating pressures up to 20 mm of mercury within the lumen.[25] The lymph flow coincides with and is proportional to the strength and frequency of the contractions. When the vessels are distended with lymph, the contractions of the vessels are greater, but little is known of humoral or neural factors that may influence the activity. Passive transmission of pressure from muscular contractions or arterial pulsations may help propel the lymph toward the heart.

The rate of flow of lymph is also dependent on those factors that influence the formation of tissue fluid and on the movement of the fluid into the terminal lymphatic capillaries. A local increase in pressure, such as with massage, enhances the movement of the fluid into the lymphatic capillaries, while the rate of formation of lymph is low in extremities immobilized as in plaster casts.[41]

REFERENCES

1. Ahmad, A.: Response of the blood vessels of the upper extremity to prolonged local heat. Clin. Sci., *15*:609-616, 1956.
2. Allwood, M. J.: Blood flow in the foot and calf in the elderly: a comparison with that in young adults. Clin. Sci., *17*:331-338, 1958.
3. Allwood, M. J. and Burry, H. S.: The effect of local temperature on blood flow in the human foot. J. Physiol. (London), *124*:345–357, 1954.
4. Barcroft, H.: Circulatory changes accompanying the contraction of voluntary muscle. Aust. J. Exp. Biol. Med. Sci., *42*:1-16, 1964.
5. Barcroft, H. and Dornhorst, A. C.: The blood flow through the human calf during rhythmic exercise. J. Physiol. (London), *109*:402-411, 1949.
6. Barcroft, H. and Edholm, O. G.: The effect of temperature on blood flow and deep temperature in the human forearm. J. Physiol. (London), *102*:5-20, 1943.
7. Barcroft, H., Edholm, O. G., McMichael, J. and Sharpey-Schafer, E. P.: Posthaemorrhagic fainting. Study by cardiac output and forearm flow. Lancet, *1*:489-491, 1944.
8. Bayliss, W. M.: On the local reactions of the arterial wall to changes of internal pressure. J. Physiol. (London), *28*:220-231, 1902.
9. Bevegard, B. S. and Shepherd, J. T.: Changes in tone of limb veins during supine exercise. J. Appl. Physiol., *20*:1-8, 1965.

10. Blair, D. A., Glover, W. E. and Kidd, B. S. L.: The effect of continuous positive and negative pressure breathing upon the resistance and capacity blood vessels of the human forearm and hand. Clin. Sci., *18*:9-16, 1959.
11. Blair, D. A., Glover, W. E., Greenfield, A. D. M. and Roddie, I. C.: Excitation of cholinergic vasodilator nerves to human skeletal muscles during emotional stress. J. Physiol. (London), *148*:633-647, 1959.
12. Brick, I., Hutchinson, K. J. and Roddie, I. C.: The vasodilator properties of noradrenaline in the human forearm. Brit J. Pharmacol., *30*:561-567, 1967.
13. Clarke, R. S. J. and Hellon, R. F.: Hyperaemia following sustained and rhythmic exercise in the human forearm at various temperatures. J. Physiol. (London), *145*:447-458, 1959.
14. Cotton, T. F. and Lewis, T.: Observations upon fainting attacks due to inhibitory cardiac impulses. Heart, *7*:23-34, 1918.
15. Downey, J. A., Frewin, D. B. and Whelan, R. F.: Vascular responses of the forearm to heating by shortwave diathermy. Arch. Phys. Med. Rehabil., *51*:354-357, 1970.
16. Duff, F., Patterson, G. C. and Whelan, R. F.: The effect of intra-arterial antihistamines on the hyperemia following temporary arrest of the circulation in the human forearm. Clin. Sci., *14*:267-273, 1955.
17. Duff, F. and Shepherd, J. T.: The circulation in the chronically denervated forearm. Clin. Sci., *12*:407-416, 1953.
18. Elsner, R. W. and Carlson, L. D.: Postexercise hyperemia in trained and untrained subjects. J. Appl. Physiol., *17*:436-440, 1962.
19. Fewings, J. D., Hyman, C., Walsh, J. A. and Whelan, R. F.: The role of forearm skin and muscle vessels in reactive hyperemia. Aust. J. Exp. Biol. Med. Sci., *48*:179-186, 1970.
20. Freeman, N. E.: The effect of temperature on the rate of blood flow in the normal and in the sympathectomized hand. Am. J. Physiol., *113*:384-398, 1935.
21. Grant, R. T.: Observations on the blood circulation in voluntary muscle in man. Clin. Sci., *3*:157-173, 1938.
22. Green, H. D. and Kepchar, J. H.: Control of peripheral resistance in major systemic vascular beds. Physiol. Rev., *39*:617-686, 1959.
23. Greenfield, A. D. M.: The circulation through the skin. *In*: Field, J. (ed.): *Handbook of Physiology.* Washington, American Physiological Society, 1963, Sec. 2, Vol. 2, pp. 1325-1351.
24. Greenfield, A. D. M., Shepherd, J. T. and Whelan, R. F.: The part played by the nervous system in the response to cold of the circulation through the finger tip. Clin. Sci., *10*:347-360, 1951.
25. Hall, J. G., Morris, B. and Wooley, G.: Intrinsic rhythmic propulsion of lymph in the unanaesthetized sheep. J. Physiol. (London), *180*:336-349, 1965.
26. Hellon, R. F. and Lind, A. R.: The influence of age on peripheral vasodilation in a hot environment. J. Physiol. (London), *141*:262-272, 1958.
27. Hockaday, T. D. R., Downey, J. A. and Mottram, R. F.: A case of McArdle's syndrome with a positive family history. J. Neurol. Neurosurg. Psychiat., *27*:186-197, 1964.
28. Keatinge, W. R.: The return of blood flow to fingers in ice-water after suppression by adrenaline or noradrenaline. J. Physiol. (London), *159*:101-110, 1961.
29. Kerslake, D. M. and Cooper, K. E.: Vasodilatation in the hand in response to heating the skin elsewhere. Clin. Sci., *9*:31-47, 1950.
30. Lever, A. F., Mowbray, J. F. and Peart, W. S.: Blood flow and blood pressure after noradrenaline infusions. Clin. Sci., *21*:69-74, 1961.
31. Lewis, T.: Observations upon the reactions of the vessels of the human skin to cold. Heart, *15*:177-208, 1930.
32. Pickering, G. W.: The vasomotor regulation of heat loss from the human skin in relation to external temperature. Heart, *16*:115-135, 1932.
33. Roddie, I. C. and Shepherd, J. T.: The effects of carotid artery compression in man with special reference to changes in vascular resistance in the limbs. J. Physiol. (London), *139*:377-384, 1957.
34. Roddie, I. C. and Shepherd, J. T.: The reflex nervous control of human skeletal muscle blood vessels. Clin. Sci., *15*:433-440, 1956.
35. Roddie, I. C., Shepherd, J. T. and Whelan, R. F.: A comparison of the heat elimination from the normal and nerve-blocked finger during body heating. J. Physiol. (London), *138*:445-448, 1957.
36. Roddie, I. C., Shepherd, J. T. and Whelan, R. F.: Evidence from venous oxygen saturation measurements that the increase in forearm blood flow during body heating is confined to the skin. J. Physiol. (London), *134*:444-450, 1956.
37. Roddie, I. C., Shepherd, J. T. and Whelan, R. F.: The contribution of constrictor and dilator nerves to the skin vasodilatation during body heating. J. Physiol. (London), *136*:489-497, 1957.

38. Sharpey-Schafer, E. P.: Venous tone. Brit. Med. J., *2*:1589–1595, 1961.
39. Scroop, G. C. and Whelan, R. F.: A central vasomotor action of angiotension in man. Clin. Sci., *30*:79–90, 1966.
40. Skinner, S. L. and Whelan, R. F.: The circulation in forearm skin and muscle during adrenaline infusions. Aust. J. Exp. Biol. Med. Sci., *40*:163–172, 1962.
41. Trueta, R. J.: *The Principles and Practices of War Surgery, With Special Reference to the Biological Method of Treatment of Wounds and Fractures,* 3rd ed. London, William Heinemann Ltd. (medical books), 1946.
42. Wood, J. E.: *The Veins. Normal and Abnormal Function.* Boston, Little, Brown and Company, 1965, pp. 91–101.
43. Wilkins, R. W. and Eichna, L. W.: Blood flow to the forearm and calf. I. Vasomotor reactions: role of the sympathetic nervous system. Bull. Johns Hopkins Hosp., *68*:425–449, 1941.

Chapter 9

EXERCISE

by Robert C. Darling, M.D.

INTRODUCTION

In broadest terms *exercise* can be defined as *purposeful motion*, which involves many systems of the body in varying degrees. The muscular, skeletal and nervous systems are always involved and may be considered a single system—the neuromusculoskeletal system. The circulatory and respiratory systems are the most important of the other systems contributing to and being affected by all but the most isolated physical activities. In fact, the exercising animal requires regulatory changes in almost all systems as compared with the animal in resting or basal state.

In a single chapter we can only summarize some of the many physiological changes that accompany exercise. For clarity it is necessary to deal with reactions of the separate body systems, provided one recognizes that necessary simplifications are made. Most of the other chapters of this book relate somewhat to exercise, especially those dealing with the architecture and functions of muscles and nerves. Even the psychologically oriented chapters are related, since physical movement is such an integral part of human function and experience.

A fundamental characteristic of the systems involved in exercise is that they adapt to meet the new condition of exercise. Most of this essay will deal with these adaptive mechanisms. The adaptations in exercise occur at two levels. First, there are immediate changes during and after a bout of exercise. Second, there is the set of adaptive changes which permit the organism to improve function during later bouts of exercise. These latter may be called training effects and are the basis for the use of exercise as therapy.

167

The factors of load, rate, intensity, complexity, coordination and extent of the muscles involved are all important variables in the physiological responses to work and in the results of the training or therapy. Underlying the various types of exercises and the physiological responses to them there can be formulated a general rule which states that *the type of stress imposed by the exercise points to the function which will be enhanced.* Here the word *stress* may designate classic physiological stress such as heavy work load, or cardiovascular load, or it may refer to more subtle neurological stresses such as the development of dexterity and skill. A corollary of this rule is that exercise with negligible stress or difficulty does not enhance any function.

An analogy to the modern computer is useful in designating subdivisions to be discussed. A computer involves various input devices that receive information, a processing unit that manipulates this information according to instructions built in as well as instructions imposed on it, a variety of output devices that produce results, a power and temperature regulating system that maintains a stable internal environment and certain external hardware that render the results practical and useful. The computer's input system is analogous to the sensory reflex stimuli and voluntary efforts in the body. The processing unit is the central nervous system. The output devices are the final common neurological path to the muscles and the muscles themselves. The power and cooling system may be considered as the metabolic and circulatory systems in the body, and some of the external hardware may be considered analogous to the joints and periarticular tissues. As in the computer, the various subdivisions of the body have separate characteristics, but all are mutually dependent. Exercise of a specific type will put stress primarily on one or another of the subdivisions of the exercise system, but one or more other divisions are always affected to some degree.

STRENGTH EXERCISE

The function of muscle is to produce tension appropriate to the demand. Tension is a single dimensional value and is synonymous with the term strength. It should not be confused with the terms work and power, which introduce the additional parameters of distance, and distance-time respectively. The commonly measured index to assess strength is the maximum tension produced under voluntary effort. What is actually measured in the intact human is the torque around a joint produced by maximum effort, which in a purely mechanical sense depends upon the angle of pull and the distance of attachment from the axis of the joint. Aside from these mechanical aspects, there are important relationships between the maximum tension and the length of the muscle.

To understand these distinctions it is well to define certain terms. The term static contraction will be used when there is no joint movement. This term is preferred to the term isometric contraction since in contractions without joint motion there is some muscle shortening to take up the elastic properties of the tendons and other noncontractile tissues. When a muscle contracts and causes joint motion in the direction of pull, it will be called a "shortening contraction"

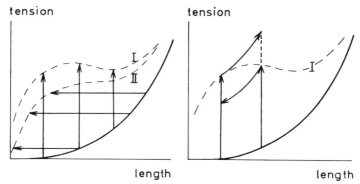

Figure 9–1 Left: Length-tension curves of resting muscle fiber (unnumbered curve), of isometric maxima (I) and isotonic shortening maxima (II). Right: Similar type of relationship during stretching (upper arrow) and shortening (lower arrow) of tetanized fiber. (From Asmussen, E.: Muscular performance. In Rodahl, K., and S. M. Horwath, eds.: *Muscle as a Tissue.* McGraw-Hill Book Co., New York, 1962.)

which is preferred to "concentric contraction" as more easily visualized. A muscle contraction which occurs during lengthening of the muscle to resist this lengthening will be called a "lengthening reaction"; this is preferred over the term "eccentric contraction."

These terms are important to a consideration of the relationship between length of the muscle and its strength, as pictured on a length-tension diagram[4] (Fig. 9-1). If the static tension produced by maximum stimulation is related to length, the maximum tension occurs at a length about 10 per cent longer than the resting length, i.e., at slight stretch. At lengths shorter or longer than this the maximum contractile tension decreases, to reach zero at points of full fore-shortening and maximum length respectively. This property of muscle can be logically explained, but not proved, by our knowledge of the ultrastructure of muscle (see Chapter 4). The length-tension relationships are important in understanding the most effective ways of utilizing muscular strength.

When the contraction occurs with motions of shortening or lengthening, the level of the tension is changed, although the maximum point is still at a length near the resting length. If there is shortening, the curve of maximum tension is below the static curve, probably because some of the energy is utilized in overcoming internal visco-elastic resistance. Maximum tension, produced during lengthening, is found to be significantly greater than when static or shortening. These conditions are those of so-called negative work, which will be discussed later. This property of muscle is utilized in many types of exercise in which a short preliminary lengthening ("a windup") is utilized to precede a maximum muscular effort.

Let us next consider the attributes which distinguish a strong muscle from a weak one. The most obvious property is muscle size, or cross sectional area to be more exact; this has been scientifically documented for nearly a century[34] and recognized since antiquity. This is obvious in the short, thick, antigravity muscles of the body such as the glutei, as well as in the relatively large muscles of highly trained weight lifters. The number of muscle fibers in a given muscle does not vary greatly from one person to the next, but the size of the muscle fibers is greater in the trained person. Recent work suggests that a relative and absolute increase in contractile protein (fibrillar protein) occurs.[8, 9, 27]

Size is an index of potential strength, but the actual tension produced by a muscle may depend on several other factors. These concern the degree to which the motor units are brought into action. As noted in greater detail in Chapter 6, increased strength is brought about by recruiting additional motor units rather than by more rapid firing of units. The number of units that can be brought into action may depend on (1) the motivation and voluntary effort expended, (2) the integrity of the central nervous connections, and (3) the degree of synaptic inhibition in (a) multisynaptic pathways, (b) the anterior horn cell synapses and (c) possibly at the motor end plate. More is known specifically of the existing balance between inhibition and excitation of the anterior horn cell than in the other areas.[21] The repeated observations that muscles may increase in strength without hypertrophy is evidence that these neurological factors exist and in some instances are the major changes in developing strength.[32, 33]

Circulatory factors are not important in explaining strength. It is well known that temporary arterial occlusion does not reduce the maximum tension possible over short periods of time, but strength will be reduced by previous prolonged exercise depleting available sources of energy and upsetting the acid-base balance. Extreme malnutrition may also have effects beyond the depletion of contractile protein.

Neurological or muscle disease introduces changes in muscle function that go beyond the major emphasis of this chapter. However, it is important to note that effective strength requires that antagonist muscles be relaxed and that there be no serious local inhibiting factors such as pain or contracture. Even in normals it has been demonstrated that primitive reflexes, such as the tonic neck reflexes, may be utilized to enhance the force of a maximum effort.[28, 43] In some pathological conditions spasticity and rigidity may cause muscular opposition to the strength which is being assessed. Pain is a powerful inhibitor of local muscular action as may be seen in arthritis and after joint surgery.

Having gained some understanding of strength, we can now turn to a discussion of methods by which strength can be increased. Exercise to enhance strength must tax this quality by maximum or near-maximum contractions. Some unanswered questions about the form of the exercises concern the details of number of repetitions, the questions of static versus dynamic exercise and the duration of exercise.

The so-called "progressive resistance exercise" techniques, popularized by deLorme,[18] are rhythmic dynamic exercises prescribing a near-maximum load, which is upgraded as the muscle improves, and several series of 10 repetitions per day. Further requirements are that the motion be carried through full range and that positioning be obligatory so that only the muscle groups being treated are the prime movers. Subsequent modifications of this system have reduced the requirements of the number of repetitions. One report states that contractions of 25 per cent of maximum are as effective as those near maximum.[17] However, the data from the more recent reports is not extensive, and the effectiveness of the original regimen has generally stood the test of time.

The use of static or isometric exercise has had considerable vogue and has many potential physiological advantages. It is difficult to design dynamic exer-

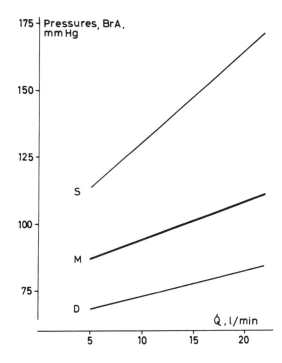

Figure 9−2 Brachial arterial pressures (BrA) in relation to cardiac output (Q̇) during exercise. S, systolic; M, mean; D, diastolic. (From Ekelund, L. G. and A. Holmgren: Central hemodynamics during exercise. Circulation Res., *20* (suppl. 1) *1*:41, 1967.)

cises that utilize near-maximum tension throughout the range. Static exercises can easily utilize maximum tension and require relatively simple apparatus. Enthusiastic supporters report optimum strength building exercises which require only one to three contractions per day, but these results have not been widely confirmed. From a practical point of view, static exercises have their greatest usefulness where motion is contraindicated or impossible.

Striking differences between static and dynamic exercise are to be seen in the hemodynamic responses. Rhythmic dynamic exercises produce changes in blood pressure primarily in the systolic level (Fig. 9-2). This indicates that in spite of the markedly increased total blood flow there is an almost completely compensatory decrease in peripheral resistance.

On the other hand, sustained static exercises, even of small muscles and of as little as 15 per cent of maximum contraction, cause considerable elevation of both systolic and diastolic pressure[2, 20, 38] (Fig. 9-3), which persists only during the period of exercise. Evidence for the mechanism of these remarkable changes points to a reflex initiated in the working muscle by some product of anaerobic metabolism. The rapidity of the response requires that it be neurologically mediated. Further facts bearing on the phenomenon are (1) that it occurs even though breath holding and the Valsalva phenomenon is avoided; (2) that it occurs during static contractions which are much less intense than those necessary to cause vascular obstruction by the forcefully contracting muscle (75 per cent of maximum); and (3) that it is produced equally well by a sustained single muscle contraction as by the contraction of multiple muscles.

Attempts to combine features of static with rhythmic dynamic exercises are the basis of some practical strength building programs. One approach, called

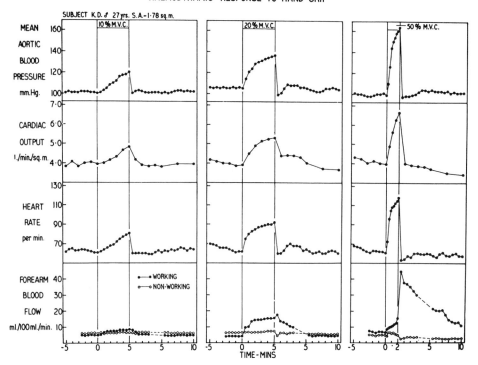

HAEMODYNAMIC RESPONSE TO HAND-GRIP

Figure 9 – 3   Cardiovascular response in a normal subject during and after sustained handgrip contractions at 10, 20 and 50 per cent of maximum voluntary contraction (MVC). (From Donald, K. W., A. R. Lind, G. M. McNicol, P. W. Humphreys, S. H. Taylor and H. P. Staunton: Cardiovascular responses to sustained (static) contractions. Circulation Res., *20* (suppl. 1) *1*:18, 1967.)

isokinetic, utilizes an apparatus in which speed of motion is kept constant, maximum tension is applied throughout the cycle and the actual tension or torque is continually recorded.[39] This device demonstrates the fallacy of using the term isotonic to apply to most rhythmic exercises, since the recordings show variable tension with a peak at the middle of the cycle and reduced values at points of less effective muscle action. With a cooperative subject it allows maximum tension throughout a range and seems to avoid the hypertension of static exercises. Although a few reports show more striking gains in strength by this device, its use has not been sufficiently studied to permit firm conclusions to be drawn.

The preceding discussion of exercises for strength applies most strictly to conditions in which strength is low because of nonuse or immobilization.[23] The term "disuse atrophy" describes a spectrum from extreme atrophy from prolonged immobilization to relative weakness for a weight lifter out of training. Estimates of possible hypertrophy from normal or nontrained conditions are on the order of 50 per cent, but the total spectrum of muscle size and strength in relation to training is much broader. The basic principles of resistive exercise apply to the entire range in normal muscles, although in the case of a muscle markedly weakened by disuse the resistance is very small. Probably the principles also apply to states of partial denervation, such as after poliomyelitis, where there is a net loss of motor units, the remaining units being normal or potentially so. As presented in Chapter 6, the situation in partial denervation also allows enlargement of motor units by terminal nerve branching.

Much less is known about redevelopment of strength after other forms of pathological damage. There is evidence that most myopathic muscles cannot be strengthened. In upper motor neuron disease the defect in strength is not a loss of the potential contractile tension of the muscle, but is a lack of controlled central impulses reaching the anterior horn cells. Although atrophy of disuse may occur in time after the onset of upper motor neuron damage, the resistive principle does not apply early in the training of these muscles. Resistance, if used in such cases, is useful because it causes an increase in sensory feedback and not because of its effect on muscle hypertrophy.

POWER EXERCISES

The terms strength and power of muscle are sometimes confused even though the physiological changes induced in power exercises involve predominantly different mechanisms and systems. The term power implies the performance of work in a definite period of time. It requires of muscle the ability to obtain metabolic ingredients for its action, to replenish stores of energy sources and to remove waste products of metabolism. These are functions of the circulatory system, and considerations of both local and general circulation are paramount. It is impossible to discuss power in a very weak muscle, yet experience has shown the muscles with maximum power capacity are rarely those with the greatest strength. It is useful to consider power as synonymous with metabolic capacity, both aerobic and anaerobic, even though each term implies a process involving different methods of adaptation.

The circulatory changes that occur during exercise are extensive, especially when the exercise is strenuous and prolonged.[12, 35] Since the total blood volume does not change rapidly, there are rapid redistributions in flow through the vascular beds. First and most striking of these is the increased volume and flow in the exercising muscles, as a result of local vasodilation and the opening of vascular channels which were previously closed. The stimulus to these changes is uncertain. It is not primarily a sympathetic neural stimulus since its magnitude is too great and it occurs after sympathetic denervation or blockade. It is not any one of the common products of metabolism, although one investigator believes that a combination of local potassium and oxygen changes could explain it.[37] It is not due to the level of lactic acid, CO_2 or pH alone.

As the muscle blood volume and the flow increase, circulation to other systems of the body is reduced owing to vasoconstriction. Constriction of vessels to nonworking muscles is moderate but significant, and constriction of the splanchnic and renal blood flows is probably the main area of compensation. Cerebral blood flow is not changed until near-total exhaustion, as the metabolic demands of the brain are unchanging. The blood flow to the skin depends on the needs for thermal regulation. Exercise in cold or nonstressful thermal environments is accompanied by vasoconstriction of the skin. Exercise in hot

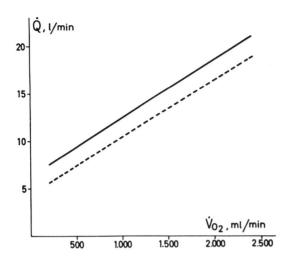

Figure 9—4 Relationship between cardiac output (Q) and oxygen consumption (V_{O_2}) in resting and exercising healthy men. Solid line = supine; broken line = sitting. (From Ekelund, L. G. and A. Holmgren. Central hemodynamics during exercise. Circulation Res., *20* (suppl. 1) *I*:35, 1967.)

environments adds a circulatory stress because the need increases for vasodilation of the skin for sweating and thermal loss.

Discussion of the redistribution of circulating blood volume has been presented before a discussion of the central or cardiovascular effects to highlight its importance and to explain the fact that some patients with cardiovascular disease can exercise moderately without an increase in cardiac output. The changes in the heart pump are usually dramatic and primary.[3] In all exercise the pulse rate rises. In exercises in a supine position the stroke output changes very little, but in those in an upright position the stroke output may more than double.

The linear relationship between O_2 consumption and cardiac output is shown in Figure 9-4. On the same figure the greater cardiac output in the supine position is shown by a comparison of the two graphs. The combination of increase in venous tone, increased ventilatory effort and the pumping action of the working muscles insures an adequate venous return to parallel these changes.

The net effect of increased pulse rate and stroke volume is an increase in cardiac output, which in maximum exercise may be up to five to sevenfold. The pulmonary ventilation readily meets this increased need for gas exchange, as voluntary hyperventilation can exceed the need for ventilation in exercise, and diffusion of the normal lung is sufficient. Thus, the arterial O_2 saturation is not reduced even in exhausting exercise. The manner by which the stimulus in exercise achieves effective adjustments of ventilation is the subject of much physiological study.[5, 15, 16] The usual humoral regulatory agents, such as CO_2, pO_2 and pH, cannot explain the changes in moderate exercise; in severe, exhausting exercise changes in pH may be a possible explanation. There is general agreement that a neural reflex mechanism is necessary to explain the rapid onset and the rapid reduction in ventilation on cessation of exercise.

The ventilatory regulation needed to meet demand in moderate exercise is illustrated in Figure 9–5, in which the linear relationship between ventilation and O_2 consumption with a near-constant pCO_2 is close even when the exercise is

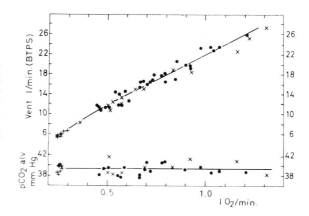

Figure 9–5 Ventilation and alveolar P_{CO_2} in relation to oxygen consumption during exercise. Dots = voluntary work; crosses = electrically induced work. (From Asmussen, E.: Exercise and the regulation of ventilation. Circulation Res., *20* (suppl. 1) *I*:133, 1967.)

performed involuntarily by electrical stimulation. At higher rates of exercise (not shown) there is a proportionally larger increase in ventilation owing to changes in pH. It is not known whether the regulation in moderate exercise occurs through proprioceptive neural pathways or via a local humoral agent which stimulates reflex neural action. An additional ventilatory stimulus during prolonged exercise is the elevation in core body temperature, which is a function of the metabolic level of the exercise.

Increased cardiac output and local circulatory redistribution cannot fully account for the increase in aerobic metabolism that occurs in strenuous exercise.[19] Maximum oxygen consumption is the best single index of exercise capacity. It varies from 2 to 5 liters per minute in relation to the work capacity of the individual, and these values represent greater increases in O_2 consumption than the changes in cardiac output. The additional adjustment is achieved by a marked decrease in the mixed venous oxygen content. The arteriovenous oxygen difference is often increased to several times the resting value; Figure 9–6 demonstrates this relationship between arteriovenous difference (A-V O_2 difference) and the oxygen consumption. This change multiplied by the five

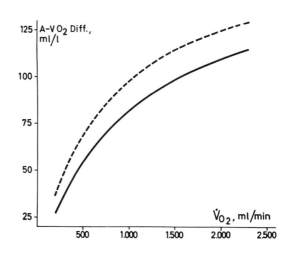

Figure 9–6 Arteriovenous O_2 difference (A-VO_2 difference) in relation to oxygen consumption (V O_2). Solid line = supine; broken line = sitting. (From Ekelund, L. G. and A. Holmgren: Central hemodynamics during exercise. Circulation Res., *20* (suppl. 1) *I*:36, 1967.)

to sevenfold increase in cardiac output gives values for the relative increase in O_2 consumption.

Exercise at an oxygen consumption of 50 per cent of maximum is regularly accompanied by a significant dependence on anaerobic metabolism in the muscles.[14] Measurements of anaerobic metabolism are expressed in terms of the equivalent O_2 which would be required if the metabolism were aerobic, while actual measurements are based on the extra O_2 consumed during recovery to remove or convert the anaerobic products. This figure, called the oxygen debt, may be in the order of 20 to 30 liters in a highly trained person. In strenuous exercise the oxygen debt can be accounted for principally by the lactic acid accumulated during the exercise. In mild exercise there is an oxygen debt which is not accompanied by accumulation of lactic acid and is termed the "alactacid" debt. There is no exact chemical explanation for the alactacid debt, but it probably represents the energy necessary to reconvert the high energy phosphate bonds, mainly creatine phosphate, in muscle. The alactacid mechanisms are likely important in the explanation of interval training, which will be discussed later.

Both aerobic capacity and the anaerobic capacity can be increased by appropriately chosen exercise. These exercises have been studied primarily in young and athletic subjects, but several recent investigations have shown that older individuals and even those who have had myocardial infarctions can significantly increase these capacities.[6, 13] Older individuals, however, start at a lower capacity level and increase less dramatically.[40, 41] Evidence that increased cardiovascular fitness in older individuals can prevent subsequent coronary disease has been suggested, but this is not yet conclusive.[26, 31]

The metabolic changes that occur during the lengthening contraction of muscles illustrate a rather special situation. In exercises such as bicycling down hill the phenomenon is called negative work[5] (Fig. 9-7). Although the muscles are called upon to produce the same tension for the same time as in bicycling up hill (positive work), the energy cost is only one-seventh of the up hill climb. The metabolic economy of such exercise is apparent. Since many muscle actions in gait and other practical activities are decelerating lengthening contractions, this type of exercise is of practical importance. At a more fundamental level, A. V. Hill[29] has produced evidence for the conversion of mechanical energy into chemical energy, a remarkable biological occurrence.

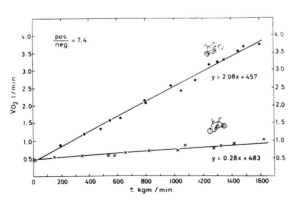

Figure 9-7 Oxygen consumption at different rates of work. Dots = bicycling uphill (positive work); crosses = bicycling downhill (negative work). (From Asmussen, E. Exercise and the regulation of ventilation. Circulation Res., 20 (suppl. 1) I:135, 1967.)

Exercises to increase metabolic capacity must be those which put stress on metabolic functions. This means that the exercise must (1) be of sufficient intensity and duration to raise cardiac output to near-maximum, (2) be sufficiently intense to utilize anaerobic mechanisms, and (3) involve large muscle groups, thereby taxing both local and general circulation. The absolute level of the exercise must be related to the present capacity of the exercising individual and must be progressively increased in intensity as the individual gains capacity from the exercise. Exercises primarily for circulatory and metabolic functions need not, and probably should not, involve great amounts of skill. Walking, running, bicycling and climbing stairs are common examples, as exercises of these types are carried on with equal efficiency by trained and untrained individuals. Changes in efficiency seem to be possible only in relation to skill. For unexplained reasons heavy metabolic exercises involving only the upper extremities involve more circulatory stress than those involving the lower extremities.

These exercises are often called "conditioning exercises." Most frequently conditioning programs include some exercises to increase strength, speed or mobility, but the other portions of the programs must involve high metabolic intensity if circulatory changes are to result. Recently, however, the new principles of "interval training" have introduced modifications of classic procedures. Here short bursts of high intensity exercise are followed by periods (usually of equal length) of rest. Åstrand et al.[7] found that the best intervals to demonstrate the benefits are only $\frac{1}{2}$ minute in duration, and other investigators have used even shorter periods.[25] Under these conditions the lactic acid anaerobic pathways are utilized very little, the alactacid debt accumulated is paid back in the rest intervals and large amounts of high intensity work can be accomplished with lactic acid levels only slightly above the resting figure. One should not assume that interval exercises permit larger amounts of work per unit time; working at half the intensity does the same amount of work per unit of time with slightly lower indices of stress. What is important in interval exercises is the high intensity level that is tolerable. These principles are being applied in the training of populations of handicapped individuals and are useful in a practical sense, although physiological explanations are not at hand. It is probably true that workmen in occupations involving heavy labor have long practiced interval exercises as an unconscious approach to high intensity tasks. Although recovery from exhausting work can be enhanced by carrying on low intensity work during early recovery, the work on interval exercises has shown that the rest interval is best spent in total rest.

So far we have emphasized the increases in aerobic capacity with exercise, but anaerobic capacity can also be increased with training. After training, the individual can tolerate higher levels of lactic acid and more marked deviations in acid-base balance. Various explanations of this have been suggested. Some mechanism must be operable to increase intracellular capacity for anaerobic metabolic turnover—either in energy sources or in enzymes. Recent simple techniques of needle biopsies performed during work have somewhat clarified matters.[1, 11, 30] The pre-exercise levels of glycogen are higher in trained individuals than in untrained; in heavy work the glycogen in the muscle is markedly reduced to near zero values at the time of complete exhaustion. Evidence

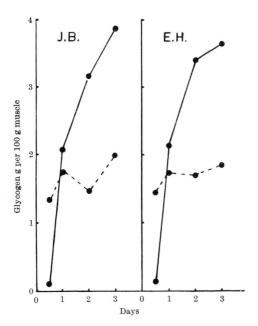

Figure 9—8 Glycogen content in biopsies of muscles from heavily exercised leg (solid line) and unexercised leg (dotted line). (From Bergstrom, J. and E. Hultman: Muscle glycogen synthesis after exercise: an enhancing factor localized to the muscle cells in man. Nature, *210*:309, 1966.)

linking these two facts together lies in the finding that the muscle, after depletion of glycogen by exercise, has the capacity to reaccumulate glycogen to much higher levels in the 2 to 3 days after depletion than it had initially (Fig. 9–8). This super-accumulation is enhanced by a high carbohydrate diet and persists at the high level for days. These findings, although we do not know the long-term effects, may explain (1) the increased anaerobic capacity after maximum training and (2) the relatively long time necessary for recovery from physical exhaustion, but they do not readily explain the gains in anaerobic capacity seen after more moderate training programs.

SKILL OR CONTROL EXERCISES

The role of the central nervous system in exercise is complicated, yet it is important that we understand it. Our original analogy with the parts of the computer is pertinent, although an oversimplification. The number of neurons in the central nervous system is many times the number of units in the central processor of the most complicated computer. The analogy is fair, however, in that each neuron can respond only in an on-off manner similar to the corresponding electrical components of the computer. In order to understand the role of the central nervous system we are forced to develop more simplified conceptual models. One of these is that of cybernetics, which emphasizes feedback and servo mechanisms whereby there is a built-in self-correction mechanism. Likewise the concepts of conditional reflexes and conditioning mechanisms are useful, in part, in that they emphasize the manner in which motor patterns can be modified by learning processes.[22, 24, 43] The work of Basmajian[10] on training for specific single motor unit activity reveals the degree of control possible, as he trained his subjects to fire single motor units upon demand and to carry across this training to later sessions.

The attributes that the central nervous system imparts to exercise can be called coordination, smoothness or direction, depending on the context of the description. The term "control" is the most general term and carries the most comprehensive description. Under usual conditions, the central nervous system is organized not in terms of individual muscle function, but rather in terms of motions or combinations of motions. The first movements of the fetus are total body motions. The newborn infant has almost all of the reflex machinery but very little of the precise control achieved by maturation and experience. Diseases and deprivation limit both normal maturation and the opportunities for experience. Commonly, the highest levels of skill are acquired only if the individual starts the skill early in life.

It is not surprising that this complicated field is an open area for proponents of "pseudo-sciences" and completely unscientific systems of exercise. In our present state of knowledge it is best to highlight those facts which are reasonably well-established and not attempt a comprehensive explanation.

1. Basic reflexes are present in the spinal cord and brain stem which
   A. affect reactions to noxious stimuli.
   B. are almost complete in the regulation of posture.
   C. facilitate reciprocal patterns of motion.
   D. may modify voluntary motor patterns.

2. Sensory information is necessary for coordinated motor activity. It involves information from the periphery of the body and through the special senses. It requires extensive organization in the brain to guide motor patterns.

3. Although the primary motor centers of the cortex are the most effective source of motor activity, there is considerable plasticity in the organization of the central nervous system which allows motor performance, although in a less precise manner, after widespread extirpation experimentally[42] or disease clinically.

4. Motor learning behaves like conditioned learning of autonomic responses in that it is acquired by repetition and reinforcement and is extinguished by nonuse and by reinforcement of other patterns.

Even these few guidelines allow us to utilize exercise as a tool in promoting skilled muscle function. For skill and control alone, exercise need not be laborious or against heavy loads. It does however require many repetitions. Exercise that is interesting and productive is more likely to be completed and successful. It can and should be monitored for error and corrected, thus the importance of the teacher and of self-criticism. In the area of skill, it is possible to increase mechanical efficiency by the smoother utilization of muscles. The underlying primitive reflex patterns play at least a minor role in facilitating motor training.

The general principles outlined are most directly applicable to persons with intact nervous systems, but they also apply to patients with central nervous system disease for training of those parts of the body not impaired by the disease. Rehabilitation is often faced with situations in which skills are lost through disuse in the course of protracted immobility and illness. Upon loss of effective use of one or more extremities the patient must be taught extra and precise skills of the remaining limbs. The ability to tie shoe laces with one hand is an example of the high degree of skill and control required. Loss of function of one or more muscles will require retraining so that other muscles may be used in a compensatory motor pattern. Retraining after muscle transplants often requires a complete reversal of the normal motor pattern for an act. Experience shows that after muscle transplants new patterns can be acquired but that they require continued reinforcement by practice. In a similar manner, artificial limbs require new patterns of skill. New electric arm prostheses, although they utilize action potentials from residual muscles, still require modification of patterns. No prosthesis to date has been made with effective reproduction of sensory input from the limb, so other sensory clues from the eyes or the stump must be utilized in the new pattern. These several examples all depend on intact nervous system or intact portions of a damaged nervous system. There is abundant evidence that older individuals acquire new skills less readily than young individuals. When possible, it is easier to retrain previously acquired skills than to develop new skills. For example, a previously trained typist or piano player can often learn most readily with these instruments.

In attempts to retrain the parts of the body directly affected by central nervous system disease or damage, the application of general principles is more difficult. A few statements can be made which are applicable.

1. Motor patterns can rarely be made as precise as when the central nervous system is intact but can serve gross function. The situation parallels that of monkeys after step-wise decortication.[42]

2. If the central motor apparatus is totally destroyed or the connections are severed, training for skill and control is not applicable.

3. The ability to effect motor patterns may be nearly intact but may be inhibited or actually mechanically impeded by the abnormal neurological manifestations of spasticity and dyskinesia or by peripheral pain. In these cases attention might well be directed toward elimination or lessening of these impeding influences.

4. Other things being equal, reinforcement of sensory clues to affect motor patterns is useful.

We have emphasized the evidence that exercise acutely adapts the body to meet the specific nature of the stress which the exercise imposes. Also, repeated attempts to overcome these particular stresses enhances the ability of the body to meet similar stresses. We have discussed the subdivisions of exercise in relationship to strength (or tension), to stamina (or metabolic capacity) and to skill (or central nervous system control).

RANGE OF MOTION EXERCISES

In a similar way the quality of joint mobility is one which varies in response to demand and can be modified by choice of exercise. In this case we are dealing less with coordination of several systems and more with local tissue modification. It is a common observation that joints become stiff if immobilized or not regularly moved. It is possible that the almost reflex pattern of stretching after sleep is an attempt to combat this natural tendency. Two proved changes occur with immobilization. First is adaptive shortening, which occurs in muscles or periarticular tissues when they are maintained in a foreshortened position. The ultimate in such changes occurs after tenotomy. In the absence of other limiting factors these changes of adaptive shortening are reversed by gradually restretching to the original length. Since pain frequently occurs in restretching, and since protective spasm of antagonist muscles may thus be produced, such exercises should be carried on actively as far as possible, taking advantage of the normal relaxation of antagonists that accompanies active contraction of the agonists. Long-continued limitations from the adaptive shortening may be accompanied by permanent fibrous replacement in the foreshortened condition. Situations in disease, where inflammatory edema and subsequent fibrosis occur, introduce a new element which modifies the normal process.

A second normal factor adding to mobility limitations is the loss of lubrication between moving planes which occurs. Even less of this mechanism is known, but one can postulate changes in the viscosity of the fluids in these moving planes, perhaps of the polymerization of the mucopolysaccharides. In the absence of disease these lubrication changes are readily reversible by re-establishing motion. On occasion, re-establishment of motion is accompanied by slight snapping noises which are spoken of as "breaking of adhesions." Even less is known with certainty about the lubrication changes in disease.

Disease and trauma introduce added factors in restricting joint motion that are peculiar to the disease process and not pertinent here. Spasticity is a process which commonly restricts motion. Since there is no peripheral pathology in this condition, the principles of the changes from joint disuse apply here if the process is not too long-standing. Permanent restrictive changes can be prevented by mobility exercises. In children the process of growth while the joint is in an abnormal position adds a more permanent influence.

CONCLUSION

The subject of exercise warrants an entire volume or even a set of volumes if it is to be covered in depth. Even excluding those parts which are pseudoscientific or parts of folklore, the physiological information is formidable. Since much of the data was acquired in young individuals and related to athletic performance, bridging the age and performance gap to apply them to the problems of loss of function in the aged and infirm is sometimes risky. Fortunately there is a growing set of data which indicates that the earlier data are qualitatively applicable, but that the variations are in degree and extent. In general, there is no way of increasing exercise performance without inducing stress. The problem is to regulate the stress so that it is not endangering and is applicable to the capabilities of the individual. The rewards to be gained would seem to justify some risk, since mobility and physical performance are such an essential part of living. No valid claim can yet be made that exercise prolongs duration of life. However, life without functional living is a sterile existence.

REFERENCES

1. Ahlborg, B. J., Bergström, J., Ekelung, L.-G., and Hultman, E.: Muscle glycogen and muscle electrolytes during prolonged physical exercise. Acta Physiol. Scand., 70:129-142, 1967.
2. Alam, M., and Smirk, F. H.: Observations in man upon a blood pressure raising reflex arising from voluntary muscles. J. Physiol. (London), 89:372-383, 1937.
3. Asmussen, E., and Nielsen, M.: Cardiac output during muscular work and its regulation. Physiol. Rev., 35:778-800, 1955.
4. Asmussen, E.: Muscular performance. In: Rodahl, K., and Horvath, S. M. (eds.): Muscle as a Tissue. New York, McGraw-Hill Book Co., Inc., pp. 161-175, 1962.
5. Asmussen, E.: Exercise and the regulation of ventilation. Circulation Res., 20 (suppl. 1):I132-I145, 1967.
6. Åstrand, I.: Aerobic work capacity in men and women with special reference to age. Acta Physiol. Scand., 49 (suppl. 169), 92 pages, 1960.
7. Åstrand, I., Åstrand, Per-Olof, Christensen, E. H., and Hedman, R.: Intermittent muscular work. Acta Physiol. Scand., 48:448-453, 1960.
8. Barnard, R. James, Edgerton, V. R., and Peter, J. B.: Effect of exercise on skeletal muscle. I. Biochemical and histochemical properties. J. Appl. Physiol., 28:762-766, 1970.
9. Barnard, R. James, Edgerton, V. R., and Peter, J. B.: Contractile properties. J. Appl. Physiol., 28:767-770, 1970.
10. Basmajian, J. D.: Control and training of individual motor units. Science, 141:440-441, 1963.
11. Bergström, J., and Hultman, E.: Muscle glycogen synthesis after exercise: an enhancing factor localized to the muscle cells in man. Nature, 210:309-310, 1966.
12. Bevegård, Sture B., and Shepherd, J. T.: Regulation of the circulation during exercise in man. Physiol. Rev., 47:178-213, 1967.
13. Christensen, E. H.: Physical working capacity of old workers and physiological background for work tests and work evaluations. Bull. Wld. Hlth. Org., 13:587-593, 1955.
14. Christensen, E. H.: Muscular work and fatigue. In: Rodahl, K., and Horvath, S. M. (eds.): Muscle as a Tissue. New York, McGraw-Hill Book Co., Inc., pp. 176-189, 1962.
15. Cunningham, D. J. C.: Regulation of breathing in exercise. Circulation Res., 20 (suppl. 1):I122-I131, 1967.
16. Dejours, P.: Neurogenic factors in the control of ventilation during exercise. Circulation Res. 20 (suppl. 1):I146-I153, 1967.
17. DeLateur, B. J., Lehmann, J. F., and Fordyce, W. E.: A test of the DeLorme axion. Arch. Phys. Med. Rehabil., 49:245-248, 1968.
18. DeLorme, T. L., and Watkins, A. L.: Progressive Resistance Exercise. Appleton, Century-Crofts, Inc., New York, 1951.
19. Dempsey, J. A., and Rankin, J.: Physiological adaptation of gas transport systems to muscular work in health and disease. Am. J. Phys. Med., 46:582-647, 1967.
20. Donald, K. W., Lind, A. R., McNicol, G. W., Humphreys, P. W., Taylor, S. H., and Staunton, H. P.: Cardiovascular responses to sustained (static) contractions. Circulation Res., 20 (suppl. 1):I15-I32, 1967.
21. Eccles, J. C.: Excitatory and inhibitory synaptic action. Harvey Lectures, series 51:1-24, 1955-1956.
22. Fischer, E.: Conditioned reflexes. Am. J. Phys. Med., 46:370-378, 1967.
23. Fischer, E.: Use and disuse of neuromuscular mechanisms. Am. J. Phys. Med., 46:563-574, 1967.
24. Fischer, E.: Factors affecting motor learning. Am. J. Phys. Med., 46:511-519, 1967.
25. Fox, E. L., Robinson, S., and Wiegman, D. L.: Metabolic energy sources during continuous and interval running. J. Appl. Physiol., 27:174-178, 1969.
26. Fox, S. M., III, and Haskell, W. L.: Physical activity and the prevention of coronary heart disease. Bull. N. Y. Acad. Med., 44:950-967, 1968.
27. Gordon, E. E., Kawalsky, K., and Fritts, M.: Changes in rat muscle fiber with forceful exercise. Arch. Phys. Med. Rehabil., 48:577-582, 1967.
28. Hellebrandt, F. A., Schade, M., and Carns, M. L.: Methods evoking the tonic neck reflexes in normal human subjects. Am. J. Phys. Med., 41:90-139, 1962.
29. Hill, A. V.: Production and absorption of work by muscle. Science, 131:897-903, 1960.
30. Hultman, E.: Physiological role of muscle glycogen in man, with special reference to exercise. Circulation Res., 20 (suppl. 1):I99-I112, 1967.
31. Katz, L. N.: Physical fitness and coronary heart disease. Circulation, 35:405-414, 1967.
32. Liberson, W. T., and Asa, M. M.: Further studies of brief isometric exercises. Arch. Phys. Med. Rehabil., 40:330-336, 1959.

33. Liberson, W. T., Dondey, M., and Asa, M. M.: Brief repeated isometric maximal exercises. Am. J. Phys. Med., *41*:3-14, 1962.
34. Morpurgo, B.: Über Aktivitaets-Hypertrophie der willkuerlichen Muskeln. Arch. Path. Anat., *150*:522-554, 1897.
35. Ouellet, Y., Poh, S. C., and Becklake, M. R.: Circulatory factors limiting maximal aerobic exercise capacity. J. Appl. Physiol., *27*:874-880, 1969.
36. Schleusing, G.: Der Einfluss des elektrischen Trainings auf den skeletal Muskel. Int. Z. Angew. Physiol., *18*:232–241, 1960.
37. Skinner, N. S., and Powell, W. J.: Regulation of skeletal muscle blood flow during exercise. Action of oxygen and potassium. Circulation Res., *20* (suppl. 1):159-167, 1967.
38. Staunton, H. P., Taylor, S. H., and Donald, K. W.: The effect of vascular occlusion on the pressor response to static muscular work. Clin. Sci., *27*:283-291, 1964.
39. Thistle, H. G., Hislop, H. J., Maffroid, M., and Lowman, E. W.: Isokinetic contraction: A new concept of resistive exercise. Arch. Phys. Med. Rehabil., *48*:279-282, 1967.
40. Tlustý L.: Physical fitness in old age. I. Aerobic capacity and the other parameters of physical fitness followed by means of graded exercise in ergometric examination of elderly individuals. Respiration, *26*:161-181, 1969.
41. Tlustý, L.: Physical fitness in old age. II. Anaerobic capacity, anaerobic work in graded exercise, recovery after maximum work, performed in elderly individuals. Respiration, *26*: 287–299, 1969.
42. Travis, A. M., and Woolsey, C. N.: Motor performance of monkeys after bilateral partial and total cerebral decortications. Am. J. Phys. Med., *35*:273-310, 1956.
43. Waterland, J. C., and Hellenbrandt, F. A.: Involuntary patterning associated with willed movement performed against progressively increasing resistance. Am. J. Phys. Med., *43*:13-30, 1964.

Chapter 10

ENERGY EXPENDITURE DURING AMBULATION

by Paul J. Corcoran, M.D.

INTRODUCTION

Since medical rehabilitation usually requires work on the part of the patient, we are concerned here with (1) how to increase the amount of work the patient can do with the residual functional parts of his body and (2) how to decrease the amount of work required by the use of adaptive devices and environmental manipulation.

In order to set realistic goals for his patients, the rehabilitation worker must know how much work normal persons do in the course of everyday activities, how much these work requirements increase for the disabled person and how much this increase can be lessened by exercise, training and assistive devices.

TERMINOLOGY

Work is equal to force times distance (Table 10–1). In walking, the *force* is primarily gravity and friction plus the inertia of acceleration and deceleration. The *distance* is the up-and-down motion of the body and its separate parts. To diminish the work required for a task such as walking, the force needed is decreased (e.g., by using lighter weight materials for prosthetics), or the distance lifted is shortened (e.g., by providing knee flexion in a prosthesis to decrease the vertical excursion of the center of gravity). If the patient has the

185

TABLE 10–1 EQUIVALENT UNITS OF SPEED, WORK AND POWER

EQUIVALENT UNITS OF SPEED

	1	mi/hr
=	88	ft/min
=	26.822	m/min
=	1.609	Km/hr
=	1.467	ft/sec
=	0.447	m/sec

EQUIVALENT UNITS OF WORK

	1	Kcal Cal (kilocalorie or "large calorie")
=	4184	watt-sec (joules)
=	3086	ft-lbs
=	1000	cal (gram calorie or "small calorie")
=	427	Kg-m
=	3.968	BTU (British thermal units)
=	0.00156	hp-hr
=	0.00116	Kw-hr

EQUIVALENT UNITS OF POWER

	1	Kcal/min (Cal/min)
=	3086	ft-lbs/min
=	1000	cal/min
=	427	Kg-m/min
=	69.733	watts (joules/sec)
=	3.968	BTU/min
=	0.0935	hp
=	0.0697	Kw

energy or capacity for doing the work required, he may succeed in walking.

Power is the rate of doing work:

$$\text{Power} = \frac{\text{Force} \times \text{Distance}}{\text{Time}} \qquad (1)$$

The power available, i.e., the rate at which a patient can expend energy for the work of walking, usually limits walking speed. Thus, the rate of energy expenditure in handicapped (and normal) persons is kept at a tolerable level by decreasing the force or distance, or both (the numerator of Equation 1), or by increasing the time spent on the task (the denominator).

The only source of energy that the human body can use is the chemical energy contained in complex food molecules.[6] The oxidation of these to simpler substances such as water and carbon dioxide is an exothermic reaction:

$$C_6H_{12}O_6 + 6\,O_2 = 6\,CO_2 + 6\,H_2O + 686\ \text{Kcal/mole}$$
$$\text{Glucose} + \text{Oxygen} = \text{Carbon dioxide} + \text{Water} + \text{Energy} \qquad (2)$$

This overall chemical reaction is in fact the sum of a multitude of individual steps in the reaction, some of which are coupled in the body to other reactions that produce chemical or physical work. The upper limit of possible efficiency is determined by the proportion of these steps that can be usefully coupled. The actual efficiency is always much less than this since a proportion of the work produced is non-useful work, and is thence converted to heat. At rest the available work energy is spent to purchase the displacements from equilibrium that are necessary for life: the maintenance of a pressure gradient in the arterial system, the intrathoracic pressure variations, which move air in and out, and the ionic gradients across cell membranes, which permit their survival and chemical functioning. The efficiency of muscle action rarely exceeds 25 per cent and averages closer to 10 per cent, so most of the energy expended during physical exertion is lost as heat; the rest is used to do external work on the environment, which is the object of the exercise.

UNITS OF MEASUREMENT

The following units of measurement are used in this chapter: Miles per hour is used as the unit for speed because it is the unit most familiar in the English speaking world. Conversion factors are given in Table 10-1 for other units. The kilocalorie (Calorie, kilogram calorie or "large calorie") is used to express work or energy. Only one kilocalorie is required to lift 3086 lbs 1 foot, or 1 lb 3086 feet, a rather formidable amount of work. Assuming 20 per cent to 10 per cent muscle efficiency, it would require 5 or 10 Kcal to do this much work, the amount in half a sugar lump.

The *rate* of work, which is power (Eq. 1), is expressed in kilocalories per minute. One Kcal per min is approximately the basal metabolic rate for an average sized adult. This unitary value is convenient in comparing values during work, which then are read directly as multiples of the basal rate. Conversion factors are given in Table 10-1 for some other units of energy that

TABLE 10–2 ENERGY COST OF LIGHT ACTIVITIES IN ADULTS

Activity	Average Energy Cost (Kcal/min/70 Kg)
Sleeping	0.9
Lying quietly	1.0
Lying quietly doing mental arithmetic	1.04
Sitting at ease	1.2 –1.6
Sitting, writing	1.9 –2.2
Sitting, playing cards	1.9 –2.1
Sitting, playing musical instrument	2.0 –3.2
Standing at ease	1.4 –2.0
Walking, 1 mph	2.3
Standing, washing and shaving	2.5 –2.6
Standing, dressing and undressing	2.3 –3.3
Light housework	1.7 –3.0
Heavy housework	3.0 –6.0
Office work	1.3 –2.5
Typing, mechanical typewriter	1.26–1.57
Typing, electric typewriter	1.13–1.39
Walking, 2 mph	3.1
Light industrial work	2.0 –5.0
Walking, 3 mph (average comfortable walking speed)	4.3

are frequently encountered in the literature on "work physiology" or "ergonomics."

In many people a work rate greater than 5 times the BMR, or 5 Kcal per min, usually results in the accumulation of an oxygen debt, with a rise in the serum lactic acid level. Five Kcal per min is about the maximum that one can maintain for several hours. It is this physiological fact that probably sets the limit on "light" industrial work or "comfortable" walking speed (Table 10-2). Brown and Brengelmann[6] have written an excellent, more general discussion of energy metabolism and units.

METHODS OF MEASUREMENT OF ENERGY EXPENDITURE

The most obvious way to study energy expenditure is to measure the actual work performed, i.e., the force produced and the distance through which it moves. Although this would be difficult for most daily activities, a number of ergometers have been devised to measure human work in such units as foot-pounds. These measure the physical work done but do not indicate the energy cost because of the unknown variable of efficiency. It is these human energy demands during adaptation to physical impairments that are the primary concern in rehabilitation.

Actual energy expenditure during ordinary activities could be determined by measuring any of the elements of Equation 2. For example, the amount of food consumed and metabolized correlates with daily work levels but cannot be measured on a minute-by-minute basis. Variations in eating habits further complicate this method.

Direct Calorimetry

If no external work is done on the environment, the energy produced (Eq. 2) is dissipated as heat and can be measured accurately in a human calorimeter. This is a large, sealed, insulated chamber within which the subject rests or works on an ergometer. The total energy he expends is measured as the calories of heat which must be removed from the chamber to maintain a constant temperature. This technique is impractical for day-to-day clinical studies because of the technical difficulties involved.

Indirect Calorimetry

The estimations of energy expenditure by measurement of the oxygen consumed in Equation 2 was introduced by Atwater at the end of the nineteenth century. An average of 4.83 Kcal of energy are released when 1 liter of oxygen is consumed to oxidize an ordinary diet. This "caloric equivalent" value varies slightly and depends on the specific food molecule in question, averaging 5.05 for carbohydrates, 4.74 Kcal for fats, 4.46 Kcal for proteins and 4.86 Kcal for ethyl alcohol. The use of the standard average value of 4.83 Kcal per liter for the caloric equivalent of oxygen causes inaccuracies no greater than a few per cent in a subject having a mixed diet.

Measurement of the oxygen consumption rate under specified resting conditions constitutes the familiar basal metabolism rate test. At rest, body surface area is the body size dimension that provides the most accurate correlation with energy expenditure. Surface area can be predicted from tables or nomograms of height and weight. However, most activities in rehabilitation involve moving all or parts of the body against gravity. During exercise, the total weight of the subject, plus clothing and equipment carried, correlates better than surface area with the energy costs of the activity. Therefore, values used in this chapter for energy costs will be expressed per unit of body weight rather than per unit of surface area.

In most systems used to measure human oxygen consumption the expired air is collected, its volume measured, the expired O_2 concentration determined and the expired volume of O_2 subtracted from the O_2 in the inspired ambient air (20.93 per cent of inspired volume, unless altered by conditions of the experiment). The volume is corrected to conditions of standard temperature (37°C), pressure (760 mm Hg) and relative humidity (zero or dry)—STPD—and expressed per unit of body weight.

The simplest method of collecting expired air is in a large floating bell spirometer if the subject is working in one place, or in a rubber-impregnated canvas "Douglas bag" or neoprene bag if the subject is moving. The bell spirometer provides a direct reading of gas volume; if a bag is used, its contents are later squeezed out through a gas meter to determine expired volume.

Kofranyi and Michaelis (1940) described a small portable respirometer that could be carried on the subject's back like a knapsack. It stored an aliquot of the total expired air in a rubber bladder. This "Max Planck respirometer" has permitted many studies of energy expenditure in actual field situations in industry, athletics and the home. With improvements in the meter and with careful calibration, variability is about ± 4 per cent; breathing resistance increases the inaccuracy at ventilation rates above 30 to 40 liters per min.[23] A similar device with lower breathing resistance and higher accuracy has been reported by Wolff.[35] The expired air is analyzed for oxygen content by chemical or physical means.

Carbon dioxide production (Eq. 2) also correlates with energy expenditure, but the relationship varies more with dietary differences. In addition, the body's bicarbonate buffer system allows significant amounts of the gas to be stored during exercise or hypoventilation, causing variations in carbon dioxide output that are unrelated to the instantaneous metabolic level. For these reasons, oxygen consumption is simpler to use as an indirect measure of energy expenditure.

Heart Rate

Although studies of oxygen consumption provide the most accurate estimation of human energy expenditure, it can be measured only a limited number of times on one subject in one day. In studies in which a large number of observations are more important than accuracy, heart rate has often been used as an index of energy expenditure.[21] For a given subject at a given time, heart rate bears a linear relationship to oxygen consumption and correlates with work measurements such as speed of walking or running, work on a bicycle ergometer and rate of stepping up and down (the basis for the Master two-step exercise test[21]). The measurement of heart rate is simple and no special equipment is necessary. It has been suggested as a routine measurement whenever elderly, debilitated or cardiac patients are given therapeutic exercise.[1] The method is also suitable in field situations in which oxygen uptake studies might be impractical. In long-term studies in a remote location, small heart rate counters can be worn by the subject.[3]

The usefulness of heart rate as an index of work level in clinical medicine is limited because the data on which the norms are based were derived from studies of high work rates in healthy young people, trained athletes or physical laborers. These results are not necessarily applicable to sedentary, elderly or physically handicapped subjects. Indeed, the heart rates of subjects during standardized work are used as an index of physical fitness. The heart rate nomogram of Astrand, which relates O_2 consumption in submaximal exercise to an extrapolated maximum O_2, underestimated actual maximum oxygen consumption by 27 per cent in a group of sedentary adults.[31] The inaccuracy increases at the lower work loads characteristic of handicapped persons. At low work levels, heart rate can vary independently of energy expenditure, under the influence of such factors as cardiac disease, drugs, fatigue, emotion, time since last meal, total circulating hemoglobin, hydration, ambient temperature, posture, body build and per cent body fat.[31]

Heart rate, as well as blood pressure, rises more when a given rate of work is being done by the upper extremities (e.g., crutch walking) than by the lower extremities (e.g., normal walking). This is probably due to the fact that when a muscle contracts with a given percentage of its maximum force, the effect on blood pressure is approximately the same as during the same percentage contraction of any other muscle.[19] Thus the smaller arm muscles contract more markedly and have a greater stimulating effect on the cardiovascular system than do the larger leg muscles doing the same work. This should be borne in mind when patients having cardiovascular disease are being considered for training with hand-held ambulation aids, wheelchairs[16] or any forceful arm and hand exercises. Sustained isometric exercises also produce more cardiovascular effects than isotonic exercises and may be dangerous in certain conditions in which cardiovascular stress must be minimized.

Pulmonary Ventilation

Pulmonary ventilation rate correlates fairly closely with energy expenditure at medium work rates, if a predetermined regression line for each subject is used.[13] A simple flow meter mounted on a face mask has been described for long-term recording of pulmonary ventilation to estimate caloric expenditure.[5] However, as with heart rate, ventilation rate is mainly useful when the need for simplicity outweighs the need for accuracy.

Control of Speed

Energy expenditure varies directly with the rate or speed of performance of an activity. Therefore, data on energy costs mean little without a known, constant rate of work. A metronome may be used to control the speed of a repetitive activity such as stair climbing, weight lifting, or shoveling. For work on an ergometer, speedometers or resistance gauges indicate the work rate. In walking, the rate may be controlled by a motor driven treadmill.[12] However, many patients in rehabilitation cannot use the treadmill because of locomotor handicaps. Most studies of the energy cost of handicapped ambulation have been done on smooth level floors, and the average speed determined by dividing distance walked by elapsed time. Fatigue toward the end of such a test is likely to decrease the speed of the subjects. Since the relation between energy cost and walking speed is not linear, energy cost determined under conditions of varying speed does not truly correspond to the average speed. In studies in which two different modes of ambulation are compared, any improvement in walking skill, as with a better prosthesis, may allow the subject to increase his walking speed, but the energy expenditure at the higher speed may be the same or even higher when utilizing the improvement. To avoid this and to control the variable of speed, a velocity-controlled cart has been developed which accurately controls walking speed at preset rates over any type of terrain while measuring oxygen consumption.[8] This system has been used to evaluate the energy advantage of brace modifications in hemiplegia, to compare paraplegic crutch-walking with wheelchair ambulation at the same speed, and to study prosthetic modifications, crutch and wheelchair ambulation in amputees.[9, 10, 34]

ENERGY EXPENDITURE BY NORMAL PERSONS

Rest

The basal or resting metabolism per unit of body size is low at birth, reaches its peak around age two, declines by 30 per cent during the growing years and by another 10 per cent during adulthood. At every age females tend to have about a 10 per cent lower metabolic rate, whether at rest or during work. This probably results from the female's higher proportion of body fat, which has a lower metabolic rate than most other tissues. The metabolic rate increases about 10 per cent for every degree centigrade rise in body temperature above normal. Cooling of the body initiates shivering and thereby an increased metabolic rate as the body attempts to restore or maintain normal temperature. Extreme shivering can increase the metabolic rate to as much as 6 Kcal per min for short periods.

During sleep the metabolic rate is 5 to 10 per cent lower than basal, while energy expenditure during sitting or standing is somewhat higher (Table 10–2).

The metabolic rate increases after eating owing to the "specific dynamic action" (SDA) of foods. Proteins have an SDA of about 30 per cent of their caloric value; for fats and carbohydrates the effect is transient and only about 5 per cent of their caloric values. The SDA is unrelated to digestion or absorption of the foods and is probably associated with their intermediary metabolism.[6] To avoid variations caused by SDA, metabolic studies are customarily performed on fasting subjects.

Ambulation

In the past half-century, studies of the energy cost of walking have produced surprisingly similar data. McDonald[22] has tabulated and analyzed data on the energy cost of walking in 8600 subjects from the world literature between 1912 and 1958. Heavy persons use more energy at a given walking speed, but when corrected for the weight of the subjects plus clothing and any equipment carried, the metabolic cost of walking is similar to lighter, normal subjects. Age and height have no effect, but female subjects usually show about 10 per cent lower energy expenditures at a given speed.

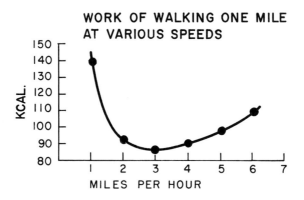

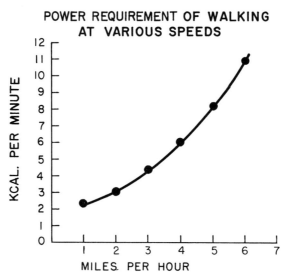

Figure 10−1 The work of walking (upper curve) decreases to a minimum around 3 mi/hr, the average walking speed of normal subjects. However, the power, or work *per unit of time* (lower curve), increases steadily as walking speed increases. Values given are for a 70-kg man.

The energy demands of walking increase as walking speed increases. This relationship is curvilinear; at faster walking speeds a further increment in speed will necessitate a greater increase in oxygen consumption than at lower speed.[8, 28]

$$E = W(.03 + .0035V^2) \tag{3}$$

where E = energy cost in Kcal per min, W = body weight in Kg and V = walking speed in mi per hr. For each sex McDonald[22] has published other equations which are more cumbersome, but provide greater accuracy at speeds above normal walking speed.

The amount of work done in walking a given distance is greater at very slow speeds than at ordinary walking speeds. The curves in Figure 10-1 are derived from Equation 3 and show that the caloric cost of walking a given distance is lowest at a walking speed of around 3 mi per hr. Several studies show that people spontaneously select this walking speed, presumably because it is

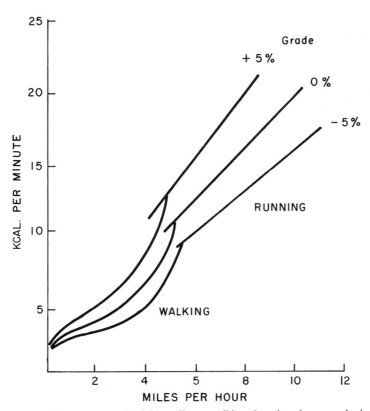

POWER REQUIRED FOR WALKING AND RUNNING

Figure 10–2 The power required for ordinary walking rises sharply at speeds above 5 mi/hr, and running becomes less demanding than walking. Note that the relationship is nearly linear for running. The limit to running speed is set by the maximum rate of energy conversion which the subject can attain. (After Margaria, et al.: Energy cost of running. J. Appl. Physiol., *18*:367, 1963.)

the most economical in caloric cost and does not exceed the 5 Kcal per min limit for sustained work without accumulating an oxygen debt.

Persons with abnormal ambulation also tend to select the walking speeds at which the work of walking the desired distance is minimal.[4] This optimal speed may not be possible if the energy cost exceeds 5 Kcal per min, or if the cardiovascular or respiratory capacity is diminished.[9]

The upper limit of normal walking speed is 5 to 6 mi per hr; beyond this speed one breaks into a run. The energy cost of running is lower than that of walking at speeds above 5 mi per hr. At speeds under 5 mi per hr walking requires less energy than running. The curve of the energy cost of running at various speeds, if superimposed on the non-linear curve for walking in Figure 10–1, intersects the walking curve near the speed of 5 mi per hr[20] (Fig. 10–2). Running on a speed-controlled treadmill provides a way to administer precise doses of work to patients on a cardiovascular reconditioning program.

The energy cost of walking on a 10 to 12 per cent grade is approximately double the energy cost of walking on the level; on a 20 to 25 per cent upgrade the rate is tripled. On downgrades the energy cost is lowest at a 10 per cent grade and rises again on steeper downgrades. Comparable data for handicapped persons are unavailable except for wheelchair use.[16]

Adding weight to the subject—either extra body weight or clothing and equipment—causes a linear increase in the energy cost of walking. Added loads are carried most efficiently on the head, somewhat less efficiently on the back, still less in the hands, and least efficiently on the feet. The addition of 2-1/2 lbs to shoe weight can increase the energy cost of walking by 5 to 10 per cent. This may be due to the greater gravitational force exerted during the up-and-down excursions of the feet during the gait cycle, as well as to the greater mass that must be accelerated and decelerated at the end of the limb. The implications for prosthetic and orthotic design are obvious.

Soft or uneven ground can increase the energy demands by 40 per cent or more; the wearing of high heels (3 inches) can cause a 10 to 15 per cent increase. A tight skirt will cause greater work. Handicapped persons usually learn to avoid these unnecessary sources of additional work. Climbing stairs requires from 6 to 12 Kcal per min, depending on body weight and speed. Descending stairs requires only one-third as much energy.

Differences Between Upper and Lower Extremity Work

Physically handicapped persons are frequently trained to adapt to lower limb impairments by using upper limb muscles with aids such as canes and crutches. Assuming equal efficiency, a given amount of mechanical work requires the same oxygen uptake whether performed by the upper or the lower extremities. Nevertheless, upper extremity work is more stressful in several respects. The smaller muscles of the arm must exert a larger percentage of their maximum contractile force, resulting in anaerobic metabolism at lower work loads and a greater blood pressure response.[19] Hard work with the upper limbs may also require forced breathing against a closed glottis and other interruptions of normal breathing patterns.

In a comparison of work performed on a hand-cranked ergometer with that done on a bicycle ergometer, the work and recovery pulse was significantly higher on the hand-cranked ergometer, although the work loads and mechanical efficiencies were the same for both.[2] Similar increases in heart rate were found in crutch-walking versus prosthetic ambulation (39 per cent),[11] and in wheelchair propulsion versus normal ambulation (33 per cent),[16] although the energy expenditures were about the same.

All these factors are compounded when the upper extremities are weakened by disuse or disease, which underscores the importance of maintaining and increasing upper extremity strength during the acute stages of such lower extremities diseases as amputations or fractures.

ENERGY EXPENDITURE IN HANDICAPPED AMBULATION

Immobilization of Body Segments

Immobilization and deformity of the joints of the trunk and lower extremities interferes with the harmonious movements of gait.[32] The effects of these deformities are summarized in Table 10–3. The extra energy cost is reduced only slightly by use of lifts to equalize leg length. The angle of a joint fixation is important, and the optimum angles should be sought whenever hip or knee immobilization is unavoidable.[30]

Lower Extremity Amputation

Below-knee amputees have about the same increase in the energy cost of walking as persons with ankle immobilization (about 10 per cent). Little data is available for bilateral below-knee prosthetic users.

The energy cost of walking with above-knee prostheses is 10 to 15 per cent above normal in younger patients, and 25 to 100 per cent above normal in older amputees. The energy cost is increased by heavier prostheses, by a more distal placement of the center of gravity and by decreases in alignment stability ("trigger setting" of the knee joint, requiring greater muscular effort to prevent knee flexion in the stance phase of gait).[26] The energy cost of walking with the

TABLE 10–3 INCREASED ENERGY COSTS CAUSED BY
IMMOBILIZATION AND DEFORMITY

IMMOBILIZATION OR DEFORMITY	APPROXIMATE % INCREASE IN ENERGY COST
Arms taped to sides	N.S.
Body cast	10
Hip spica cast—180°	20
—150°	0–10
—120°	30
Hip arthrodesis (140–160°)	
slow walking speed	0–10
fast walking speed	25
Knee immobilized in cast	
180°, 165°, or 150°	5–10
135°	25–35
One ankle immobilized in cast	6
Both ankles immobilized in cast	9

prosthetic knee locked is about the same as with a free knee in a group of older above-knee amputees at slower speeds.[34]

The alternatives to prosthetic ambulation are crutch-walking and wheel-chair use. Crutch-walking requires nearly as much energy as prosthetic use, while wheelchair ambulation by amputees requires no more energy than normal walking at the same speeds.[11, 34] The above-knee amputees who succeed in walking usually select lower speeds (average 1.86 mi per hr), but their energy expenditure (3.5 to 4.0 Kcal per min) is about the same as for normal walking at the usual 2.5 to 3.0 mi per hr.[29]

A hydraulic knee unit requires the same energy as a constant friction knee joint at comfortable walking speeds (2.1 mi per hr), but about 10 per cent less energy at 2.7 mi per hr, and permits a higher maximum walking speed (3.3 mi per hr) than is possible with the constant friction knee (2.7 mi per hr).[27] The speed of an above-knee amputee is limited by the resonance frequency of the prosthesis. Patients automatically select the step length at which the energy cost is minimal.[24]

Paraplegia

The energy cost of paraplegic ambulation using crutches is two to four times greater than that of a normal person walking at the same speed and increases rapidly with small increases in speed.[7, 10, 15] Top speed for most paraplegics is 1 to 2 mi per hr. At a given speed, energy cost of ambulation is greater for paraplegics with higher neurologic levels. The minimum energy requirement is reached after four to six weeks of training, and again rises significantly after a few months' lack of practice.[7] By contrast, wheelchair ambulation requires no more energy than normal walking and allows the paraplegic to maintain the normal speed of other pedestrians.[10, 16]

Modification of braces can influence the energy cost of walking. The use of a rigid ankle brace with a firm sole plate lowers energy costs appreciably when compared with a brace allowing free dorsiflexion. The rigid brace lifts the center of gravity passively at the end of the stance phase, so that 1 to 1-1/2 inches less lifting is required by the arms during the swing phase.[18] In another study one patient was found to expend 20 per cent more energy when the spinal extension of his pelvic band was removed.[15] In our laboratory, preliminary studies of removal of the pelvic band showed little effect on energy expenditure. Paraplegics seem to select the gait pattern (4-point or swing-through) that for them requires the least energy expenditure.[10]

Hemiplegia

In one series, the energy cost of hemiplegic ambulation averaged 64 per cent greater than normal for a given speed, but this could be reduced to 51 per cent above normal by use of a short leg brace.[9] The net effect of hemiplegia is to decrease the walking speed to a point at which the energy demands are tolerable. At comfortable walking speeds, which varied from 1 to 2 mi per hr (average 1.8 mi per hr), the hemiplegics expended almost the same amount of energy as normal subjects at 3 mi per hr. On stairs, hemiplegic subjects use 18 to 35 per cent more energy *per step* than normals, but expend approximately the same energy *per minute* because they select slower rates of climbing.[17]

Wheelchair Ambulation

The finding that wheelchair use on a smooth, level surface requires the same or slightly less energy than normal walking explains why "wheelchair independence" is a desirable reality for many persons who are too handicapped to walk.

Slight inclines cause marked increases in the energy requirements. Placement of the large wheel in the rear results in greater steering accuracy, higher efficiency, lower energy expenditure and a smaller rise in heart rate. The average heart rate rises from 90 to 130 beats/min as speed increases to 2.5 mi per hr; this rise is even greater in those patients with involvement of upper extremity or shoulder girdle muscles.[16] Thus upper extremity strengthening is an important part of wheelchair training.

DISCUSSION

A large body of data is available on the energy costs of many everyday activities, occupations and sports in normal persons.[14, 25, 33] Use of this information allows the prescription of known amounts of work, either to increase physical fitness in the healthy or to restore it to normal after illness.

Much less information can be found to guide the rehabilitation practitioner in the management of physical disabilities. When the patient also suffers from cardiovascular or pulmonary disease, the need for objective energy cost data is even more acutely felt. Should this amputee be given a locked knee or a free knee? Would crutches or a walker be better for that hip fracture patient? How wise is it to embark on bracing and crutch-walking for this middle-aged paraparetic?

It is hoped that the guidelines given in this chapter will encourage the acquisition of more of this needed information.

REFERENCES

1. Anderson, A. D.: The use of the heart rate as a monitoring device in an ambulation program: a progress report. Arch. Phys. Med. Rehabil., *45*:140–146, 1964.
2. Asmussen, E. and Hemmingsen, I.: Determination of maximum working capacity at different ages in work with the legs or with the arms. Scand. J. Clin. Lab. Invest., *10*:67–71, 1958.
3. Baker, J. A., Humphrey, S. J. E. and Wolff, H. S.: Socially acceptable monitoring instruments (SAMI) (abstract). J. Physiol., *188*:4P–5P, 1967.
4. Bard, G. and Ralston, H. J.: Measurement of energy expenditure during ambulation, with special reference to evaluation of assistive devices. Arch. Phys. Med. Rehabil., *40*:415–420, 1959.
5. Bloom, W. L.: A mechanical device for measuring human energy expenditure. Metabolism, *14*:955–958, 1965.
6. Brown, A. C. and Brengelmann, G.: Energy metabolism. *In:* Ruch, T. C. and Patton, H. D. (eds.): *Physiology and Biophysics*, 19th ed. Philadelphia, W. B. Saunders Company, 1965, pp. 1030–1049.
7. Clinkingbeard, J. R., Gersten, J. W. and Hoehn, D.: Energy cost of ambulation in the traumatic paraplegic. Am. J. Phys. Med., *43*:157–165, 1964.
8. Corcoran, P. J. and Brengelmann, G. L.: Oxygen uptake in normal and handicapped subjects, in relation to speed of walking beside velocity-controlled cart. Arch. Phys. Med. Rehabil., *51*:78–87, 1970.
9. Corcoran, P. J., Jebsen, R. H., Brengelmann, G. L. and Simons, B. C.: Effects of plastic and

metal leg braces on speed and energy cost of hemiparetic ambulation. Arch. Phys. Med. Rehabil., *51*:69-77, 1970.

10. Dubo, H. and Corcoran, P. J.: Paraplegic crutch-walking versus wheelchair propulsion: A comparison utilizing oxygen consumption, speed control and other physiological parameters. In preparation.

11. Erdman, W. J., II, Hettinger, T. and Saez, F.: Comparative work stress for above-knee amputees using artificial legs or crutches. Am. J. Phys. Med., *39*:225-232, 1960.

12. Erickson, L., Simonson, E., Taylor, H. L., Alexander, H. and Keys, A.: The energy cost of horizontal and grade walking on the motor-driven treadmill. Am. J. Physiol., *145*:391-401, 1946.

13. Ford, A. B. and Hellerstein, H. K.: Estimation of energy expenditure from pulmonary ventilation. J. Appl. Physiol., *14*:891-893, 1959.

14. Gordon, E. E.: Energy costs of activities in health and disease. Arch. Intern. Med., *101*:702-713, 1958.

15. Gordon, E. E. and Vanderwalde, H.: Energy requirements in paraplegic ambulation. Arch. Phys. Med. Rehabil., *37*:276-285, 1956.

16. Hildebrandt, G., Voigt, E.-D., Bahn, D., Berendes, B. and Kröger, J.: Energy costs of propelling wheelchair at various speeds: cardiac response and effect on steering accuracy. Arch. Phys. Med. Rehabil., *51*:131-136, 1970.

17. Hirschberg, G. G. and Ralston, H. J.: Energy cost of stair-climbing in normal and hemiplegic subjects. Am. J. Phys. Med., *44*:165-168, 1965.

18. Lehmann, J. F., DeLateur, B. J., Warren, C. G., Simons, B. C. and Guy, A. W.: Biomechanical evaluation of braces for paraplegics. Arch. Phys. Med. Rehabil., *50*:179-188, 1969.

19. Lind, A. R.: Cardiovascular responses to static exercise (Isometrics anyone?) (editorial). Circulation, *41*:173-176, 1970.

20. Margaria, R., Cerretelli, P., Aghemo, P. and Sassi, G.: Energy cost of running. J. Appl. Physiol., *18*:367-370, 1963.

21. Master, A. M. and Oppenheimer, E. T.: A simple exercise tolerance test for circulatory efficiency with standard tables for normal individuals. Am. J. Med. Sci., *177*:223-243, 1929.

22. McDonald, I.: Statistical studies of recorded energy expenditure of man. II. Expenditure on walking related to weight, sex, age, height, speed and gradient. Nutr. Abstr. Rev., *31*:739-762, 1961.

23. Montoye, H. J., van Huss, W. D., Reineke, E. P. and Cockrell, J.: An investigation of the Müller-Franz calorimeter. Intern. Z. Angew. Physiol., *17*:28-33, 1958.

24. Müller, E. A. and Hettinger, T.: Effect of the speed of gait on the energy transformation in walking with artificial legs. Germ. Zschr. Orthop., *83*:620-627, 1953.

25. Passmore, R. and Durnin, J. V. G. A.: Human energy expenditure. Physiol. Rev., *35*:801-840, 1955.

26. Peizer, E.: On the energy requirements for prosthesis use by geriatric amputees. In: Conference on the Geriatric Amputee, Washington, 1961 (a report). Washington, National Academy of Sciences – National Research Council, 1961, (Publication 919), pp. 146-150.

27. Radcliffe, C. W. and Ralston, H. J.: Performance characteristics of fluid controlled prosthetic knee mechanisms. San Francisco, 1963. (University of California, Biomechanics Laboratory, Report no. 49).

28. Ralston, H. J.: Energy-speed relation and optimal speed during level walking. Intern. Z. Angew. Physiol., *17*:277-283, 1958.

29. Ralston, H. J.: Some observations on energy expenditure and work tolerance of the geriatric subjects during locomotion. In: Conference on the Geriatric Amputee, Washington, 1961 (a report). Washington, National Academy of Sciences – National Research Council, 1961, (Publication 919), pp. 151-153.

30. Ralston, H. J.: Effects of immobilization of various body segments on the energy cost of human locomotion. Proceedings of the Second International Ergonomics Association Congress, Dortmund, 1964. Suppl. to Ergonomics, 1965, pp. 53-60.

31. Rowell, L. B., Taylor, H. L. and Wang, Y.: Limitations to prediction of maximal oxygen intake. J. Appl. Physiol., *19*:919-927, 1964.

32. Saunders, J. B. de C. M., Inman, V. T. and Eberhart, H. D.: The major determinants in normal and pathological gait. J. Bone Joint Surg., *35-A*:543-558, 1953.

33. Seliger, V.: Energy metabolism in selected physical exercises. Intern. Z. Angew. Physiol., *25*:104-120, 1968.

34. Traugh, G. H., Corcoran, P. J., and Reyes, R. L.: Energy expenditure of above-knee amputees. In preparation.

35. Wolff, H. S.: The integrating motor pneumotachograph: A new instrument for the measurement of energy expenditure by indirect calorimetry. Quart. J. Exp. Physiol., *43*:270-283, 1958.

Chapter 11

FATIGUE

by Robert C. Darling, M.D.

The study and understanding of fatigue has been hindered by the lack of a precise definition of the word. The word, of course, antedates the development of the science of physiology. As physiology developed, especially in the study of isolated tissue preparations, fatigue came to mean a diminished response of a tissue to an unchanging stimulus, or the requirement of a larger stimulus to reproduce the response. These fatigue changes were in many cases explainable by metabolic events such as a reduction in available oxygen or in fuel stores. At the same time the word was commonly used to describe, as a subjective symptom, an unpleasant sensation. With further studies of the function of the intact animal and as the science of psychology emerged, the earlier physiological definition relating stimulus to response became less clear.

The situation was not unlike the study of pain, in which it was recognized that pain could not be described from the noxious stimulus alone because the response was complicated by the environment and by the status of the central nervous system. Scientists now recognize that pain must be considered from both the psychological and physiological points of view.

The study of fatigue has seen a less effective merging of disciplines. The psychologists tend to use other terms to describe the physiologists' data and to hold firmly to their concept of fatigue as a "sensory-cognitive" phenomenon.[1, 2] Most commonly they call the physiological decrements "impairments," which they recognize may underlie and predispose to the symptom of fatigue, but are distinctly separable from fatigue itself.

For the purposes of this discussion it seems fruitless to carry the semantic dispute further. Dill[6] presents the physiologists' definition in its broadest terms: " . . . the various unmistakably different disagreeable sensations commonly referred to by the word fatigue are in fact the accompaniments of a great variety of different physiological conditions which have in common only this, that the physiological equilibrium of the body is somewhere breaking down." This will be the basis for the discussion to follow.

First it is necessary to dismiss with brief discussion certain different and inexact, and sometimes erroneous, uses of the word. Most of these arise from clinically inexact descriptions of symptoms. Frank pain is sometimes described as fatigue, as is shortness of breath, abdominal discomfort and anxiety. Experienced clinicians recognize the need to obtain more precise descriptions of symptoms. We can only decry the use of the word fatigue to lump together all forms of distress.

There is one form of sensory phenomenon described by a few neurologists which is fairly precise and which does not meet our criteria of fatigue—a decreasing response to a stimulus. The fatigue that they describe is a sensation akin to pain which occurs after excessive muscular use. In fact, from studies on a few cases of impairment of pain sensation (in syringomyelia) they describe an absence of fatigue sensation. In order to adhere to our original definition of fatigue, it would seem preferable to say that these symptoms are associated with fatigue, rather than to designate them as fatigue itself.

LOCAL MUSCULAR FATIGUE

The phenomena that follow prolonged use of local muscle groups are called local muscular fatigue, as distinguished from more general fatigue in which general circulatory adaptations are the main area of stress. Local fatigue can be demonstrated and measured after prolonged static contracture of muscles or after rhythmic exercises which produce external work.

Fatigue in such conditions can be due to malfunction anywhere along the path by which a voluntary effort is communicated to the muscle or in the muscle itself. Although in isolated preparations it is possible to show fatigue in the transmission of nerve impulses along axons in the spinal cord or in peripheral nerves, these tissues have a much higher threshold to fatigue than the other links in the chain—the synapses in the cord and brain, the special synapse at the myoneural junction and the muscle itself. Therefore nerve transmission fatigue can be dismissed as not pertinent to whole-body physiology.

The common experimental approach used to fix the location of fatigue is to voluntarily exercise a muscle until it is fatigued and then to compare its response to a maximal electrical stimulus (via the nerve or at the motor point) with its response to further voluntary effort. A normal or near normal response to the electrical stimulus indicates that the failure is proximal to the stimulating point, whereas equal decrements caused by the two methods of stimulation would indicate a peripheral site for the cause of fatigue. Such experiments have produced variable results.[3, 4] In general one can derive from these variable results the conclusion that after static contraction or contraction under ischemic conditions, the failure to contract lies in the muscle itself. Fatigue after rhythmic contractions is either mainly in the nervous system proximal to the motor nerve or in both the muscle and the upper nervous system. In no case is there convincing evidence of block at the myoneural junction under normal conditions. Of course in the disease myasthenia gravis or after use of curariform drugs, the limiting factor is clearly myoneural transmission.

In those instances in which the failure in fatigue is found in the muscle itself (static and ischemic contraction), the mechanism of the failure to contract is not fully explained.[14, 16, 17, 18, 22] There is a partial depletion of intracellular potassium, but this alone is probably insufficient to account for the failure to contract.[23] Under conditions of exhaustion of large muscle groups, fatigue is definitely correlated with the depletion of the stores of glycogen, but this has not been measured in the fatigue of small muscles. Furthermore the recovery of local muscle fatigue is much more rapid than the restoration of glycogen, which takes hours to days.

It may be significant that those conditions causing failure of muscle contraction are similar to those causing maximal blood pressure rise in exercise (i.e., ischemia and static exercise). The mechanism for the blood pressure changes is presumed to be a humoral factor setting up a reflex that produces vasomotor effects.

After rhythmic exercises to exhaustion, electrical stimulation can still cause a forceful contraction,[20, 24] which suggests that the mechansim of the fatigue is central. Further localizing evidence, placing the neuromotor failure in synaptic transmission, is largely indirect. Eccles[7] has described the dynamic balance between inhibitory and excitatory influences at the synapses of the anterior horn cell. Work on training for strength has shown gains in strength without muscle hypertrophy, which implies the involvement of more motor units and a decrease in pretraining inhibition.[11] Another point of evidence comes from observations on the fatigue in reflexes, which show that ease of fatigue is proportional to the number of synapses that are involved in the reflex. However,

Figure 11–1 Maximum strength, measured by voluntary effort and by electrical stimulation, in the course of local muscle fatigue. (From Ikai, M., K. Yabe and K. Ischii: Muskelkraft und muskuläre Ermüdung bei willkürlicher Anspannung und elektrischer Reizung des Muskels. Sportarzt und Sportmedizin, 5:201, 1967.)

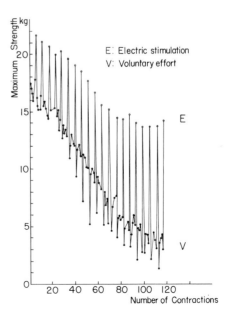

E: Electric stimulation
V: Voluntary effort

one study (Ikai, et al.[12]) demonstrated a diminution in response to electrical stimulation of lesser magnitude than the drop in voluntary contraction (Fig. 11-1). This suggests that under some conditions there may be blocks in both peripheral and the neuromotor apparatus.

Electromyographic data adds little clarity to the picture, but may be important in itself. One regular finding is an increase in the integrated electrical potential produced in the face of a decrease in muscular tension.[13, 15, 21] This is produced most clearly in static contractions and emphasizes peripheral failure. At the same time the motor unit potentials tend to lose some of their asynchronous timing and develop a synchrony which may be seen as visible tremor. This suggests a change in the more central mechanisms such as might occur with synaptic fatigue.

GENERAL MUSCULAR FATIGUE

Fatigue in general exercises such as running, climbing, rowing or bicycling is due to failure of the circulatory and metabolic adaptations rather than to a local failure.[5] If the oxygen consumption of such exercise is more than 50 per cent of maximum, anaerobic mechanisms become significant in carrying on the exercise. If these conditions are made even more stringent, the limits of anaerobic metabolism may be approached. These limits are characterized by lactic acid blood levels of greater than 100 mg/100 ml and oxygen debt figures of above 10 liters of oxygen. These upper limits of anaerobic metabolism are increased in individuals who have been trained for cardiovascular fitness but after training still do not exceed double the preceding figures. It is significant that the highest lactic acid figures produce an uncompensated acidosis with a serum pH of 7.0 or slightly lower. Such low values are comparable to the lowest figures reported in diabetic and renal acidosis. We might consider the limitations under these conditions as "acidotic fatigue."

As the anaerobic metabolic capacity is being taxed, and often before the acid changes are extreme, the circulatory system is put under stress to supply oxygen for the greatly increased aerobic metabolism of the muscles. The circulatory adaptations to exercise are discussed more fully in Chapter 9. In summary, they are an increase in cardiac output (an increase in both pulse rate and in stroke volume) and a shunting of circulating blood into the working muscles. In addition, a drop in the mixed venous oxygen content adds to the efficiency of oxygen transport. As these adaptive mechanisms approach their upper limits, fatigue becomes evident; this we might call "circulatory fatigue."

Age and cardiovascular fitness are important factors in circulatory fatigue. Maximum pulse rate is closely related to age, being 190 to 200 in young adults and decreasing approximately 10 beats per decade in older adults. Cardiovascular fitness can be defined as a condition of efficient cardiovascular adjustments leading to a high level of maximum oxygen consumption. The fit individual, who has a high ceiling for oxygen consumption, performs moderate work with less fatigue and less disturbance of equilibrium than an unfit individual. Furthermore, the fit individual having a high capacity restores his equilibrium more rapidly toward the resting state after cessation of exercise. Figure 11-2

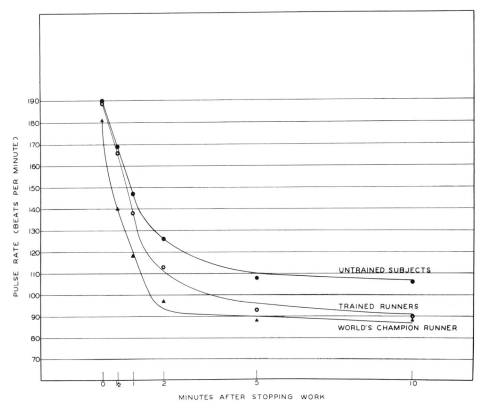

Figure 11–2 Pulse rate during recovery after exhausting exercise in relation to degree of cardiovascular fitness. (From Johnson, R. E., Brouha, L., and Darling, R. C.: A test of physical fitness for strenuous exertion. Rev. Canad. de Biol., *1*:491 (June) 1942.)

illustrates this difference in recovery rate with respect to pulse rate. Such measurements in recovery are, in part, the basis for many of the tests for cardiovascular fitness.

The fuel of moderate or moderately severe exercise may be up to 70 per cent fat, but in severe and exhausting exercise the fuel must be carbohydrate, and the available carbohydrate is the glycogen in the muscle. Muscle biopsies under such conditions have demonstrated the almost total disappearance of glycogen.[10] This is restored slowly, but a greater capacity is achieved for subsequent loading from the diet. Fatigue with depletion of glycogen may be considered as "metabolic" or "fuel" fatigue.

In prolonged exercise at low intensity the limiting factors may be somewhat different, although the lack of carbohydrate still seems to be a determining factor. In this type of exercise the liver stores of carbohydrate, as well as the blood sugar, may be reduced. Intake of food is important in very prolonged exercise, although it has been demonstrated repeatedly that glycogen in the muscle cannot be replenished or its depletion prevented by carbohydrate intake during exercise.

GENERAL FATIGUE

All sorts of activities, if continued, lead eventually to a decrement in performance, and this fatigue usually does not involve a failure of muscle contraction or an exhaustion of circulation or metabolic supply. Many subtle factors such as interest, reward and motivation determine the time of onset of this fatigue. A physiological explanation must lie in the function of the central nervous system. Our knowledge of the reticular formation of the midbrain and medulla suggests that this is the most likely site,[9] and the concept is expressed pictorially in Figure 11-3. Most knowledge of this area relates to consciousness and unconsciousness, to arousal and depression, and to sleep and wakefulness. It can be argued that general fatigue is the opposite of arousal. The known multiple connections of this part of the brain to higher and lower centers could explain the many modifying effects on general fatigue. The fact that sleep can overcome general fatigue points to a common area of action. Early work suggested the presence of an extractable factor produced in the midbrain by sleeplessness, and this has been confirmed by recent and rigorous work of Pappenheimer et al.[19] Results of current study to determine its chemical nature will be most important.

Decrements in performance associated with lack of sleep are a form of fatigue in themselves and have a specific character. There is a delay in their maximum effect; thus lowered performance in various tasks is most clearly evident the second day after a sleepless night even though a good night's sleep has intervened.

This brief observation on daily sleep rhythms raises the question of how various rhythms affect human performance and emphasizes the need for various restorative processes to occur in the body before further effective activity can be undertaken.[25] The shorter-term restoration of acid-base bal-

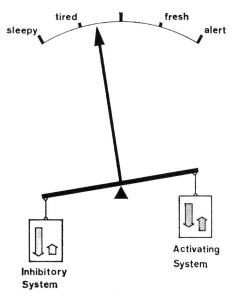

Figure 11–3 Scheme for the neurophysiological concept of general fatigue. The activating and inhibitory systems refer to the reticular formation and its connection. (From Grandjean, E.: Fatigue: Its physiological and psychological significance. Ergonomics, *11*:429, 1968.)

ance, of circulatory adjustment and of carbohydrate stores has already been mentioned. Several observations and experiments in industrial situations have shown that a work week longer than 5 or 6 days leads to a drop in production. Even longer cycles may exist.

SPECIAL FORMS OF FATIGUE

Effort Syndrome

This term is the latest in a series of descriptive names (soldier's heart, neurocirculatory asthenia) used to describe a condition in certain individuals whose capacity for general muscular work is limited by distressing circulatory manifestations: excessive pulse elevation, breathlessness and near-collapse. There is some evidence that these individuals have a constitutional inadequacy in their cardiovascular system and vasomotor capacity to adapt, but most authorities believe that the syndrome is produced by deep-seated psychological factors. Very little success has been reported in treating these people either psychologically or by progressive exercise training. Individuals with effort syndrome are similar to other individuals who have a marked loss of cardiovascular conditioning from prolonged inactivity and so represent the lower end of the spectrum of cardiovascular fitness.

Tropical Fatigue

The physical performance of many individuals deteriorates after prolonged residence in the deep tropics. The difficulties imposed by a hot climate on the performance of physical work are important sources of stress, but the progressive character of this disorder is also due to social and psychological factors, which are often complicated by medical disease.[8] These difficulties can be reduced by acclimatization, i.e., by graded work in the heat prior to prolonged exposure.

During general muscular work in the heat, the body's adaptations must not only support the working muscles but also provide for the more difficult elimination of the heat caused by the increased metabolism. Although the blood volume increases during acclimatization to heat and there is more effective cooling by sweating after acclimatization, the extra circulatory stress and decreased work capacity are evident. In a cooler climate the blood vessels to the skin constrict and help shunt blood to the working muscles. In the heat there must be a peripheral vasodilation to supply the sweat glands and allow greater heat loss by radiation. Another factor tending to reduce performance is the great loss of water (and salt) in the sweat. Total replacement of this water loss does not occur in response to thirst alone, so dehydration (and decrease in performance, which is fatigue) may occur even though water is available in unlimited quantities. These difficulties in adaptation by acclimatized man are magnified in the working man in a temperate climate during the first hot days of summer.

Altitude Fatigue

The subject of performance of work at high altitude is so vast that only brief mention can be made here. The primary effect of decreased oxygen pressure at high altitudes is complicated in the early stages of exposure by hypocapnia from relative overbreathing. In spite of adaptations in the control of pH, the work capacity is reduced since the amount of oxygen transportable per volume of blood is decreased. Compensatory polycythemia at high altitude can correct this only to a minor degree. Individuals living at high altitudes have higher capacities for muscular work than transients even after some months. Their special adaptations have never been adequately explained.

Sensory Fatigue

Decreasing response to a loud noise, an example of sensory fatigue, fits our crude definition of fatigue, but in fact it may represent a useful adaptation rather than a signal of maladaptation. Various visual tests, especially flicker fusion, have been studied extensively as indices of general fatigue. They have not proved their merit as well as the proponents of the tests originally proposed.

FATIGUE IN RELATION TO DISEASE

Fatigue is reported as a significant symptom in almost all acute and in many chronic diseases. In many instances the symptom, if more precisely described, is not fatigue; in others it is only an accompaniment of other and more localizing symptoms. However, in a few diseases it is the predominant or sole symptom.

Most striking of these is the rare disorder of glycogen metabolism, McArdle's syndrome, in which there is a specific lack of muscle phosphorylase. Here the muscle cannot utilize anaerobic breakdown of glycogen and is limited to aerobic metabolism for maintenance of muscle activity. The disease is important as a demonstration of the potential for purely aerobic muscle metabolism, since individuals with this disease can carry on moderate activity without difficulty.

Hypothyroidism is another disease in which fatigue is often the predominant symptom. Fatigue and sleepiness often go together. The general depression of body metabolism with decreased thyroid hormone not only lowers the voluntary drive to work but also impedes the cardiovascular adjustments necessary to carry on work. Hypofunction of other endocrines may also manifest fatigue as one of the main symptoms, as in Addison's disease (hypofunction of the adrenals) but usually the other manifestations are preponderant.

CHRONIC FATIGUE. This syndrome occurs in a wide variety of psychological or psychiatric derangements. The common characteristic is that the fatigue is not related to work performed. The symptom is likely to be greatest after sleep and may abate as the day progresses. It can be considered as a pathological deviant of normal "general fatigue."

DANGERS OF FATIGUE?

Frequently in both medical and general thinking, fatigue is looked upon as something to be avoided entirely. Aside from the fact that such an avoidance is practically impossible, it is certainly undesirable except in certain acute medical conditions. According to the physiological definition by Dill, quoted earlier, fatigue is not an index of breakdown of physiological adaptations, but rather an index of early stress on these adaptations. As described in Chapter 9, most increases in neuromuscular function can be achieved only by practice in the area of stress and fatigue. As a corollary, it can be stated that total avoidance of fatigue would lead in time to extreme loss of neuromuscular function and circulatory adaptability.

When is fatigue undesirable and possibly dangerous? If one considers fatigue as a sign that rest is necessary to restore equilibrium, then it logically follows that it is dangerous only when insufficient rest is allowed to restore the original status. Under conditions of brief static contractions the restoration time may be measured in seconds. Circulatory adjustments after moderate work may take minutes or hours. Glycogen replenishment takes days, and other more subtle adjustments may take longer. The test of inadequate rest lies in evidence of accumulation of losses of function. Progressive decrement of function on successive bouts of activity indicates that rest and restoration has been inadequate. Evidence of accumulative fatigue requires alertness to possible danger.

REFERENCES

1. Bartley, S. H.: Fatigue and inadequacy. Physiol. Rev., 37:301-324, 1957.
2. Bartley, S. H.: Fatigue Mechanism and Management. Springfield, Ill., Charles C Thomas, 1965.
3. Bourguignon, A., and Scherrer, J.: La capacité de travail au cours de la fatigue chez l'homme. Rev. de Path. Gén. et Physiol. Clin. 60:347-355, 1960.
4. Brown, G. L., and Burnes, B. D.: Fatigue and neuromuscular block in mammalian skeletal muscle. Proc. Roy. Soc. B, 136:182-195, 1949.
5. Christensen, E. H.: Muscular work and fatigue. In: K. Rodahl and S. M. Horvath. (eds.): Muscle as a Tissue. New York, McGraw-Hill, Book Co., Inc., 1962, pages 176-189.
6. Dill, D. B.: The Harvard Fatigue Laboratory: Its development, contributions and demise. Circulation Res. 20 (suppl. 1): 1161-1170, 1967.
7. Eccles, J. C.: The Physiology of Synapses. Berlin, Springer-Verlag, 1964.
8. Ellis, F. P.: Tropical fatigue. In: W. F. Floyd and A. T. Welford (eds.): Symposium on Fatigue. London, Lewis, 1953.
9. Grandjean, E.: Fatigue: Its physiological and psychological significance. Ergonomics, 11:427-436, 1968.
10. Hermansen, L., Hultman, E., and Saltin, B.: Muscle glycogen during prolonged severe exercise. Acta Physiol. Scand., 71:129-139, 1967.
11. Ikai, M., and Steinhaus, A. H.: Some factors modifying the expression of human strength. J. Appl. Physiol., 16:157-163, 1961.
12. Ikai, M., Yabe, K., and Ischii, K.: Muskelkraft und muskuläre Ermüdung bei willkürlicher Anspannung und elektrischer Reizung des Muskels. Sportarzt und Sportmedizin, 5:197-204, 1967.
13. Kogi, K., and Hakamada, T.: Slowing of the surface electromyogram and muscle strength in muscle fatigue. Rep. Inst. Sci. Labour (Tokyo), 60:27-41, 1962.
14. Kuroda, E., Klissouras, V., and Milsum, J. H.: Electrical and metabolic activities and fatigue in human isometric contraction. J. Appl. Physiol., 29:358-367, 1970.
15. Lippold, O. C. J., Redfearn, J. W. T., and Nugo, J.: The electromyography of fatigue. Ergonomics, 3:121-131, 1960.

16. Merton, P. A.: Voluntary strength and fatigue. J. Physiol. (London), *123*:553-564, 1954.

17. Naess, K., and Storm-Matheson, A.: Fatigue of sustained tetanic contractions. Acta Physiol. Scand., *34*:351-366, 1955.

18. Myers, S. J., and Sullivan, W. P.: Effect of circulatory occlusion on time to muscular fatigue. J. Appl. Physiol., *24*:54-59, 1968.

19. Pappenheimer, J. R., Miller, T. B., and Goodrich, C. A.: Sleep-promoting effects of cerebrospinal fluid from sleep-deprived goats. Proc. Nat. Acad. Sci., *58*:513-517, 1967.

20. Reid, C.: The mechanisms of voluntary fatigue. Quart. J. Exp. Physiol., *19*:17-42, 1928.

21. Scherrer, J., and Bourguignon, A.: Changes in the electromyogram produced by fatigue in man. Am. J. Phys. Med., *38*:148-158, 1959.

22. Scherrer, J., Bourguignon, A., and Monod, H.: La fatigue dans le travail statique. Revue de Path. Gén. et Physiol. Clin., *60*:357-367, 1960.

23. Scherrer, J., and Monod, H.: Le travail musculaire local et la fatigue chez l'homme. J. Physiol. (Paris), *52*:419-501, 1960.

24. Schwab, R. S.: Motivation in measurements of fatigue. In: W. F. Floyd and A. T. Welford (eds.): *Symposium on Fatigue*. Lewis, London, 1953, pages 143-148.

25. Soula, C., Scherrer, J., Moynier, R., Bourguignon, C., Bourguignon, A., and Monod, H.: Aspects musculaire, sensoriels, psychologique et sociaux de la fatigue. Arch. des Malades Professionelles, *22*:419-445, 1961.

Chapter 12

METABOLIC EFFECTS OF INACTIVITY AND INJURY

by Calvin L. Long, Ph.D., and Luis E. Bonilla, M.D.

The human body may be viewed as a number of metabolic compartments which interact with each other. Each of these compartments is affected in a particular way by changes in physical activity, illness or trauma. These changes complicate injury or illness and may become greater problems than the primary disease.

The biochemical changes in metabolism caused by trauma are compounded by inactivity. Inactivity is defined as a decreased or restricted muscular activity and is often required in the management of trauma and chronic illness. Inactivity causes alterations in the fluid compartments, in electrolyte balance and in the circulation. It contributes to an increased nitrogen loss and muscular wasting, to a change in mineral content of bone and a decrease in resting metabolic expenditure.

Metabolic expenditure is increased by any injury. The decrease in energy requirements associated with inactivity is rarely adequate to counteract the increased energy requirements caused by the trauma. The increase in metabolism after trauma is proportional to the severity of the trauma and may also be accompanied by secondary complications. The frequent observation of weight loss after trauma illustrates the heavy drain on body reserves and is a measure of the metabolic mixture burned following trauma and inactivity. An increased catabolic state occurs at a time when the exogenous fuel is greatly reduced owing to restriction in eating.

THE WATER COMPARTMENT

Water comprises 50 to 60 per cent of the body weight of an adult man; this figure is slightly less in women and in the elderly. Man obtains water from the liquid he ingests and from the oxidation of food materials. A 3000 Kcal diet provides from 750 to 900 ml of water, of which 450 ml are contained in the solid food and the rest is obtained from oxidation.

The total obligatory loss of water approaches 1400 ml per day. Under normal circumstances, a 70 kg man loses about 850 ml per day, which is evaporated from lungs and through the skin as "the insensible perspiration"; this is the actual amount determined by metabolic activity, and not reducible by any control mechanism. Water is also lost by sensible perspiration (sweating), but the amount depends on the heat stress and humidity. Loss of water in the feces accounts for about 150 ml per day. A regular diet requires the excretion of about 600 milliosmoles of solutes per day per square meter of body surface. The kidneys have only a limited ability to concentrate (0.7 cc of water per milliosmole), so a minimum of about 420 ml of water per day is eliminated in the urine, which prevents the accumulation of metabolic waste products in the blood.

Distribution of Water in the Body

Approximately 55 per cent, or 330 ml per kg body weight, of the body water is in the cellular compartment; the remainder is in the extracellular space. The extracellular space is a heterogeneous compartment and is divided into plasma, interstitial fluid, interstitial lymph, connective tissue, cartilage and bone.

Composition and Tonicity of the Body Fluids

The solute content of each compartment determines the osmotic pressure. The most important solutes for the distribution and retention of water within a compartment are the inorganic electrolytes, sodium and potassium. Nonelectrolyte solutes, to which cells are freely permeable, such as urea, contribute to total osmolality but not to water distribution. By contrast, an acute increase in concentrations of solutes to which cells are only slowly permeable, such as glucose, will temporarily add to the extracellular osmolality and volume.

The content of water and solutes differs markedly between the extracellular and intracellular fluids. The osmolality of the intracellular fluid is determined by the potassium content, and the extracellular fluid by its sodium concentration. An active mechanism (sodium pump) is required at the cellular membrane level to maintain the extracellular position of sodium and the corresponding intracellular position of potassium. Constancy of osmolality in either compartment requires a proportional relationship between the volume of fluid and the combined concentration of sodium and potassium. The osmolality of the body fluids normally ranges between 270 and 300 milliosmoles per kg of water.

Fluid and Protein Exchange Between the
Capillaries and the Tissues

The passage of fluid from the blood to the tissues is determined by the balance of hydrostatic pressure, the colloid osmotic pressure and the tissue pressure across the capillary wall. Fluid enters the tissues at the arteriolar side of the capillary, and most of this fluid re-enters the circulation at the venular end of the capillary. The rest is brought back to the circulation through the lymphatics.

Regulation of the Water Volume and the Solute Content

Normally the intake of water and electrolytes is in excess of the needs of the body. Metabolic and neuroendocrine mechanisms determine the retention or elimination of water and electrolytes by the kidneys. The concentration of the extracellular fluid is maintained by antidiuretic hormone secreted by the neurohypophysis. Once in the bloodstream, this hormone enters the kidneys where it regulates the absorption and the excretion of water at the distal tubule.

The regulation of volume of the extracellular fluid depends on the action of aldosterone, which controls the sodium concentration. Extracellular fluid volume is dependent upon the extracellular sodium concentration, whereas the water content of the intracellular compartment is dependent on the intracellular potassium content.

BLOOD VOLUME

The average healthy adult man has a blood volume of five liters, a value which remains within 5 to 10 per cent of a mean value over periods of weeks or months. The mean plasma volume (approximately 60 per cent of blood volume) of men is 77.7 ml per kg body weight and for women 66.1 ml. per kg body weight.[64] Blood and plasma volumes vary directly with the metabolically active body cell mass, and when the body weight increases because of deposition of fat, the blood volume per kilogram of body weight decreases.

Approximately 20 per cent of the total blood volume is within the high pressure arterial system and only 5 per cent is contained in the capillaries. The remaining 75 per cent is distributed in the low pressure venous system.

The Body Fluids and Physical Activity

In man, blood volume increases from 10 to 19 per cent following a period of physical training,[36] and conversely decreased blood volume occurs in physically incapacitated individuals.[64, 72] Blood volume values also decrease in healthy men after prolonged bed rest.[16]

The maximum reduction in blood volume during bed rest occurs from the second to the sixth day of recumbency and no further reduction occurs after a month.[25] The larger blood volumes seen in physically active individuals are probably associated with an adjustment of the vascular system to meet the circulatory requirements determined by external conditions. The change in blood volume seen during prolonged bed rest seems to be due to the reduced hydrostatic pressure in the recumbent position, but it is certain that decreased physical activity also contributes to the loss of plasma fluid. Fuller et al.[25] report that the blood volume reduction of prolonged bed rest could be partly prevented when the patient exercised in bed.

Influence of the Supine Posture on the Body Fluids

As a person lies down, approximately 500 ml of blood shifts to the thorax,[69] and there is an immediate fall in heart rate and an increase in cardiac output by 24 per cent. Stroke volume increases and the calculated cardiac work is increased by approximately 30 per cent.[11, 30] As the hydrostatic pressure decreases in the extremities during recumbency, a hypotonic expansion of the blood volume is produced. This disturbance of the osmolality of the body fluids triggers neuroendocrine mechanisms that inhibit release of the antidiuretic hormone and aldosterone, with resultant sodium and water diuresis. The sodium excretion increases from 0.075 mEq per min when upright to 0.15 mEq per min excretion lying down.[22] The diuresis observed during recumbency is a temporary occurrence lasting for about one hour.

INFLUENCE OF TRAUMA ON THE BODY FLUIDS

Trauma alters the content and distribution of body fluids as a result of hemorrhage, edema and disturbed fluid intake. The loss of 500 ml of blood from a normal man has little effect, and even a removal of a liter of blood may not embarrass the circulation if the individual remains recumbent. A greater loss of blood reduces the venous return to the heart and lowers the right atrial pressure, the ventricular filling pressure and the cardiac output. The immediate response to a large blood loss is a reflex arterial and venous constriction and a liberation of epinephrine and norepinephrine, which reinforces the peripheral vascular constriction. In small concentrations catecholamines, especially epinephrine, increase blood flow through the vital organs at the expense of the peripheral tissues. This may be efficacious initially, but in prolonged hypotension the peripheral vasoconstrictive action is so severe that anaerobic metabolism occurs and a large amount of metabolic acids are formed and released into the systemic circulation.

Angiotensin released by the kidneys also contributes to restoring the plasma volume. A decrease in the renal blood flow results in release of renin, which acts as a proteolytic enzyme to form angiotensin II, a powerful vasoconstrictor as well as a stimulator of aldosterone secretion. Angiotensin thus directly increases the peripheral resistance and indirectly affects the excretion of sodium and water. Hypovolemia stimulates the secretion of antidiuretic hormone, thus promoting water retention and, because of this, expansion of the plasma volume.

The neuroendocrine vasoconstriction is accompanied by other responses which serve to restore the volume loss. Almost immediately after hemorrhage fluid enters the intravascular space through the lymphatics, thus expanding the plasma volume with protein-poor fluid.[62]

PHYSICAL ACTIVITY AND POSTURAL CIRCULATORY CHANGES

A normal individual tilted from the supine to the upright posture shows a decrease in systolic blood pressure and an increase in heart rate. This is followed by a redistribution of blood volume, since the intravascular pressure decreases in the parts of the body above the hydrostatic indifferent point (HIP) and increases in the dependent parts of the body.[26] The venous pressure at the ankle, for instance, increases from 15 cm of water in the supine position to 120 to 130 cm of water in the upright position. The inflow of blood to the legs when the foot is tilted down has been estimated to be 500 ml.[74]

The pooling of blood in the lower extremities produces a rapid increase in the volume in the leg, which increases further if passive standing is maintained. This pooling causes an extravasation of plasma into the tissues that may result in a decrease in blood volume of about 11 to 15 per cent.[64] Plethysmographic studies indicate that most of the blood entering the dependent regions of the body comes from the thoracic vascular bed.[63] This displacement of blood reduces the end diastolic ventricular volume, the stroke volume and lowers the cardiac output to 60 or 80 per cent of the pretilting value. The heart rate increases 10 to 20 strokes per minute.[5] The systemic blood pressure changes are moderated by constriction of the arterioles in the muscular bed.

Further compensatory mechanisms are activated to restore central blood volume and maintain blood pressure. Standing causes a decreased renal blood flow and glomerular filtration rate[7] and an increase in aldosterone excretion.[22] Increased secretion of antidiuretic hormone is thought to occur, but no direct measurements have been made. The circulatory response to the upright posture is much less effective even in normal subjects after a few days of bed rest[71] or sitting immobile in a chair 11 hours a day.

ENERGY EXCHANGE IN TRAUMA AND INACTIVITY

A normal individual maintains a constant body weight that fluctuates less than 1 per cent around a mean. This constancy is due to a balance between the caloric intake and output. The average energy expenditure of a normal sedentary adult male is about 1800 Kcal per day; this would increase to about 2500 to 3000 Kcal per day if he performs light to moderate work.

Weight loss after trauma can be due either to a restriction of food intake or to an increase in resting metabolism or both. Resting metabolic expenditure after major surgery is within ± 10 per cent of preoperative levels if there are no major complications.[34] However, after long bone fractures the metabolism is usually 10 to 25 per cent above the normal resting level. Severe sepsis produces a further increase of 20 to 40 per cent above resting value. Severe trauma, such as third-degree burns over a large portion of the body surface, produces the largest increase in resting metabolic expenditure, being up to 100 per cent above the predicted normal value.[12] Much of this increase is associated with the obligatory loss of water from the burned surface. The insensible water loss in burned patients has been found to be as high as 5000 to 6000 ml. Approximately 0.5 Kcal per gm of water is expended on evaporation and can account for as much as 3000 Kcal of energy in 24 hours. This loss requires excessive amounts of metabolic fuel and increases in ventilation and circulation. These increases added to a high resting expenditure greatly increase the metabolic needs of the critically ill patients.

Fever alone causes an increase in resting metabolic expenditure. It is commonly accepted that for each rise of 1.0° C in body temperature, a 10 per cent rise in energy expenditure is required. Other metabolic stimuli associated with trauma can add greatly to the increase in heat production and heat loss. The elevated resting metabolic expenditure caused by fever or trauma enhances protein breakdown in spite of adequate caloric intake. Conversely, a decrease in resting metabolic expenditure, such as during starvation, causes a decreased protein breakdown.

The changes in body composition following inactivity and injury are best understood when compared to body composition of a normal healthy man. An arbitrary division of the whole normal adult body into its various compartments is graphically presented in Figure 12-1. The whole compartment represents a 70 kg man; this is divided into smaller compartments which represent the areas under discussion. Twenty-two per cent of the body weight is fat, which in a 70

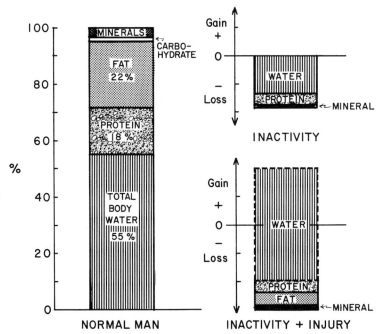

Figure 12–1 Approximate composition of the adult body under normal conditions and its derangement following inactivity and injury. In the illustration showing direction of changes, the magnitudes noted are not proportional to the normal values.

kg man would be about 15.4 kg. of his body stores. The protein mass represents about 18 per cent of the body weight, or about 13 kg. The carbohydrate content of the body, mainly in the form of glycogen, is very small and represents only a few hundred grams.

A normal man maintains a constant weight on a diet composed of 50 per cent carbohydrates, 30 per cent fat and 20 per cent protein. If the caloric intake equals the caloric expenditure, any variation in body weight will usually be the result of changes in fluid intake or output.

The body can adapt to caloric deficits and protect the protein mass by changing the fuel mixture it burns. When an individual goes from a normal to a starvation diet, there is a shift to a fat-rich fuel mixture owing to the mobilizing of the fat stores of the body. Thus protein breakdown by the body does not represent the major source of calories in the starvation state of an otherwise normal individual or in patients after severe trauma.[18] Even in the most severe forms of nitrogen wastage following injury more than 80 per cent of the energy demands are met by nonprotein fuel.

In starvation, the urinary nitrogen decreases over a few days from a normal value of 10 to 12 gm of nitrogen excreted per day to 5 to 6 gm of nitrogen. In extremely prolonged starvation, less nitrogen is excreted until a level of 1 to 3 gm nitrogen per day is reached. Initially glycogen is metabolized, and thereafter the body's requirement for glucose is mainly from amino acids, glycerol or recycled lactate. Even the brain, which normally requires about 120 gm glucose per day, uses less, based on C^{14}-glucose turnover rates. These and other adaptive mechanisms allow the conservation of up to 50 gm of endogenous protein per day.

The loss in weight of postoperative patients has important clinical implications.[68] In 46 patients who sustained operations for chronic peptic ulcer, the weight loss was the only factor that correlated well with operative mortality rates. The mortality rate was 33 per cent in those patients who had lost more than 20 per cent of their preoperative body weight, and 3.5 per cent in those who had lost less than 20 per cent.

The losses during the postoperative period are approximately half fat and half lean tissue.[46] In starvation the proportion of fat burned is considerably greater. Kinney et al. have studied the body composition and weight loss in 10 elective operative patients.[34] In 10 days the female patients lost an average of 17 gm of protein and 68 gm of fat per day and the males 34 gm of protein and 45 gm of fat per day. The fat loss appeared to be a direct effect of caloric deficit due to limited food intake during the early postoperative period.

The caloric content, or caloric equivalent of weight loss, depends on the nature of caloric restriction.[28] In the absence of injury or infection, the caloric equivalent of each kg of weight loss is 2000 to 3500 Kcal during the first week of caloric restriction, but increases twofold within three weeks. Thus the average caloric equivalent per kg in the elective postoperative male patient was found to be 1584 Kcal and 3105 Kcal for the female.[33] The lower figure in man is the result of greater protein and less fat breakdown than in the female group. The total stores of protein and fat are about equal on a weight basis, but the caloric content of fat is much higher; therefore, fat plays a very important role in relation to body energy sources.

Many alternate pathways are available to metabolize protein, fat and carbohydrate. The metabolic map shown in Figure 12-2 is provided to indicate general sequences of interrelationships of metabolism. It is important to recognize that in any discussion of cellular changes one must keep in mind the general restrictions on the interchange in certain reactions.

BODY CELL MASS

In spite of the seemingly stable and inert protein supporting structure, a large portion of body protein has a relatively rapid turnover rate, which has been referred to as the active or labile pool.[49] This dynamic aspect of body protein was well illustrated by Schoenheimer, Ratner and Rittenberg,[59] who, in 1939, employed a technique using labeled N^{15}-amino acids. They found that less than 50 per cent of the labeled amino acid ingested was excreted in the urine, while the body weight remained unchanged and the nitrogen balance was maintained. Approximately one-third of the N^{15} incorporated into the tissues was still linked to the same amino acid, while the remainder had been incorporated in other amino acids. Labeled ammonium salts administered to animals are recovered in all amino acids with the exception of lysine.[24] Radioactive methionine is incorporated into the protein of many organs in animals during starvation,[69] indicating a continuing breakdown and resynthesis of body protein.

In 1953, San Pietro and Rittenberg, using N^{15}-amino acids, measured the rate of protein synthesis in man. They found that approximately 1.3 gm of protein per kg of body weight was synthesized each day. A 70 kg man, therefore, synthesized about 100 gm of protein per day; about the same amount is broken down. The metabolic amino acid pool was estimated to represent about 0.5 gm of nitrogen per kg of body weight or, at the most, about 35 gm of nitrogen total in a normal adult.

The supporting "nonmetabolic" protein component resists wear and tear and is of little importance in the total energetics in the human body. This supporting structure consists of skeleton, tendon, fascia, collagen, elastin and dermis; it uses almost no oxygen. Inactivity and injury largely affects the active mass or labile protein pool. It is also accepted that there is no identifiable tissue protein pool that serves exclusively as a storage depot.

When a normal healthy adult is injured, a number of metabolic changes in protein metabolism occur which clinically appear as anemia and hypoproteinemia and which signal loss of body cell mass. The laboratory evidence of abnormal protein metabolism is seen as excessive urinary excretion of nitrogen and other constituents including sulfur, phosphorus, potassium and creatine.[14] A healthy, well-nourished subject usually consumes 10 to 15 gm of protein nitrogen daily and is in positive nitrogen balance (i.e., in an anabolic state). During total starvation, his nitrogen excretion will fluctuate around prestarvation levels for the first two to four days and then slowly drop to a basic level of 5 to 6 gm. of urinary nitrogen per day.[47] A serious injury superimposed on starvation causes an additional nitrogen loss that is proportional to the severity of the trauma. The nitrogen loss usually starts on about the third or fourth day and reaches a peak in about eight days. The upper limit of nitrogen loss following severe trauma is unknown, but it is not uncommon for 20 to 40 gm of nitrogen to be lost per day. Losses may persist for several weeks.

A large part of the negative nitrogen balance that follows trauma is the result of the decreased food intake. Changes in the resting caloric expenditure following weight reduction are related to the composition of the body tissue that is lost.[52] When weight is reduced at the expense of fat alone, the metabolism diminishes in proportion to surface area, and the relation of metabolic rate to surface area is maintained; but if the tissue lost is largely protein, the metabolic rate falls more rapidly.

Negative nitrogen balance, along with an increase in the plasma nonprotein nitrogen, occurs in patients who have been burned.[48, 70] Nardi studied the urinary amino acids in severely burned patients and in patients undergoing conventional surgical procedures.[51] Both essential and nonessential amino acids are excreted in the urine of patients after trauma or burns, the quantity and nature of the amino acids excreted being related to the severity of the injury.

Rats suffering from hemorrhagic shock show an increase in blood α-amino nitrogen[21] owing in part to an increased breakdown of protein in the peripheral tissue[56, 57] and to a decreased ability of the liver to deaminate amino acids[20] and to form urea.[73]

Some investigators have reported lowered total amino nitrogen and decreased plasma levels of amino acids.[23, 39, 43] However, it seems that the apparent reduction in plasma amino nitrogen is really an increased uptake by the amino acids into the cells, as various types of trauma have been shown to influence the distribution of amino acid between erythrocytes and plasma.[6]

The biological significance of increased nitrogen loss after injury is poorly understood. Amino acids represent the major source for conversion to carbohydrate in the body under fasting conditions, and fatty acids cannot serve as an alternate source of glucose. At the time of actual or relative loss of exogenous carbohydrate, it is reasonable to consider the excess nitrogen breakdown as a reflection of a mechanism to increase the supply of carbohydrate intermediates. The changes in protein breakdown in muscle tissue may be in response to the liver's need of the essential and nonessential amino acids for the synthesis of certain proteins during the increases in hepatic protein synthetic activity after trauma.[31, 38] The increased nitrogen loss might then represent the deamination of amino acids mobilized and brought to the liver in excess of the organism's needs for synthetic purposes.

The rise in metabolic rate that is associated with the nitrogen excretion after injury may be due in part to the specific dynamic action of protein,[10] as animals deficient in dietary protein fail to increase their metabolism or protein breakdown in response to injury.[50] Other factors also play an important role in the increased metabolic activity after injury. Normal body temperature is accomplished by a balance of heat production and heat loss. In a cool environment this balance can only be effected by raising resting heat production through increased metabolism; animal studies have shown that recovery from injury is slower and metabolic derangements are greater when the animals are kept in a cool environment.[8]

The metabolic response to severe trauma is complicated by inactivity. In the face of severe demand for calories, decreased activity is often assumed to be an asset; however, inactivity also causes a loss of nitrogen and wasting of muscle mass. During strict bed rest, nitrogen equilibrium can only be maintained with a diet rich in protein.[65] Keys, in 1944, found that a subject performing normal activities required 54 gm of protein to maintain nitrogen balance, but after a three week period of bed rest he required 110 gm a day to maintain equilibrium.[32]

Although a number of studies have been made of people confined to bed as a result of skeletal trauma, only a few studies are known of healthy normal subjects immobilized in a cast. Cuthbertson's studies involved several normal subjects of both sexes and of different ages each with one leg immobilized by splints for 10 to 14 days.[13] The subjects consumed the same amount of food during the study as they did prior to the study. Within one or two days they showed increased excretion of sulfur, followed by nitrogen, phosphorus and calcium, which suggested a loss of muscle protein and bone substance. Deitrick et al. reported on four normal healthy young men immobilized in casts from the toes to the umbilicus for a period of six to seven weeks.[16] These men showed an average decline in basal energy expenditure of 2.4 Kcal per m[2] per hr (range 1 to 4.3 Kcal per m[2] per hr), which represents an average reduction in basal oxygen consumption of 6.9 per cent. These findings persisted for three to four weeks after bed rest was discontinued. Nitrogen excretion increased by the fifth day of bed rest, resulting in the loss of approximately 50 gm per subject during the experimental period. Creatine tolerance was decreased, presumably because of a decreased ability of the muscle to store creatine. The circumference of the thigh and calf was decreased owing to loss of muscle substance. Whedon et al. later showed that some of the effects of immobilization could be reduced by using an oscillating bed.[75]

The mechanism that causes an increased nitrogen loss after bed rest and immobilization is not known. The negative nitrogen balance may be due to decreased tissue repair while tissue breakdown continues at normal rate or to an increased tissue breakdown at a normal rate of protein synthesis. In an attempt to determine the mechanism of nitrogen loss following inactivity, a quantitative study of nitrogen dynamics using N^{15}-glycine was reported by Schønheyder et al.[60] They found that the negative nitrogen balance occurred after a lag of about five days and reached a maximum about the tenth day after cast immobilization. In this study a reduced synthesis of tissue proteins occurred while the breakdown remained unchanged.

CARBOHYDRATE

The carbohydrate fuel reserves of the body are very small and exist mainly as glycogen. The average body glycogen content, including liver and muscle, represents only a few hundred grams of glucose. This small storehouse of fuel presumably serves as a buffer between meals and is replenished at the next meal. If no food is eaten, the glycogen stores are largely depleted in a day.

Certain organs and cells, including the brain, red cells, leukocytes, adrenal medulla and bone marrow, have an obligatory glucose requirement, while others use either glucose or fatty acid substrates for energy, although under severe starvation conditions ketone bodies may also be used by the brain. The brain's absolute carbohydrate requirement of approximately 120 gm per day is supplied from glycogen stores and gluconeogenesis from amino acids, lactate and pyruvate.

Prior to glucose synthesis the amino acids are deaminated and the carbon skeleton then is made available for energy purposes. With a limited carbohydrate intake, the hormonal and neuroendocrinal response shifts amino acid carbon to glucose (gluconeogenesis). The ketosis and increased gluconeogenesis associated with carbohydrate-free intake can be modified by feeding as little as 25 to 50 gm of carbohydrate per day.

The regulation of carbohydrate metabolism will not be discussed here except to indicate that interrelationships to other fuels may be mediated by insulin and other mechanisms. Low carbohydrate intake causes a decrease in insulin production, allowing the insulin sensitive lipase to mobilize fat. The increased fatty acid and also the low insulin levels tend to promote gluconeogenesis.

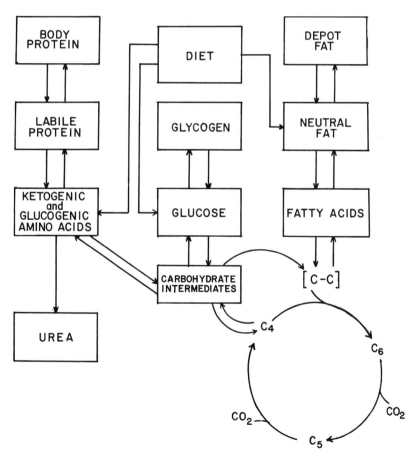

Figure 12—2   Intermediary metabolic pathways of clinical significance.

The glucose from the diet or from gluconeogenesis is either stored as glycogen or burned for energy. An excess of calories over the daily caloric expenditure will be stored as depot fat; however, this fat can then only be used as calories and cannot be resynthesized to glucose. Fatty acid carbon can be converted to glucose, but there is no net gain in glucose, as this conversion can only take place through decarboxylation of oxalacetic acid to phosphoenolpyruvate.[37] Figure 12-2 shows that for each two carbon acetate fragments from fatty acid breakdown that enter the cycle and condense with oxalacetic acid, two carbons are lost as CO_2 with each turn of the cycle.

The carbohydrate content in the body is important in determining the response to injury. For example, there is greater resistance of well-fed rats to ischemic injury than fasted ones.[66] However, once the response to injury is underway, the animal cannot be protected by supplying exogenous glucose. Rats on a high carbohydrate diet have an exaggerated catabolic response to injury as compared to those on a high fat diet.[27] The reason for this difference is not clear but it may be because this diet is advantageous for tissue repair after injury, or it may merely serve as a less fluctuating source of fuel.

The glycogen content in the liver and hind limb muscle is reduced following fracture of the hind limb owing to muscular disuse, tissue damage and alterations in the overall metabolism.[76] Although glycogen is not stored after hind limb ischemia, its synthesis from glucose in liver and muscle continues.[67] Immediately after bilateral hind limb ischemia, rats develop hyperglycemia with a fall in heat production before general circulatory failure. During this time glucose production, as measured with C^{14}-labeled glucose, shows no change, but the oxidation rate decreases by 30 per cent. It is concluded that the most important effect on carbohydrate metabolism following hind limb ischemia is an inhibition of the oxidation of pyruvate to carbon dioxide.[3]

The changes in glycogen metabolism suggest, but do not necessarily show, the degree of glucose utilization following injury. The metabolic response of the body evidently changes as glucose tolerance is decreased following injury in both man and animals, and hyperglycemia tends to be proportional to the severity of injury and may lead to glycosuria. The reduced peripheral utilization of glucose after injury is largely an assumption, although it is correct to say that glucose tolerance is lowered.[19]

Hyperglycemia following injury occurs in man, the amount varying directly with the severity of injury and inversely to the decreased plasma amino nitrogen level. Abnormal carbohydrate metabolism, in the form of the diabetic type of glucose tolerance curve, appears to be more marked following severe injuries than following minor injuries.

The glucose and insulin responses have been studied after abdominal operations of moderate severity[2, 55] and were found to show high fasting blood glucose level and a reduced tolerance to intravenous glucose, which persisted for at least 72 hours following the operation. Fasting plasma insulin levels were increased 24 hours after the operation and suggested that the changes in glucose tolerance were due either to increased insulin antagonists in the blood or to resistance to insulin activity at a cellular level. The level of growth hormone, a powerful insulin antagonist,[40] is raised after surgery. Further data on the effect of injury on carbohydrate metabolism show that in the early shock phase after burns, glucose tolerance is reduced, plasma insulin levels after glucose are low and free fatty acids are high.[1] These changes are related to the severity of the burn, and it was suggested that they may correspond to the high level of epinephrine secretion, as epinephrine can suppress insulin response to glucose infusion in normal subjects.[53]

In the succeeding days after severe burns, patients show a higher level of fasting insulin and an insulin response to glucose characteristic of insulin resistance. The development of insulin resistance after trauma is striking, but the mechanism of the response is not known. Severe starvation will produce such a picture, but this is not usually encountered in patient care. Impairment of hepatic function has been seen in severe battle casualties, but it would not be expected to produce this kind of picture, although it does produce a decreased sensitivity to insulin.

The initial alteration in energy metabolism following blood loss is due to release of neuroendocrine hormones. Recently, Bauer et al. reported a rise in catecholamines following hemorrhage.[4] This response enhances the vasomotor reaction in maintaining blood pressure, but may also be essential for immediate survival as it occurs at a time when energy demands are increased. The increased secretion of catecholamines may, however, eventually compromise homeostasis by increasing the drain on energy metabolism.[17] Glycogen and other substrates are mobilized by epinephrine, causing hyperglycemia and a stimulation of insulin.[44] The metabolic alterations become progressively more severe even as the catecholamine concentration falls, which suggests that changes in energy metabolism in prolonged shock reflect more than just the activity of the sympathetic nervous system.

Hyperglycemia following trauma has often been attributed to a decreased glucose oxidation rate. A similar condition of high blood sugar following injury could also be due to an increased synthesis of glucose with a normal or slight increase in oxidation rate. Recent studies reported by Long et al.[41, 42] on glucose metabolism in patients who have sustained major injury, such as third degree thermal burns, major sepsis and peritonitis, indicate greatly increased glucose oxidation and turnover rates during hyperglycemia. A two- to threefold increase in the size of the glucose pool was also noted. Minor changes were noted in glucose metabolism in patients before and after elective operation.[41] The combination of an increased oxidation rate and an increased size of glucose pool in injury suggests that the body is responding to the injury by synthesizing additional amounts of glucose. Thus the body requirements for carbohydrate may in part be due to increased needs for glucose during wound healing and tissue repair.

FAT

The fat compartment of the body represents about 22 per cent of the body weight in a normal individual, and this compartment is the largest caloric store (Figure 12-1); but loss of body weight will reduce the size of this compartment. The average man eats 25 to 160 gm of lipid per day, mostly triglyceride, with small quantities of phospholipid, cholesterol and fat soluble vitamins. Triglyceride is hydrolyzed at the adipose cell membrane to free fatty acids (FFA) and glycerol. Most of the free fatty acids penetrate the endothelium and enter the adipose tissue cell, but some of the free fatty acids and all of the glycerol are removed by the blood. Upon entering the cell, the free fatty acids are converted to fatty acyl-CoA, which reacts with L-α-glycerophosphate that is derived from glucose or glycogen in the adipose cell to form triglyceride. In this way the adipose tissue adds dietary fatty acids to the larger pool of triglycerides, increasing the size of the major energy reservoir. Adipose tissue plays a very important role in stabilizing the fuel supply. Its accumulation during periods of feeding and overfeeding and its release during starvation provides the necessary delicate balance in day to day activity.

The availability of glucose L-α-glycerophosphate influences lipid mobilization and the formation of triglycerides. Since free fatty acids are not used by the adipose tissue cell of fasting animals for triglyceride biosynthesis, they are mobilized from the tissue into the blood stream. In severe starvation the FFA's are broken down to form ketone bodies (acetoacetic and β-hydroxybutyric acids). In addition to the L-α-glycerophosphate, the increased lipid mobilization is also related to the low insulin levels during fasting. In the absence of the inhibitory effect of insulin on triglyceride lipase and when the rate of triglyceride biosynthesis in the adipose tissue is low, fat mobilization occurs at high rates in fasting mammals.

Lipid or fat mobilization is defined as the net release of FFA's from triglycerides stored in adipose tissue. Carbohydrate, as previously indicated, plays an important role in regulation of fat mobilization. In addition to this regulation, fat mobilization is also influenced by the endocrine system. Catecholamines promote fat mobilization by activating the hormone sensitive triglyceride lipase, which is a rate-limiting enzymatic step in adipose tissue breakdown that is mediated through increased concentration of 3' 5'-cyclic adenosine monophosphate in the adipose cell. The catecholamine response requires thyroid and adrenocortical hormones to function permissively in fat mobilization. Glucagon is also able to increase the concentration of cyclic adenosine monophosphate in adipose tissue, thus activating the hormone sensitive triglyceride lipase.

The FFA's supplied for energy needs through lipid mobilization come mainly from adipose tissue, although the triglycerides within any cell are capable of satisfying this need. This delicately balanced total lipid mobilization can be altered by many processes acting on different controlling mechanisms. Large increases in the lipid content of the liver have been shown to be caused by cold exposure, excessive muscular exercise and in surgical trauma. In 1966, Ross reported on an increase in plasma nonesterified fatty acids following abdominal operation in man.[55] In studying the effect of glucose loading during operation and after myocardial infarction, Allison et al. also observed increases in free fatty acids.[2]

In severe trauma, such as burns, gross fatty infiltration of the liver has been recognized.[61] This is accompanied by reduced levels of cholesterol, but with no change in the triglyceride level.[9]

The cause for the post-traumatic increase in lipid mobilization is unknown, but it may be related to an increased activity of the sympathetic nervous system.

For instance, in burns there is a marked increase in the urinary excretion of catecholamines, especially norepinephrine. In severe cases, the catecholamine excretion may be elevated for more than a week. The increased lipid mobilization after trauma may be made useful by supplying calories to different organs of the body; however, there is some evidence that the rate of lipid mobilization is greater than the concomitant caloric need.

There is indirect evidence which suggests that increased oxidation rates of fatty acids follow fat mobilization in injury, as seen, for example, in the loss of body fat that results from serious burns.[54] The changes in body composition, particularly with reference to water and fat, following surgery caused Moore to conclude that increased rates of fat oxidation occur.[46] Direct measurement of fatty acid oxidation in shock was made by Heath and Stoner using radioactive fatty acids.[29] They did not find a change in the rate of removal of 1-C^{14}-palmitate from the plasma nor in its distribution in the tissues after severe trauma, but they did note a depressed rate of $C^{14}O_2$ excretion. The authors suggested that inhibition of plasma nonesterified fatty acid oxidation by the tricarboxylic acid cycle occurred rather than poor perfusion of the fat depots.

The critically ill and poorly fed patient is dependent on mobilizing fat reserves to meet increased energy demands. Lipid mobilization may be useful as increased energy demands have to be met, but when excessive and under certain conditions, this may be harmful, as seen in a large infiltration and deposits of fat in the liver after trauma.

The role of fat in inactivity is not too different from that in the resting state. Decreasing the work will cause the expenditure to fall to resting levels. The contribution of fat to calories during inactivity is dependent in part on the postabsorptive state. In the immediate postabsorptive state (or within a 24 hour interval following food intake) changes in lipid metabolism are evident. The free plasma fatty acids become elevated, causing increased uptake by the liver, heart, skeletal muscle and other tissues. It is interesting to note that these same tissues almost completely lose the capacity to metabolize glucose even though the concentration of glucose in the plasma is not markedly lowered by the 24 hour fast. The liver increases production of ketone bodies, acetoacetic and β-hydroxybutyric acids, which diffuse out into the extracellular fluid and are transported to other organs for use as fuel. Biosynthesis of fatty acids is stopped after a 24 hour fast. The needs of organs which continue to use glucose as the primary fuel are met by a vigorous gluconeogenesis by the liver and renal cortex. Because of these changes, it can be seen that the adipose tissue becomes a major source of calories.

THE DECONDITIONING SYNDROME

The concept of deconditioning has been used to describe the deleterious effects that attend the lack of physical activity and exercise regardless of the presence of disease. These changes are magnified in the case of patients who have recovered from extensive injuries or prolonged illness. Here deconditioning is manifested by intolerance to the upright position and by an altered response to muscular exercise as seen in response to slight and moderate work loads and during tilting of the body from the supine to the upright position.

The response of a well-conditioned individual to a submaximal work load is characterized by a slow pulse rate, and an elevated stroke volume. The conditioned individual thus tends to maintain the various internal equilibria as close as possible to the resting state during strenuous exercise; upon completion of work, he tends to restore promptly any equilibria which have been disturbed.[15]

The deconditioned individual, on the other hand, responds to a slight to moderate work load with increased heart rate, blood pressure and the slower return of each parameter to the resting level. The work capacity in a deconditioned individual is further limited by the attending reduction in blood volume, reduced hemoglobin content and muscle weakness.

In conclusion, the intense manifestations of altered body composition discussed in this chapter, resulting from injury and inactivity, decrease the physical competence of the individual to satisfy the metabolic demands of the active tissues.

Circulatory maladaptations, metabolic derangements, loss of muscle and other tissue, as well as derangements in more general homeostatic and adaptive functions, all contribute to malfunction in man after inactivity and trauma. The maintenance of the various body compartments as close to their average values as possible should reduce the manifestations of the deconditioning syndrome.

REFERENCES

1. Allison, S. P., Hinton, P., and Chamberlain, M. J.: Intravenous glucose-tolerance, insulin, and free-fatty-acid levels in burned patients. Lancet, 2:1113-1116, 1968.
2. Allison, S. P., Prowse, K., and Chamberlain, M. J.: Failure of insulin response to glucose load during operation and after myocardial infarction. Lancet, 1:478–481, 1967.
3. Ashby, M. M., Heath, D. F., and Stoner, H. B.: A quantitative study of carbohydrate metabolism in the normal and injured rat. J. Physiol. (London), 179:193–237, 1965.
4. Bauer, W. E., Levene, R. A., Zachwieja, A., Lee, M. J., Menczyk, Z., and Drucker, W. R.: The role of catecholamines in energy metabolism during prolonged hemorrhagic shock. Surg. Forum, 20:9-11, 1969.
5. Bevegård, S., Holmgren, A., and Jonsson, B.: The effect of body position on the circulation at rest and during exercise, with special reference to the influence on the stroke volume. Acta Physiol. Scand., 49:279-298, 1960.
6. Björnesjö, K. B., Kinwall, B., and Waller, Å.: Effect of surgery on protein metabolism with special attention to distribution of amino nitrogen between erythrocytes and plasma. Acta Chir. Scand., 128:449-459, 1964.
7. Brun, C., Knudsen, E. O. E., and Raaschou, F.: The influence of posture on the kidney function. Acta Med. Scand., 122:332-341, 1945.
8. Caldwell, F. T., Jr.: Metabolic response to thermal trauma II. Nutritional studies with rats at two environmental temperatures. Ann. Surg., 155:119-126, 1962.
9. Campbell, R. M., and Cuthbertson, D. P.: Effect of environmental temperature on the metabolic response to injury. Nature, 210:206-208, 1966.
10. Carlson, L. A., Boberg, J., and Högstedt, B.: Some physiological and clinical implications of lipid mobilization from adipose tissue. In: Handbook of Physiology, Sect. 5, pp. 625-644. Washington, American Physiological Society, 1965.
11. Chapman, C. B., Fisher, J. N., and Sproule, B. J.: Behavior of stroke volume at rest and during exercise in human beings. J. Clin. Invest., 39:1208-1213, 1960.
12. Cope, O., Nardi, G. L., Quijano, M., Rovit, R. L., Stanbury, J. B., and Wight, A.: Metabolic rate and thyroid function following acute thermal trauma in man. Ann. Surg., 137:165-174, 1953.
13. Cuthbertson, D. P.: The influence of prolonged muscular rest on metabolism. Biochem. J., 23:1328-1345, 1929.
14. Cuthbertson, D. P.: Observations on the disturbance of metabolism produced by injury to the limbs. Quart. J. Med., 1:233-246, 1932.

15. Darling, R. C.: The significance of physical fitness. Arch. Phys. Med., 28:140-145, 1947.
16. Deitrick, J. E., Whedon, G. D., and Shorr, E.: Effects of immobilization upon various metabolic and physiologic functions of normal man. Am. J. Med., 4:3-36, 1948.
17. Drucker, W. R., Schlatter, J., and Drucker, R. P.: Metabolic factors associated with endotoxin-induced tolerance for hemorrhagic shock. Surgery, 64:75-84, 1968.
18. Duke, J. H., Jr., Jorgensen, S. B., Broell, J., Long, C. L., and Kinney, J. M.: The contribution of protein to the caloric expenditure following injury. Surgery, 68:168-174, 1970.
19. Engel, F. L.: Metabolic aspects of hemorrhagic and traumatic shock. In: *Conference on Shock and Circulatory Homeostasis*, 2nd edition. Princeton, N. J., 1952. Transactions, pp. 26-161. New York, Josiah Macy Jr. Foundation, 1953.
20. Engel, F. L., Harrison, H. C., and Long, C. N. H.: Biochemical studies on shock. III. The role of the liver and the hepatic circulation in the metabolic changes during hemorrhagic shock in the rat and the cat. J. Exp. Med., 79:9-22, 1944.
21. Engel, F. L., Winton, M. G., and Long, C. N. H.: Biochemical studies on shock. I. The metabolism of amino acids and carbohydrate during hemorrhagic shock in the rat. J. Exp. Med., 77:397-410, 1943.
22. Epstein, F. H., Goodyear, A. V. N., Lawrason, F. D., and Relman, A. S.: Studies on the antidiuresis of quiet standing: The importance of changes in plasma volume and glomerular filtration rate. J. Clin. Invest., 30:63-72, 1951.
23. Everson, T. C., and Fritschel, M. J.: The effect of surgery on the plasma levels of the individual essential amino acids. Surgery, 31:226-232, 1952.
24. Foster, G. L., Schoenheimer, R., and Rittenberg, D.: Studies in protein metabolism. V. The utilization of ammonia for amino acid and creatine formation in animals. J. Biol. Chem., 127:319-327, 1939.
25. Fuller, J. H., Bernauer, E. M., and Adams, W. C.: Renal function, water and electrolyte exchange during bed rest with daily exercise. Aerospace Med., 41:60-72, 1970.
26. Gauer, O. H., and Thron, H. L.: Postural changes in the circulation. In: *Handbook of Physiology*, Sect. 2, v. 3, pp. 2409-2439. Washington, American Physiological Society, 1965.
27. Gilder, H., DeLeon, V., Sternberg, D., and Valcic, M.: Effect of diet on body composition changes after experimental injury in rats. Metabolism, 18:509-518, 1969.
28. Grande, F.: Nutrition and energy balance in body composition studies. In: *Conference on Techniques for Measuring Body Composition*, Natick, Mass., 1959. Proceedings edited by J. Brožek and A. Henschel, pp. 168-188. Washington D. C., National Academy of Sciences, National Research Council, 1961.
29. Heath, D. F., and Stoner, H. B.: Studies on the mechanism of shock. Non-esterified fatty acid metabolism in normal and injured rats. Brit. J. Exp. Path., 49:160-169, 1968.
30. Holmgren, A., and Ovenfors, C. O.: Heart volume at rest and during muscular work in the supine and in the sitting position. Acta Med. Scand., 167:267-277, 1960.
31. Jarnum, S., and Lassen, N. A.: Albumin and transferrin metabolism in infectious and toxic diseases. Scand. J. Clin. Lab. Invest., 13:357-368, 1961.
32. Keys, A.: Introduction to the symposium on convalescence and rehabilitation. Fed. Proc., 3:189, 1944.
33. Kinney, J. M.: Energy deficits in acute illness and injury. In: *Proceedings of a Conference on Energy Metabolism and Body Fuel Utilization*, pp. 167-188. Cambridge, Harvard University Printing Office, 1966.
34. Kinney, J. M.: The effect of injury on metabolism. Brit. J. Surg., 54:435-437, 1967.
35. Kinney, J. M., and Roe, C. F.: Caloric equivalent of fever. I. Patterns of postoperative response. Ann. Surg., 156:610-622, 1962.
36. Kjellberg, S. R., Rudhe, U., and Sjöstrand, T.: Increase of the amount of hemoglobin and blood volume in connection with physical training. Acta Physiol. Scand., 19:146-151, 1949.
37. Krebs, H. A.: Considerations concerning the pathways of synthesis in living matter; Synthesis of glycogen from non-carbohydrate precursors. Johns Hopkins Hospital Bull., 95:19-33, 1954.
38. Kukral, J. C., Riveron, E., Tiffany, J. C., Vaitys, S., and Barrett, B.: Plasma protein metabolism in patients with acute surgical peritonitis. Am. J. Surg., 113:173-182, 1967.
39. LaBrosse, E. H., Beech, J. A., McLaughlin, J. S., Mansberger, A. R., Keene, W. D., III, and Cowley, R. A.: Plasma amino acids in normal humans and patients with shock. Surg. Gynecol. Obstet., 125:516-520, 1967.
40. Levine, R.: Analysis of the actions of the hormonal antagonists of insulin. Diabetes, 13:362-365, 1964.
41. Long, C. L., Spencer, J. L., Kinney, J. M., and Geiger, J. W.: Carbohydrate metabolism in normal man and the effect of glucose infusion. J. Appl. Physiol., 31 (1):10, 1971.
42. Long, C. L., Spencer, J. L., Kinney, J. M., and Geiger, J. W.: Carbohydrate metabolism in man: effect of elective operation and major injury. J. Appl. Physiol., 31 (1):18, 1971.

43. Man, E. B., Bettcher, P. G., Cameron, C. M., and Peters, J. P.: Plasma alpha-amino acid nitrogen and serum lipids of surgical patients. J. Clin. Invest., 25:701-708, 1946.

44. McCormick, J. R., Lien, W. M., Herman, A. H., and Egdahl, R. H.: Glucose and insulin metabolism during shock in the dog. Surg. Forum, 20:12-14, 1969.

45. Milstein, S. W., and Coalson, R. E.: Depot fat depletion following thermal trauma. Am. J. Physiol., 193:75-78, 1958.

46. Moore, F. D.: Bodily changes in surgical convalescence. I. The normal sequence — observations and interpretations. Ann. Surg., 137:289-315, 1953.

47. Moore, F. D., and Ball, M. R.: The Metabolic Response to Surgery. Springfield, Ill., Charles C Thomas, 1952.

48. Moore, F. D., Langohr, J. L., Ingebretsen, M., and Cope, O.: The role of exudate losses in the protein and electrolyte imbalance of burned patients. Ann. Surg., 132:1-19, 1950.

49. Moore, F. D., Olsen, K. H., McMurrey, J. D., Parker, H. V., Ball, M. R., and Boyden, C. M.: *The Body Cell Mass and Its Supporting Environment: Body Composition in Health and Disease.* Philadelphia, W. B. Saunders Company, 1963.

50. Munro, H. N., and Cuthbertson, D. P.: The response of protein metabolism to injury. (Abstract.) Biochem. J., 37:xii, 1943.

51. Nardi, G. L.: "Essential" and "nonessential" amino acids in the urine of severely burned patients. J. Clin. Invest., 33:847-854, 1954.

52. Peters, J. P.: Protein metabolism. In: (A. Grollman, ed.) *Clinical Physiology; the Functional Pathology of Disease*, pp. 115–159. McGraw-Hill Book Co., Inc., New York, 1957.

53. Porte, D., Jr., Graber, A. L., Kuzuya, T., and Williams, R. H.: The effect of epinephrine on immunoreactive insulin levels in man. J. Clin. Invest., 45:228-236, 1966.

54. Reiss, E., Pearson, E., and Artz, C. P.: The metabolic response to burns. J. Clin. Invest., 35:62-67, 1956.

55. Ross, H., Welborn, T. A., Johnston, I. D. A., and Wright, A. D.: Effect of abdominal operation on glucose tolerance and serum levels of insulin, growth hormone, and hydrocortisone. Lancet, 2:563-566, 1966.

56. Russell, J. A., and Long, C. N. H.: Amino nitrogen in liver and muscle of rats in shock after hemorrhage. Am. J. Physiol., 147:175-180, 1946.

57. Russell, J. A., Long, C. N. H., and Engel, F. L.: Biochemical studies on shock. II. The role of the peripheral tissues in the metabolism of protein and carbohydrate during hemorrhagic shock in the rat. J. Exp. Med., 79:1-7, 1944.

58. San Pietro, A., and Rittenberg, D.: A study of the rate of protein synthesis in humans. II. Measurement of the metabolic pool and the rate of protein synthesis. J. Biol. Chem., 201:457-473, 1953.

59. Schoenheimer, R., Ratner, S., and Rittenberg, D.: Studies in protein metabolism. X. The metabolic activity of body proteins investigated with L(–)-Leucine containing two isotopes. J. Biol. Chem., 130:703-732, 1939.

60. Schønheyder, F., Heilskov, N. S. C., and Olesen, K.: Isotopic studies on the mechanism of negative nitrogen balance produced by immobilization. Scand. J. Clin. Lab. Invest., 6:178-188, 1954.

61. Sevitt, S.: *Burns: Pathology and Therapeutic Applications.* London, Butterworth, 1957.

62. Shafiroff, B. G. P., Doubilet, H., Preiss, A. L., and Co Tui: The effect of thoracic duct drainage and hemorrhage on the blood and lymph. Surg. Gynecol. Obstet., 76:547-550, 1943.

63. Sjöstrand, T.: Volume and distribution of blood and their significance in regulating the circulation. Physiol., Rev., 33:202-228, 1953.

64. Sjöstrand, T.: Blood volume. In: *Handbook of Physiology*, Sect. 2, v. 1, pp. 51-62. Washington, American Physiological Society, 1962.

65. Spence, H. Y., Evans, E. I., and Forbes, J. C.: The influence of a special high protein diet on protein regeneration in the surgical patient. Ann. Surg., 124:131-141, 1946.

66. Stoner, H. B., and Threlfall, C. J.: The effect of nucleotide and ischaemic shock on the level of energy-rich phosphates in the tissues. Biochem. J., 58:115-122, 1954.

67. Stoner, H. B., and Threlfall, C. J.: The effect of limb ischaemia on carbohydrate distribution and energy transformation. In: H. B. Stoner and C. J. Threlfall, eds.: *Symposium on the Biochemical Response to Injury*, Vienna, 1958, pp. 105-128. Oxford, Blackwell Scientific Publications, 1960.

68. Studley, H. O.: Percentage of weight loss, a basic indicator of surgical risk in patients with chronic peptic ulcer. J.A.M.A., 106:458-460, 1936.

69. Traver, H., and Schmidt, C. L. A.: Radioactive sulfur studies. I. Synthesis of methionine. II. Conversion of methionine sulfur to taurine sulfur in dogs and rats. III. Distribution of sulfur in the proteins of animals fed sulfur or methionine. IV. Experiments in vitro with sulfur and hydrogen sulfide. J. Biol. Chem., 146:69-84, 1942.

70. Taylor, F. H. L., Levenson, S. M., Davidson, C. S., and Adams, M. A.: Abnormal nitrogen metabolism in patients with thermal burns. New England J. Med., *229*:855–859, 1943.
71. Taylor, H. L., Erickson, L., Henschel, A., and Keys, A.: The effect of bed rest on the blood volume of normal young men. Am. J. Physiol., *144*:227–232, 1945.
72. Thoren, C.: Cardiomyopathy in Friedreich's ataxia, with studies of cardio-vascular and respiratory function. Acta Paediat., *53*(Suppl. 153):1–136, 1964.
73. Van Slyke, D. D., Phillips, R. A., Hamilton, P. B., Archibald, R. M., Dole, V. P., and Emerson, K., Jr.: Effect of shock on the kidney. Trans. Assoc. Amer. Physicians, *58*:119–127, 1944.
74. Waterfield, R. L.: The effect of posture on the volume of the leg. J. Physiol. (London), *72*:121–131, 1931.
75. Whedon, G. D., Deitrick, J. E., and Shorr, E.: Modification of the effects of immobilization upon metabolic and physiologic functions of normal men by the use of an oscillating bed. Am. J. Med., *6*:684–711, 1949.
76. Wray, J. B.: Alterations in muscle and liver glycogen secondary to fracture. Metabolism, *13*:551–556, 1964.

Chapter 13

OBESITY*

by E. R. Buskirk, Ph.D.

INTRODUCTION

Obesity is an accumulation of excess body fat stored in adipose tissue rather than large body size or weight. An arbitrary but useful rule is to label a man obese if more than 20 per cent of his body weight is in stored fat (a woman if more than 25 per cent).

The recommended body weight obtained from tables of height and weight and a rough description of body build does not provide an accurate assessment of body fatness, but a skilled clinical appraisal of body conformation for "soft roundness" is useful, providing it is recognized as being gross quantitation.

Obesity affects approximately one half the population of the United States and is associated with a number of health problems:

1. Changes in the regulation or regulated level of various body functions.

2. An association with a higher incidence of certain diseases, including diabetes mellitus, arteriosclerosis, coronary artery disease and hypertension.

3. An increase in the severity or complications of an established disease. As an example, the risk of surgery is heightened because of difficulty in operating through a mass of fat, anesthetic gases may have variable rates of storage or release and postoperatively the obese patient may not move or breathe as well as a normal subject.

4. An increase in psychological disorders which may alter metabolic patterns as well as adversely affect mental health.

*Original data reported in this chapter were obtained during investigations supported by PHS Research Grant No. AM 08311 from the National Institute of Arthritis and Metabolic Diseases, Bethesda, Maryland.

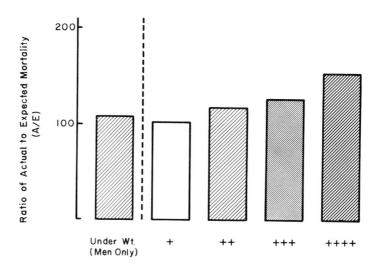

Extent of Overweight

Figure 13−1 Ratio of actual (A) to expected (E) mortality from all causes for men and women aged 15 to 69 years. Subjects were classified according to extent of overweight. (Modified from *Build and Blood Pressure Study*, Vol. 1. Chicago, Society of Actuaries, 1959.)

5. The obese person is limited in his mobility because of the added energy necessary to move his excessively fat body. This becomes a major problem in the patient with motor disorders or cardiovascular limitations in whom there is organic cause for a limited energy ceiling.

Obesity in itself may not be directly responsible for the increased morbidity and mortality associated with being overweight. Many factors contribute to the development of obesity, and the actual excess weight may not be directly correlated with the physiological and pathological status of the patient.

However, obesity can certainly contribute to disease; for example, it may serve as a respiratory stress. As adiposity develops, there is an increased effort in breathing, owing to the expanded mass of the chest wall and elevation of the diaphragm. Extra effort is also required to compress a massive abdomen. Inspiratory and expiratory capacities are reduced, as is the fast component of expiration. Increased kyphosis may develop, leading to pulmonary inefficiency and uneven ventilation-perfusion ratios in various sections of the lung. Lying down forces the diaphragm further upward and reduces the inspiratory and expiratory reserves. Breathlessness on exertion may result because the depth of breathing is compromised, and the only way increased ventilation can occur is by the patient's breathing more rapidly. Plethora, hypoxia, hypercapnia, respiratory acidosis, somnolence and pulmonary hypertension may ensue—this has been termed the "Pickwickian syndrome." Conversely, impending chronic pulmonary failure can lead to obesity because the breathlessness on exertion stimulates the afflicted to avoid exercise.[4, 7, 11, 28, 37]

In view of the above and similar considerations, it is important to consider the management of weight reduction regimens for the obese and the prevention of obesity at all ages.

FACTORS ASSOCIATED WITH THE DEVELOPMENT AND MAINTENANCE OF OBESITY

Several factors have been associated with the development and maintenance of obesity (Fig. 13-2). Obesity genes have been identified in several species, including the mouse, rat, dog and chicken, but they have not been identified in man. Obese parents tend to have obese children and thin parents tend to have thin children, but the interaction of environmental factors, such as familial cooking, eating and physical activity habits, with genetically transmitted factors makes it difficult to assess the relative contribution of each. Adopted children who are thin may not become obese even though their foster parents are obese, and twins separated from their parents or from each other when young often retain the obesity trait even though raised in an environment favorable to weight reduction. Children who are obese at birth probably have an "obesity gene." The physical characterization of obesity is not established, but according to Bjurulf[5] the number of fat cells probably reflects the inherited tendency for fat accumulation (endogenous factor), whereas the fat cell size reflects relative overnutrition (exogenous fat factor).

A defect in regulation of appetite, of satiety or of physical activity may predispose the individual to obesity. An increase in appetite or a decrease in satiety can cause overeating. A decrease in activity and energy expenditure may result in a caloric imbalance and an accumulation of fat. Regulatory defects may occur at a single meal or persist for a longer period. If over a time more calories are taken in than are consumed, accumulation of body fat occurs and obesity results. Various body areas and organs are involved in the regulation of caloric balance; these include the cerebral cortex, hypothalamus, thalamus, gastrointestinal tract, liver, pancreas, pituitary, thyroid, adrenals, adipose tissue and perhaps skeletal muscle, plus the various neural interconnections (see Figure 13-3).[20]

Figure 13–2 Interaction scheme for development and maintenance of obesity.

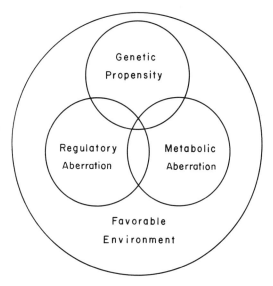

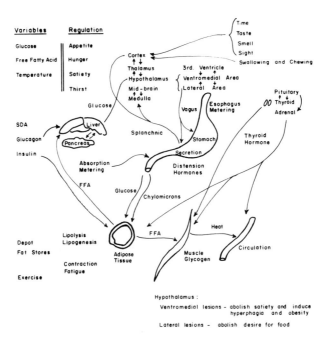

Figure 13–3   Some possible regulatory interrelationships. (Adapted from Mayer: *Overweight: Causes, Cost, and Control.* Englewood Cliffs, N.J., Prentice-Hall, 1968.)

Metabolic aberrations leading to the development of obesity have not been well defined, but various investigators have suspected that in some obese patients there are abnormalities in the rate at which fat is deposited in or mobilized from adipose tissue. Abnormalities have also been suggested in the rate of absorption of foodstuffs from the gastrointestinal tract, in the rate of the incorporation of metabolic products into adipose tissue or in the rate of metabolism of foodstuffs in the peripheral tissues, which are presumably under the influence of circulating thyroid hormone. Distinct metabolic abnormalities in man have been shown in the various types of hyperlipemias and lipoidoses and in severe adrenal malfunction or hypothyroidism.[6, 19, 25, 31]

Environment plays a role in the regulation of energy expenditure and in caloric intake. Many people are employed in sedentary occupations and avoid active recreational pursuits. On the other hand, they are continuously exposed to attractively packaged food and drink. Man is tempted to eat many readily available foods for their taste alone and to disregard satiety signals and nutritional value. If caloric intake is not watched, it is easy to add body fat insidiously. In addition, because we live in air conditioned environments and have the benefit of good clothing, we rarely need to increase metabolic heat production to maintain body temperature. Thus, both environmental and cultural factors favor accumulation of added fat stores.

CALORIC TURNOVER

Imbalance of caloric intake and output causes obesity, but the commonly held view that exercise expends relatively little energy is wrong. Exercise is the only factor that leads to a major increase in energy expenditure, and the performance of more exercise does not necessarily increase food intake. It has been demonstrated that regular participation in exercise programs results in body weight loss by fat individuals.[8, 10, 23] Tables of caloric requirements and dietary allowances list values that increase as the classification of physical activity changes. For men, the range in daily caloric requirements – depending on age, body size and physical activity – ranges from 2000 to 5000 Kcal per day. When energy expenditure exceeds 4000 Kcal per day in an occupational group, one seldom sees obesity.

Unfortunately, regular exercise has never been popular with many obese women and a number of obese men. Accumulation of excess body fat impairs movement and normal motor patterns and increases the energy required for a given task. Thus, a vicious circle is created whereby unusual or uncomfortable movement promotes inactivity and the assumption of a more sedentary way of life. Once obesity has developed and a sedentary life is assumed, body fat stores are preserved even with relatively low caloric intakes because daily energy expenditure is low. It is not unusual to observe an obese man in caloric balance at 2200 to 2400 Kcal per day or an obese woman at 1800 to 2000 Kcal per day. This achievement of energy equilibrium at low caloric intakes has led to the concept "she eats very little and doesn't lose weight." The observation is correct, but the low daily energy expenditure accounts for it.

If the active man overeats slightly, weight gain is limited by the increased energy required to move his added weight. During activity energy expenditure is directly proportional to body weight because the body mass must be accelerated, decelerated, lifted, and so on. In contrast, the inactive man does not use this weight limiting mechanism because he moves his body mass less.

The energy level at which metabolic balance occurs is proportional to the total active tissue or cell mass of the body. Under resting conditions the liver, heart, kidneys, nervous system, endocrine glands and other organs provide the major portion of metabolic activity.[16] Overeating increases the cell mass of these organs only slightly, and resting metabolic rate changes little. Increased physical activity causes skeletal muscle hypertrophy, and the resting metabolic rate increase is proportional to the increase in muscle mass. However, muscle accounts for only 25 per cent or less of the total resting metabolism, so the net effect is small.

A sudden decrease in physical activity, as may occur after a job change or as a result of trauma or illness, may cause obesity if a relatively high food intake is maintained. Many obese people begin to accumulate weight under such circumstances.

Careful studies of caloric balance in obese patients undergoing diets or exercise, or both, indicate clearly that calories can be accounted for accurately and that both caloric restriction and exercise play synergistic roles in reduction of body fat stores. It is important to realize that both diet and physical activity can be voluntarily regulated, albeit with considerable difficulty for some individuals.

The relationship of appetite, inactivity and body fatness can be observed in the very young. Infants show only a moderate association between food intake and growth but a more marked association between food intake and physical activity. Fat babies may have moderate food intakes and be inactive, whereas thin babies may have large intakes but be very active. Thus, the habit of inactivity starts at an early age and may mean development of obesity in later life.[20]

In our society many women, especially housewives, are more active than men. They shop, carry groceries, chase the children, perform housework and may be on their feet and moving most of the day. Many husbands, in contrast, are grossly inactive. They ride to work, sit at the office and watch television in the evening. Their "activities" consist of riding in a golf cart or sitting in a boat. Inactivity may well be the most important factor in the creeping deposition of body fat in the middle years.

PREVENTION OF OBESITY

Until it is possible to detect the cause of obesity in each patient, preventive measures must be based on reducing food intake and increasing energy expenditure. Prevention of obesity is easier than treatment, particularly if prevention is initiated during childhood.

Any diet selected for weight control must be nutritionally sound and yet recognize the likes, dislikes and eating practices of the individual. Overeating at night cannot be condoned, but it may be more beneficial to allow controlled food intake at the time desired than to attempt to abolish an established pattern. Breakfast is often skipped by the dieter, yet this meal is important if symptoms of hypoglycemia and hyperketonemia during the day are to be avoided. Individual differences in hunger and satiety patterns may dictate the size and frequency of meals. There is little evidence that men lose weight if they have frequent small meals, as has been suggested in some popular magazines. Many men do not feel hungry until they start eating—then they find that they cannot stop. They are obviously poor candidates for the frequent small meal routine. Others get hungry with any form of caloric restriction. Frequent small meals should satisfy this type of person, although he may have to experience a life of hunger if he attempts to control his body fatness through diet alone. Fad diets can be effective for short periods of time, but they have little long lasting worth and should be avoided. There is some merit in eating slowly to allow the satiety mechanisms, both regulatory and psychological, time to operate. Education in the nutritive and caloric values of foods is essential if obesity is to be prevented.

A person who cannot reduce his food intake enough to control his overweight can only prevent obesity by an increase in physical activity. Regular use of activities such as walking, jogging, cycling, skating, swimming distances, and so on, is most effective for weight loss. It is important that the young be encouraged to learn skills that enable them to enjoy activities that involve transport of their body weight. Hiking, tennis, cross-country skiing, skating and swimming are such skills. These activities are frequently neglected in our physical education instruction programs, whereas competitive sports that cannot be enjoyed in later life are emphasized. The goal, for purposes of weight control and prevention of obesity, is to achieve a regular exercise pattern with activities of reasonable intensity that are well within one's physical capacity.[22, 23, 35]

TREATMENT OF OBESITY

Diagnosis of the cause of obesity is important if a body fat reduction program is planned. A carefully recorded history of gain in weight is essential. In the few persons who are obese because of endocrine disorders such as hypothyroidism, hypogonadism (in men) and hyperadrenocorticism, treatment is directed at the underlying disease. Overweight caused by fluid retention, as in congestive heart failure or renal dysfunction, must also be treated.[2, 34, 35]

Hyperlipemia alone, or in association with hypercholesterolemia, can be treated by restricting dietary fat with consequent reduction to a more ideal weight. To what extent the substitution of unsaturated fats for saturated ones may reduce triglyceride levels in essentially familial hyperlipemia is not clear.[31] Obesity is associated with diabetes, so a glucose tolerance curve is important for clinical purposes.

If poor dietary habits are present in a patient, the familial, economic and psychological background for these habits should be assessed. Patterns of appetite, satiety and physical activity should also be made to determine the energy balance of the patient.

In the absence of demonstrable disease, treatment should include the use of diet, pharmacological aids and exercise.

The characteristics of a patient most likely to benefit from a weight reduction program are as follows:[35, 40]

1. Slightly or moderately overweight.

2. The patient became overweight as an adult and has not tried to lose weight before.

3. The patient desires weight reduction and is sufficiently well adjusted emotionally to pursue this goal.

Diet

In a successful weight control program the patient must match his caloric balance throughout his life. This is easier to maintain if the individual's cultural patterns and habits are taken into consideration in planning the diet.

The caloric equivalent of body weight loss increases as diet restriction is

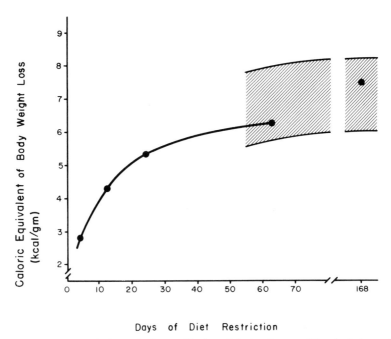

Days of Diet Restriction

Figure 13—4   Mean caloric equivalents of body weight loss in man. The shaded area indicates the equilibrium range of values with sustained negative caloric balance.

continued (see Figure 13-4). Initially the weight loss is primarily water, but as time passes progressively more fat is metabolized and the caloric equivalent approaches (but never reaches) the value for pure fat, i.e., 9.0 to 9.4 Kcal per gm. During dietary restriction, cell substance, including protein matrix, and extracellular fluid are also lost.[8, 16]

The caloric equivalent of the weight loss varies with the type and severity of diet restriction, the salt content of the diet, the length of time that diet restriction is in force, the type and duration of the exercise program and the extent of obesity.[8, 15, 16]

Diets that provide less than 1000 Kcal per day for women and 1500 Kcal per day for men are poorly tolerated over long periods of time, although successful ward or clinic regimens utilizing lower caloric intakes have been completed.[10, 18] A successful diet that leads to a weight reduction of 0.45 Kg or one pound per week yields a yearly loss of 23.2 Kg or 52 pounds. Unless patients are under careful supervision, a sustained weight loss exceeding 0.7 Kg, or about 1.5 pounds, per week may be considered excessive and the diet should be adjusted upwards. The long-term potential is frequently overlooked because of disappointment in the small weekly loss.

It is important to teach the patients what is a usual serving or portion of food and to teach them the value of restricting alcohol consumption. Vitamin supplements are not necessary when they are getting a balanced, though restricted, diet.

Many different diets have been proposed, but in the long run their success in inducing reduction of body fat stores depends on how much they induce negative caloric balance. Kekwick and Pawan[18] found that high fat diets fail to alter, except transiently, the equilibrium between lipolysis and lipogenesis. Varying the proportion of fat, carbohydrate and protein failed to produce unique weight loss patterns.[13]

Restriction of sodium chloride and the use of artificial sweeteners are commonly associated with diets. Until recently, there was little reason to prohibit artificial sweeteners, but the restriction of cyclamates and the possible restriction on saccharin may make artificial sweeteners unavailable. Although their role in weight reduction is relatively minor, they do provide a psychological crutch. If hypertension or water retention and edema is present along with obesity, sodium chloride restriction may be recommended.

The use of liquid diets or of simple convenience foods seems to be declining in popularity as a regular dietary restriction technique. Many obese patients have found that long-term employment of formulas is impractical, although these diets have helped in long-term caloric balance experiments.[10] If formulas are employed, a useful technique is to use them to replace only one meal.

Fasting has been used in several experimental investigations of weight loss. The advantages of employing fasting in a weight loss regimen, according to Drenick,[12] are as follows:

1. There is no hunger at least after the first seven days.
2. Weight loss is rapid.
3. The patient may convince himself that he can control his compulsive eating.
4. The patient feels that fasting is simpler than dieting.

However, because fasting may result in many physiological and metabolic effects careful medical supervision is necessary. The physiological effects of fasting include postural hypotension due to the sodium, potassium and water excretion, continued potassium excretion with possible depletion, reduced gastric secretory activity and bowel function, ketoacidemia and metabolic acidosis (including citric acidosis and lactacidemia), erosion of protein stores, magnesium loss with possible muscle irritability and cramping, contraction of red blood cell mass and plasma and blood volumes, hyperuricemia and acute gout.[12, 15, 34] Acute gout is thought to be due to the competition of ketoacid with uric acid for excretion by the kidney and to the retention of uric acid. Hair loss and emotional disturbances may be observed.[12]

Group Therapy

Social reinforcement of a weight reduction plan has had great success. Physicians frequently lack the time to ease the psychological burden associated with caloric deprivation, and support of a group of other patients may be helpful. Together the patients, with professional supervision, can help each other to resolve the stresses and anxiety that provoke overeating and to place the weight loss goals in perspective.[34, 36]

Exercise

Exercise can be an important factor in a successful weight reduction regimen. The largest single factor on the energy expenditure side of the energy balance equation is exercise or physical work. During peak work loads man can increase his metabolic rate up to 20 times his resting level. Above a minimum rate of energy turnover, regulation of food intake appears closely related to energy expenditure.[21] This relationship may not hold, however, for obese men and women, for it has been repeatedly shown that if obese subjects exercise the equivalent of 300 Kcal per day or more, a slow reduction in body fat stores occurs, even though the subjects have free choice of meals (see Figure 13-5).[8, 10, 23]

The ability to deliver oxygen to working muscles (aerobic capacity) and its rate of utilization by these muscles may be reduced in the obese, depending on their sex, age, disability or past exercise history. On a per kilogram basis, their aerobic capacity is definitely low. Thus, their relative fitness to perform hard work is reduced, and the obese individual voluntarily regulates his activities at relatively low levels of work intensity.[8]

The physical activity habit is hard to develop in fat people. Several studies have shown that obese subjects—especially men—are less active than the non-obese and generally do not continue to exercise when they leave a supervised program.[8]

Obese men may eat more to compensate for exercise than other men. An obese subject who is made more active during certain periods of the day often becomes less active during the remainder of the day, especially if he is on a reduced caloric intake. A combination of diet restriction and exercise may, therefore, produce a negative caloric balance that is less than would be anticipated. Even with caloric restriction, however, obese subjects lose more fat when they exercise regularly than when they do not.[10]

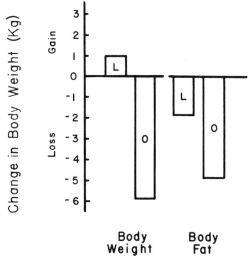

Figure 13–5   Average gain or loss in body weight and fat in sedentary young men who participated in a regular exercise program for 10 weeks (L-lean; O-obese).

Drugs and Chemical Agents

As knowledge of the regulation of food and physical activity increases, it may become possible to manufacture and utilize drugs that have specific sites of action as well as specific effects, i.e., a satiety stimulant as contrasted with an appetite depressant. The man who continues to overeat and fails to experience hunger will not be helped by an appetite depressant. Similarly, drug stimulation of a physical activity "go" center could have important therapeutic ramifications for an obese patient. At present specific drugs are not available.

The use of pharmacological aids to weight reduction cannot be viewed as a permanent tool for weight control except in specific endocrinological or metabolic disorders. The drugs that have been employed include diuretics, thyroid hormones and sympathomimetic amines. The *Physicians' Desk Reference* (1970) lists 51 different drugs in the last category that have been used to promote weight reduction.

Diuretics induce body water loss and have no effect on lipid stores in adipose tissue. A diuretic should be used only if the patient retains excess water and sodium; routine use of diuretics for purposes of weight reduction is untenable.

Thyroid function is usually normal in obese patients. Unless a definite deficiency can be established, supplementary hormone treatment has no long-term value in weight reduction and can cause unnecessary complications.

Sympathomimetic amines are administered because they suppress appetite in some patients, although the mechanism for this action is not known. Short-term effectiveness has been reported, but tolerance develops and side effects, which include irritability, tenseness, insomnia and sweating on forehead and palms, are numerous. For patients with heart disease, the mimetic effects on heart rate and work and on blood pressure make their usage hazardous.

Other Forms of Treatment

Surgical bypass or removal of a portion of the small intestine to reduce the absorption of foodstuffs into the body has been employed as a temporary or permanent cure for severe persistent obesity. These procedures have had some success but often led to complications, including vitamin and mineral deficiences. Frequently, supplementation of potassium and calcium were required.[24, 39] Surgical removal of excess adipose tissue has been employed as a cosmetic aid.

TEMPERATURE REGULATION AND OBESITY

Subcutaneous fat provides thermal insulation against cold. The insulation is about four times as effective as an equivalent amount of fat-free tissue. Performance of a fixed work task in the cold without adequate clothing is accomplished by the obese person with a lower body surface temperature but a higher core temperature than a lean person.[9]

Performance of a fixed work task, involving transport of body weight, in moderate heat causes greater thermal strain on the obese. A higher metabolic

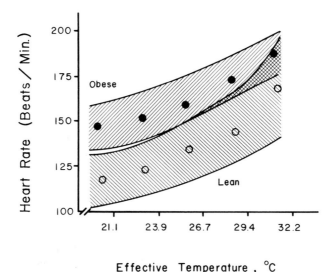

Effective Temperature , °C

Figure 13—6 Heart rate response in college women (mean ± 1 S.D.) to walking on the treadmill (3 mph, 5 per cent grade) for one hour in environmental temperatures ranging from comfortable to very warm.

heat production in the obese, along with environmental heat, produces more heat to be dissipated and results in a higher heart rate and core temperature and a greater sweat rate than in the lean patient (see Figure 13-6). The number of heat activated sweat glands on the trunk of the obese young man are fewer than in the lean man presumably because of the physical separation of the glands owing to stretching of the skin.[3] At temperatures above 37°C (98.6°F) the lean tend to gain more heat from the environment because of their larger surface to mass ratio. Under these hot conditions thermal stress tends to equalize between the lean and obese if evaporation of sweat is sufficient to insure stable core temperatures. As an example of the consequence of thermal stress in the fat subject, it has been found that many of the heat injury fatalities in football occur in large, overweight young linemen during the first one or two practice sessions before they had time to acclimatize to heat.[14]

CIRCULATION AND EXERCISE AND OBESITY

The cardiovascular hemodynamics of extremely obese men and women during rest and mild exercise have been studied.[1] In the obese at rest, cardiac output and stroke volume were somewhat higher than in the lean. The central arterial-venous oxygen difference was the same[1] or lower[32] in obese subjects presumably because of the greater blood perfusion associated with more adipose tissue. During a treadmill walk, the obese used a higher cardiac output at each work condition. The systemic and pulmonary blood pressures were frequently higher in obese than in lean subjects during exercise. The heart rate of women walking at 3 mph on a 5 per cent grade under five environmental conditions is shown in Figure 13-6. The heart rates of the obese women are higher than those of the lean women at each temperature. Similar results have been shown for obese men.

Little is known of the circulatory responses of the obese to maximal or even strenuous exercise. Maximal heart rate is presumably independent of body composition. If there is no difference in maximal heart rate between the obese and lean, the obese should tend to perform a given submaximal work task at a higher percentage of their maximal heart rate.

A major finding in autopsies of obese people is a heart weight greater than the norms for the general population, but this weight is not out of proportion to total body weight. Left ventricular hypertrophy was usual.[2]

It is apparent from the above discussion that obesity is an important factor in the predisposition to diseases of various sorts. Aside from its relationship to other diseases, it is likewise apparent that obesity is a disabling condition in its own right in that it reduces the functional performance of the afflicted individual. In the rehabilitation of patients with neuromotor or cardiovascular disorders the problem becomes compounded in several ways:

1. Their disability enforces a sedentary existence through either lack of functioning muscles or decreased exercise tolerance.

2. Their previous eating habits, established when they were able-bodied, are retained and not easily changed.

We have seen patients who, having been rehabilitated from poliomyelitis to a relatively active life many years ago, have regressed to wheel chair life because of obesity. Control of obesity in patients of this type involves to an extreme degree the problems outlined in this chapter.

REFERENCES

1. Alexander, J. K.: Obesity and cardiac performance. Am. J. Cardiol., *14*:860–865, 1964.
2. Amad, K. H., Brennan, J. C. and Alexander, J. K.: The cardiac pathology of chronic exogenous obesity. Circulation, *32*:740–745, 1965.
3. Bar-Or, O., Lundegren, H. M., Magnusson, L. I. and Buskirk, E. R.: Distribution of heat-activated sweat glands in obese and lean men and women. Human Biol., *40*:235–248, 1968.
4. Bedell, G. N., Wilson, W. R. and Seebohm, P. M.: Pulmonary function in obese persons. J. Clin. Invest., *37*:1049–1060, 1958.
5. Bjurulf, P.: Micromorphologic aspects of variation in human body fat. *In: Occurrence, Cause and Prevention of Overnutrition.* 2nd Symposium of the Swedish Nutrition Foundation. Uppsala, Almqvist, 1964, pp. 95–102.
6. Brodoff, B. N. (ed.): Adipose tissue metabolism and obesity. [papers of a conference] Ann. N.Y. Acad. Sci., *131*:1–683, 1965.
7. Burwell, C. S., Robin, E. D., Whaley, R. D. and Bickelmann, A. G.: Extreme obesity associated with alveolar hypoventilation—A Pickwickian syndrome. Am. J. Med., *21*:811–818, 1956.
8. Buskirk, E. R. Increasing energy expenditure: The role of exercise. *In*: Wilson, N. L. (ed.): *Obesity.* Philadelphia, F. A. Davis Company, 1969, pp. 163–176.
9. Buskirk, E. R., Bar-Or, O. and Kollias, J.: Physiological effects of heat and cold. *In*: Wilson, N. L. (ed.): *Obesity.* Philadelphia, F. A. Davis Company, 1969, pp. 119–139.
10. Buskirk, E. R., Thompson, R. H., Lutwak, L. and Whedon, G. D.: Energy balance of obese patients during weight reduction: Influence of diet restriction and exercise. Ann. N.Y. Acad. Sci., *110*:918–940, 1963.
11. Carroll, D.: A peculiar type of cardiopulmonary failure associated with obesity. Am. J. Med., *21*:819–824, 1956.
12. Drenick, E. J.: Starvation in the management of obesity. *In*: Wilson, N. L. (ed.): *Obesity.* Philadelphia, F. A. Davis Company, 1969, pp. 191–203.

13. Fletcher, R. F., McCririck, M. Y. and Crooke, A. C.: Reducing diets. Weight loss of obese patients on diets of different composition. Brit. J. Nutr., 15:53-58, 1961.
14. Fox, E. L., Mathews, D. K., Kaufman, W. S. and Bowers, R. W.: Effects of football equipment on thermal balance and energy cost during exercise. Res. Quart., 37:332-339, 1966.
15. Gilder, H., Cornell, G. N., Grafe, W. R., MacFarlane, J. R., Asaph, J. W., Stubenbord, W. T., Watkins, G. M., Rees, J. R. and Thorbjarnarson, B.: Components of weight loss in obese patients subjected to prolonged starvation. J. Appl. Physiol., 23:304-310, 1967.
16. Grande, F.: Man under caloric deficiency. In: Field, J. (ed.): Handbook of Physiology. Washington, American Physiological Society, 1964, Sect. 4, pp. 911-937.
17. Kannel, W. B., LeBauer, E. J., Dawber, T. R. and McNamara, P. M.: Relation of body weight to development of coronary heart disease. The Framingham study. Circulation, 35:734-744, 1967.
18. Kekwick, A. and Pawan, G. L. S.: Metabolic study in human obesity with isocaloric diets in fat, protein, or carbohydrate. Metabolism, 6:447-660, 1957.
19. Mayer, J.: Some aspects of the problem of regulation of food intake and obesity. New Eng. J. Med., 274:610-616, 662-673, 722-731, 1966.
20. Mayer, J.: Overweight: Causes, Cost, and Control. Englewood Cliffs, N.J., Prentice-Hall, Inc., 1968.
21. Mayer, J., Roy, P. and Mitra, K. P.: Relation between caloric intake, body weight, and physical work: Studies in an industrial male population in West Bengal. Am. J. Clin. Nutr., 4:169-175, 1956.
22. Mayer, J. and Thomas, D. W.: Regulation of food intake and obesity. Science, 156:328-337, 1967.
23. Moody, D. L., Kollias, J. and Buskirk, E. R.: The effect of a moderate exercise program on body weight and skinfold thickness in overweight college women. Med. Sci. Sports, 1:75-80, 1969.
24. Payne, J. H., Dewind, L. T. and Commons, R. R.: Metabolic observations in patients with jejunocolic shunts. Am. J. Surg., 106:273-289, 1963.
25. Renold, A. E. and Cahill, G. F. (eds.): Adipose tissue. In: Field, J. (ed.): Handbook of Physiology. Washington, American Physiological Society, 1965. Section 5.
26. Rodahl, K. and Issekutz, B., Jr. (eds.): Fat as a Tissue. New York, McGraw-Hill Book Company, 1964.
27. Seltzer, C. C.: Overweight and obesity: The associated cardiovascular risk. Minn. Med., 52:1265-1270, 1969.
28. Sharp, J. T., Henry, J. P., Sweany, S. K., Meadows, W. R. and Pietras, R. J.: The total work of breathing in normal and obese men. J. Clin. Invest., 43:728-739, 1964.
29. Society of Actuaries: Build and blood pressure study. Chicago, 1959, vol. 1.
30. Stallones, R. A.: Population patterns of disease and body weight. In: Wilson, N. L. (ed.): Obesity, Philadelphia, F. A. Davis Company, 1969, pp. 109-117.
31. Stanbury, J. B., Wyngaarden, J. B. and Fredrickson, D. S. (eds.): The Metabolic Basis of Inherited Disease. New York, McGraw-Hill Book Company, 1960.
32. Taylor, H. L., Brozek, J. and Keys, A.: Basal cardiac function and body composition with special reference to obesity. J. Clin. Invest., 31:976-983, 1952.
33. Thorn, G. W. and Bondy, P. K.: Gain and loss of weight. In: Harrison et al. (eds.): Principles of Internal Medicine, 3rd ed. New York, McGraw-Hill Book Company, 1958, pp. 182-197.
34. U.S. Public Health Service, Division of Chronic Diseases: Obesity and Health: A Source Book of Current Information for Professional Health Personnel. Washington, U.S. Government Printing Office, 1966.
35. Van Itallie, T. B.: Management of obesity. In: Southward, H. and Hofman, F. G. (eds.): Columbia-Presbyterian Therapeutic Talks. New York, Macmillan Company, 1963, vol. 1, pp. 163-169.
36. Weight Control Colloquium, Iowa State College, 1955. Collection of papers presented at the colloquium. Ames, Iowa State College Press, 1955.
37. Wilson, R. H. L. and Wilson, N. L.: Obesity and respiratory stress J. Am. Dietet. Assoc., 55:465-469, 1969.
38. Wilson, R. H. L. and Wilson, N. L.: Obesity and cardiorespiratory stress. In: Wilson, N. L. (ed.): Obesity. Philadelphia, F. A. Davis Company, 1969, pp. 141-151.
39. Wood, L. C. and Chremos, A. N.: Treating obesity by "short-circuiting" the small intestine. J. Am. Med. Assoc., 186:63, 1963.
40. Young, C. M.: Management of the obese patient. J. Am. Med. Assoc., 186:903-904, 1963.

Applied Physiology

Chapter 14

UROGENITAL PHYSIOLOGY

by Richard C. Mason, Ph.D.,
and John A. Downey, M.D., D.Phil. (Oxon.)

An understanding of the basic physiology of the urogenital system is important in the rehabilitation of many patients. In this chapter we will review the current status of our knowledge in this area. It should be recognized that for cultural and sociological reasons, it has been possible only recently to obtain much information about human sexual function. Earlier information had been provided primarily by comparative animal studies, and these are difficult to extrapolate to man. Studies of urinary function, however, have suffered from almost the opposite problem. As Hippocrates recommended, urinary tract disease has been treated and consequently investigated by a highly specialized group of practitioners who have tended to emphasize only the human diseases. Such exclusions have deprived clinicians of the physiological knowledge available from comparative studies of other species and physiological systems. For these and other reasons, many of the conclusions and interpretations presented in this chapter must remain tentative until confirmed by adequate descriptive and experimental studies in man. As the title of the chapter suggests, the lower urinary tract and sexual function are intimately interrelated. As evidence on this point, one need only recall the interrelationship between the expression of the micturition reflex and the level of the sex steroid testosterone in canines. The male dog micturates as a territorial marking device, but micturition is modified so that bladder emptying is not complete, as it is in the bitch. Other, but less well documented, interactions undoubtedly occur in man, such as the occurrence of nocturnal priapism and emission accompanying bladder distention, which may be examples of this type of interaction. To the authors' knowledge, they have not been described in physiological terms.

Urogenital function cannot be considered as either primarily urinary or primarily genital, nor can it be divorced from other, more general homeostatic functions. For the sake of clarity, however, the following discussion will be subdivided along more classical lines.

PHYSIOLOGY OF SEX

Endocrine research during the last half-century has succeeded in elucidating the fact that secondary sex characters are controlled by a group of sex steroids whose secretion is under the control of pituitary trophic hormones, which are in turn controlled by specific peptide releasing hormones from the hypothalamus. These discoveries, when considered in conjunction with developments in the field of cytogenetics, have explained much of the mechanism of sex determination, differentiation and function.

The chromosome complement of the normal human consists of 44 autosomes that occur in 22 pairs, and two X chromosomes in the female, giving a total of 46. In the male, the 22 pairs of autosomes are accompanied by one X and one Y chromosome.

Genetic Determination of Sex

Genetic determination occurs at the time of fertilization, when the zygote is formed by the fusion of a sperm nucleus bearing either an X or a Y chromosome with the maternal X-bearing nucleus of the ova. This event, under normal circumstances, determines whether the cell of the resulting embryo will be XX or XY in chromosome composition. The differentiation of the primary and secondary sex characters, however, is not an immutable process, as a number of clinical situations demonstrate.

Current evidence suggests that the chromosomal composition of the genital ridge of the early embryo is one critical factor. For example, a genotype with one X chromosome (XO) will result in a phenotypic female with poorly developed ovaries and certain other systemic anomalies (Turner's syndrome). On the other hand, presence of a Y chromosome in combination with an X, as in the normal male (XY), or with two X chromosomes, as in the most frequent karyotype of Klinefelter's syndrome (XXY), produces a phenotypic male with testes.

At least two X chromosomes are necessary for normal ovarian development. A single X chromosome allows for the survival of the individual but not for the normal development of the ovaries. The Müllerian duct system, however, shows the normal female pattern when only a single X chromosome is present (as in the XO patient), although it remains underdeveloped unless stimulated by exogenous female sex hormones.

Presence of a Y chromosome is essential for testicular development and for the expression of the male phenotype. One or two Y chromosomes in combination with one X chromosome (XY or XYY) results in normal male gonadal differentiation and male sex hormone (androgen) secretion, whereas excess X

TABLE 14–1 EFFECT OF HUMAN CHROMOSOME COMPLEMENT ON PHENOTYPIC EXPRESSION OF SEX

Karyotype	Phenotype	Barr Bodies	Gonads	Hormones
XX	♀ Normal	1	Normal ovary	Estrogen and progesterone
XXX	♀ ± Normal	2	± Normal ovary	Estrogen and progesterone
XO	♀ Anomalies (Turner's syndrome)	0 (Negative)	Rudimentary ovary	None
XY	♂ Normal	0 (Negative)	Normal testis	Androgens
XXY	♂ Hypogonadal (Klinefelter's syndrome)	1	Sterile testis	Low androgens
XXXY	♂ Hypogonadal (Klinefelter's syndrome)	2	Sterile testis	Low androgens
XYY	♂ Normal	0 (Negative)	Normal testis	Androgens

chromosomes in the male (XXY or XXXY) prevents normal postnatal testis function, although morphogenetic induction of male structure is normal. The embryonic differentation of male sex structure appears to depend on the early secretion of small amounts of male sex hormones.[9] These observations are confirmed by the results of gonadectomy experiments in mammalian embryos, which indicate that without male gonad activation by a Y chromosome in a presumptive male, a female sex duct system develops independently of the presence or absence of ovaries.[4, 8] During male development, under the influence of a Y chromosome, the female system is actively suppressed by embryonic androgen secretion.

Table 14-1 summarizes these interrelationships. The quantitative aspects of this analysis may become more firmly established as additional cases of extreme situations are studied. For example, it would be of interest to compare hormonal secretion rates, age of menarche and menopause, and other quantifiable parameters between individuals with two, three and four X chromosomes. At present, the evidence is only suggestive of a detrimental effect of extra X chromosomes or "Barr" or "chromatin" bodies in the cells. This latter structure is observed in the interphase nuclei of various cell types and represents the condensation of one X chromosome; thus, the number of chromatin bodies is always one less than the number of X chromosomes and provides a convenient method of providing X chromosome counts in any tissue that is euploid—i.e., that has a normal complement of 46 chromosomes. Current evidence suggests that only one X chromosome at a time is functional in terms of messenger RNA synthesis in a cell. In normal females, one Barr or chromatin body is seen as a result of the condensation of the second X chromosome. In patients with abnormal numbers of X chromosomes, each nonfunctional X is represented by a separate Barr body. In the normal male, no Barr body is seen, since there is only one X chromosome.

As yet, it is impossible to present a definitive answer to the question of how X and Y chromosomes determine sex in molecular biological terms. Evidence for a specific gene locus and nucleotide sequence in the Y chromosome specifying maleness is completely lacking. The whole chromosome appears to function as a quantitative determinant. It is interesting to speculate that the suppression of one X chromosome in females to form a Barr body may be related to sex determination.

Hormonal Sex Determination

The developing human testis elaborates secretions that act to suppress the development of the female Müllerian ducts and their derivatives. The testis also produces substances that cause the masculinization of the embryonic cloaca and its derivatives. It is probable that the main hormone of the developing testis is the principal androgen of the later gonadal secretion, testosterone, but this is not established. The role of testosterone in postnatal male development is known; its actions on male secondary sex characteristics in adolescent and mature individuals range from influencing the expression of genes that produce alopecia to lowering the pitch of the voice. The androgen-responsive secondary sex characters show different thresholds and response curves to endogenous androgens. Hence, pubic hair may be the first indication of the elevation of androgen secretion that accompanies puberty, while other structures reach the adult male condition only following years of androgen stimulation.

The initial development of the female duct system is independent of hormone secretion by the ovary. Its full development, however, depends on a synergistic action of estrogens and progesterone elaborated by the ovary beginning shortly after birth. At puberty, the development of breasts, female hair pattern, genitalia and pelvic organs to adult condition is brought about by enhanced levels of secretion of progesterone and estrogen.

Sexual Function

Sexual union requires changes in both the male and the female genital organs, which are mediated and effected by the somatic, sympathetic and parasympathetic nervous systems and which are integrated by all levels of the nervous system.

Nervous reflexes and pathways in the medulla and spinal cord can, by themselves, initiate all the reflex responses and activities essential for coitus. Spinal male animals and man can respond to manipulation of the genitalia, with erection of the penis and even ejaculation. Spinal females can become pregnant and carry a child to full term. These responses and reflexes require the integrity of the lumbosacral cord. Integrity of sympathetic outflow (T12–

L2) may also may be necessary to allow posigrade ejaculation, as will be discussed later in this chapter.

The rostral areas of the central nervous system integrate and organize the neural reflexes of the lower centers into more effective sexual activity and bring them at least partially under volitional control. The higher centers have both inhibitory and facilitatory actions on the reflexes of the lower cord. Cortical stimulation by thought, sight, sound or even electrical excitation can initiate or prepare man or woman for copulation, and in physiological terms, the effect of such cortical stimulation is to remove any inhibitory effect and to increase or facilitate local reflexes. The anterior parts of the brain thus contribute an "appetitive" element to coital activity,[2, 3] and this appetite or libido seems to be influenced by the level of circulating sex hormone (testosterone or estrogen). The site of action of the hormone is not known in man but in animals includes the anterior preoptic hypothalamus.[5, 7, 10, 13] The hormones however, do not appear to modify the activity of—or to be necessary for—the excitation of the reflexes occurring at the medullary or spinal level.[1] Damage to certain areas of the brain can influence sexual activity. For example, temporal lobectomy can result in increased sexual activity in monkeys and man. The cerebral cortex is relatively unimportant in the maintenance of sexual activity in most female animals, but it is important in the male animal in the initiation of mating activity. Information in man is lacking regarding this aspect.

The quantitative nature of sex drive is an important societal problem; although androgens in the male and estrogens in the female condition the intensity of libido, they do not prescribe direction. Homosexual behavior is not the consequence of the presence or absence of a particular hormone, but is rather the result of a complex set of psychosocial behavioral patterns that are learned and reinforced by repetition. As an example, testosterone administration to a homosexual male will only intensify his homosexual drive, and a similar situation appears with estrogen administration in the human female.

Innervation of the Genitalia

Successful coitus requires erection of the penis to allow intromission into the vagina and ejaculation of semen. In the female, sexual arousal includes engorgement of the external genitalia and lubrication of the vagina. These responses require complex integrated neurovascular reflexes.

Male

The testes and the spermatic cord are innervated through the internal spermatic, the hypogastric and the vesical (pelvic) plexuses. The internal spermatic plexus, which is associated with the internal spermatic artery, contains afferent sensory fibers and also sympathetic postganglionic adrenergic nerves originating in the T12–L2 spinal segments. The vas deferens and the seminal vesicles are innervated from both the hypogastric and vesical plexuses. The nerves from the hypogastric plexus contain afferent fibers as well as sympathetic postganglionic nerves (Fig. 14–1).

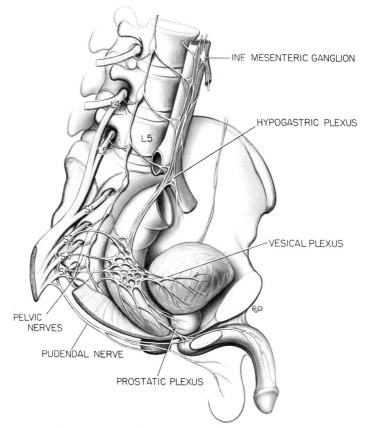

Figure 14 – 1   Anatomical relationships of the pelvic viscera and their innervation.

The nerves from the vesical plexus largely contain the parasympathetic preganglionic fibers originating in the S2–4 spinal segments and pass to the vas deferens and seminal vesicles via the pelvic nerves (nervi erigentes). Sympathetic fibers, originating in the lower thoracic–upper lumbar cord, also pass to the muscle of the vas deferens and the ductus epididymidis from the vesical plexus. The prostatic plexus of nerves lies on both sides of the prostate and innervates the prostatic urethra and the prostate gland with sympathetic and somatic afferent fibers. The sympathetic preganglionic fibers reach the prostatic plexus through the hypogastric plexus; the parasympathetic fibers arrive via the pelvic nerves. The vascular components of the penis (the corpora cavernosa and corpora urethra) are innervated through the cavernous plexus, which is intimately connected with the prostatic and vesical plexuses and contains sympathetic, parasympathetic and afferent nerves. The sympathetic and afferent nerves pass through the hypogastric plexus from the thoracolumbar spinal segments, while the parasympathetic nerves enter with the pelvic nerves.

Sensation from the skin of the penis and the glans pass to the spinal cord (S3–4) via the pudendal nerve. The motor innervation of the somatic (voluntary) muscles of the penis (the musculi ischiocavernosus and bulbocavernosus) also runs in the pudendal nerve.

Female

The ovaries receive only sympathetic innervation via the ovarian plexus, and the somatic afferent fibers mainly reach the tenth thoracic segment of the spinal cord. The fallopian tubes are largely innervated via the uterine plexus, although they also receive sympathetic and parasympathetic nerves from the ovarian and hypogastric plexuses and through the intermesenteric nerves. The somatic afferent nerves, which pass back to the spinal cord, synapse in T11–L2 segments. The uterus receives sympathetic pregangli- onic nerves from the uterovaginal plexus, which originate from the hypogas- tric plexus and the lower lumbar and sacral segments of the sympathetic trunk. Parasympathetic nerves reach the uterus via the pelvic nerves. Somatic afferent nerves from the uterus synapse at the T11–12 spinal segments. The vagina, urethra, clitoris and the labia are innervated by the lower portion of the uterovaginal plexus, consisting of both sympathetic and parasympathetic nerves. The somatic sensory fibers pass via the pudendal nerves to S2–4 of the spinal cord.

Local Responses

Male

ERECTION.   Erection of the penis is largely a vascular phenomenon. The penis consists of three cylindrical columns of erectile tissue (Fig. 14–2). The two larger masses, the corpora cavernosa penis, lie side by side above the smaller, single corpus cavernosum urethra, through which passes the urethra. At the distal end of the penis, the corpus cavernosum urethra expands to form the glans penis. Each corpus is surrounded by a dense fibrous coat, and all three are enclosed in a thick fibrous fascia. At the root of the penis, the corpora cavernosa attach to the pubic arch, and each is covered by a sheet of skeletal muscle called the ischiocavernosus. The expanded proximal portion of the corpus cavernosum urethra is covered by the bulbocavernosus muscle. The cavernous sinuses are formed by a network of vascular spaces which receive arterial blood from branches of the internal pudendal arteries. Venous blood

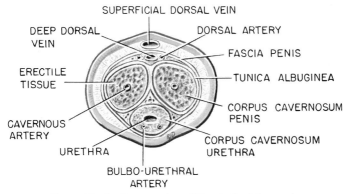

Figure 14 – 2   Cross section of the shaft of the penis.

leaves the penis by a superficial dorsal vein, which drains the glans and the corpus cavernosus urethra, while the corpora cavernosa are drained by the deep dorsal vein, which lies between the two dorsal arteries. The penis is flaccid when the vascular spaces are empty and turgid when they are filled. The arteries and vein of the penis have a dual innervation by both the sympathetic (via the hypogastric nerve) and the parasympathetic system (via pelvic nerves).

During normal erection, there is increased blood flow to the penis with engorgement and distention of the vascular channels. This increased flow is caused by dilatation of the arteries and opening of the arteriovenous shunts within the corpora as a result of activation of the cholinergic parasympathetic fibers in the pelvic nerves (S2-4). Venous return is reduced by the mechanical interference of the distended corpora and perhaps also by neurally mediated venoconstriction. Contraction of the ischiocavernosus muscle to further impede venous drainage is a minor factor in maintaining erection (Table 14-2).

After surgical sympathectomy, patients often experience impotence; this indicates the importance of the sympathetic nerves in erection, but the action of the sympathetic nerves in maintaining erection is not clear. The arterial dilatation to the corpora is mediated by the parasympathetic nerves, but it is possible that this is accompanied by a concomitant sympathetically mediated constriction of the arterioles to the rest of the penis.[15] Other explanations for

TABLE 14–2 THE MECHANISMS INVOLVED IN NORMAL ERECTION*

Sensory stimulation of genitalia → Via pudendal nerve

Psychic stimuli via cerebral cortex → Diencephalon → Spinal cord

→ Lumbosacral cord

Diminished sympathetic constrictor tone to arteries and A-V anastomosis of penis allowing dilatation → Possible constriction of blood vessels to other areas of penis

Parasympathetic efferent (S2-3-4) → Pelvic nerve (n. erigentes) → Vesical plexus → Blood vessels and A-V anastomosis of penis → Dilatation of vessels → Engorgement of corpora and possible compression of venous outflow → Erection

*(After Whitelaw, G. P. and R. H. Smithwick: Some secondary effects of sympathectomy. New Eng. J. Med., 245:121–130, 1951.)

impotence after sympathectomy include increased vascular sensitivity of the penile vascular beds to the constricting effect of circulating catecholamines, a phenomenon that is well recognized in other denervated vascular beds. Also, it is possible that sympathectomy modifies the balance of blood flow to various vascular beds, preventing appropriate constriction in one area to allow for shift and increased flow to the penile area.

Erection produced by stimulation of the penis requires an intact somatic sensory pathway (through the pudendal nerves), an intact lumbosacral cord, where a center for erection is thought to be present,[11] and the afferent parasympathetic pelvic nerves. Psychic or centrally mediated erection can occur without an intact pudendal nerve but requires an intact spinal cord.

EJACULATION AND ORGASM.   The culmination of the sexual act for the male is the propulsive expulsion of semen from the urethra, with the associated systemic and psychic phenomena. The first stage, or emission of seminal fluid, consists in the movement of spermatozoa from the vas deferens and cauda epididymidis by peristaltic contractions mediated by the sympathetic nerves. As sperm pass from the vas into the ejaculatory duct, they mix with secretions produced by the simultaneous contraction of the seminal vesicles and mix subsequently in the urethra with the prostatic contribution, the expulsion of

TABLE 14–3 THE MECHANISMS INVOLVED IN NORMAL EJACULATION*

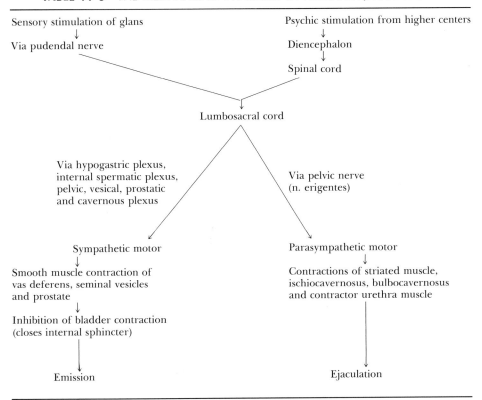

*(After Whitelaw, G. P., and R. H. Smithwick: Some secondary effects of sympathectomy. New Eng. J. Med., *245*:121–130, 1951.)

which is also dependent on sympathetic discharge. The sympathetic adrenergic nerves supply the ducts, the seminal vesicles and the prostate. When the seminal fluid distends the prostatic urethra, the bladder neck remains closed, to prevent retrograde ejaculation into the bladder.

The second stage of ejaculation begins with relaxation of the external sphincter, the passage of the seminal fluid into the penile urethra, and the spasmodic contractions of the urethra and the perineal musculature, which move the fluid to and out of the urethral meatus with propulsive force. Ejaculation is caused by stimulations of the parasympathetic motor nerves to the urethra and somatic motor fibers to the accessory muscles (compressor urethral ischiocavernosus and bulbocavernosus). Contraction of the detrusor muscle of the bladder is usually produced by activation of the parasympathetic nerves, but during ejaculation this is inhibited by activation of the sympathetic nerves to the bladder in order to: (1) avoid bladder emptying during ejaculation, and (2) prevent retrograde ejaculation through the internal sphincter into the bladder. During the sexual act, and especially during orgasm, systemic reactions occur, including hyperventilation, hypertension (both systolic and diastolic), tachycardia (up to 180 beats/min), flushing and sweating of the skin, and both local and generalized myotonia. The neurohumoral factors causing these responses have not been worked out in detail (Table 14–3).

Female

The initial response of the female genitalia to stimulation includes engorgement of the clitoris by a mechanism similar to that described for the penis, vasomotor dilation, distention and swelling of the labia (particularly the labia minora) and lubrication of the vagina by transudation of mucoid secretion through the vaginal wall. With continued sexual stimulation, the clitoris increases in diameter and length to a maximum with orgasm. The vaginal wall becomes engorged, the vault expands and elongates, and during orgasm the muscle of the vaginal wall contracts spasmodically. During the excitement phase of sexual activity, the uterus becomes engorged, elevates superiorly and anteriorly, and the cervix retracts and is directed more anteriorly. During orgasm, the woman experiences systemic muscular and cardiorespiratory changes similar to those seen in man. In both man and woman, but more so in the latter, engorgement and tumescence is seen in the breasts and nipples. The vasomotor reactions of the clitoris and labia would appear to result from inhibition of sympathetic vasoconstrictor tone and active, parasympathetically mediated vasodilation. The neural control of the vaginal secretion is not known. The motor responses of orgasm, such as contraction of the muscles of the pelvic floor and movement of the uterus, would, if analogous to the events of ejaculation in man, be mediated by both parasympathetic and somatic motor nerves from the sacral cord. In general, sexual function in women in health and disease has not been as well studied as in man. Women who have undergone sympathectomy or who have other neurological deficits can conceive and bear children, but this does not imply that these disorders have no effect on sexual function.

In summary, normal sexual function is the result of a complex, highly integrated system of neurological, physiological and psychological responses. The basic mechanical factors are partly understood, but more complex neurological and psychosocial aspects—although often they are more important—are largely unexplored.

MICTURITION

Bladder emptying in normal man comprises a highly coordinated set of reflexes controlled by various levels of the nervous sytem (Table 14-4). The fundamental basis for the reflex exists within the muscle of the bladder wall. A strip of isolated detrusor muscle responds to stretch by repeated contractions, a property it shares with other "unitary smooth muscle." The contractility in an intact bladder can be strongly facilitated or inhibited by neural influences.

The bladder usually fills slowly until it is mildly distended. A plot of pressure-volume relationships is seen in Figure 14-3. The initial introduction of fluid into a bladder causes a rather sharp increase in pressure, which quickly gives way to a flat, very slowly ascending curve. The initial pressure increase of

TABLE 14—4 THE MECHANISMS INVOLVED IN NORMAL MICTURITION

Bladder distention   Cortical Activation

(Afferents via pelvic nerve)   ←——— Brain stem ———→

                                               Inhibition   Facilitation

                              Lumbosacral cord

Somatic motor neurons   Preganglionic parasympathetic neurons

Pudendal nerve   Pelvic nerve (efferent)

External sphincter   Vesical plexus
(Ischiocavernosus)
                                         Postganglionic parasympathetic motor fibers

Inhibition of sphincter   Detrusor muscle of bladder wall

                                         Contraction of bladder

                       Micturition

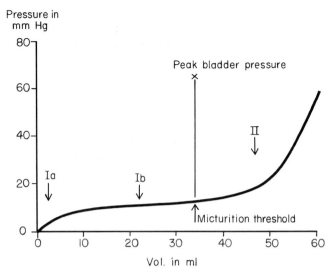

Figure 14–3 Cystometrogram showing the pressure (mm Hg) and volume (ml) in the bladder during slow filling.

the cystometrogram, phase IA, appears to be a result of purely passive physical factors. The second phase segment, IB, of the cystometrogram is almost parallel to the abscissa. The pressure during phase IB increases gradually over a wide range of filling volumes in the normal individual. This phase has been called the "tonus limb" of the cystometrogram, and the mechanisms that explain its characteristic form have been widely discussed in the classical bladder physiology literature. Presently available evidence suggests that this segment of the cystometrogram is an expression of the passive distensibility of the bladder, as it is possible to reconstruct the shape of the cystometrogram from the length-tension relationships of isolated strips of bladder muscle.

The large modulus of elasticity of bladder muscle is an important property, which accounts for the ability of the bladder to accommodate large volumes of urine. On repeated distention, the bladder wall demonstrates the property of hysteresis in that each successive filling results in a decrease in passive pressure at any given volume.[16, 20] The mechanisms by which the elastic properties of smooth muscle return to the resting state after stretch are unknown, but they do not depend on neurological or reflex mechanisms. The behavior of the detrusor muscle under these conditions is an expression of its viscosity or plastic deformation and may be intimately related to the contractile mechanism.

In the cystometrogram of a normally innervated bladder, phase IB (Fig. 14-3) is interrupted by a strong contraction of the detrusor muscle. The volume at which this contraction occurs is reproducible in any one individual and is accompanied by a strong desire to void. The initiation of voiding is prevented in conditioned individuals by strong contractions of the pelvic floor musculature or diaphragm that serves as the external urinary sphincter. Contractions of the external sphincter are involuntary at low to medium filling volumes; however, at high degrees of distension, a definite voluntary effort is required to prevent voiding whenever spontaneous detrusor contractions occupy the bladder muscle. The reflex nature of this early "guarding" can be observed in the subject with a Foley catheter in place. A gentle tug on this inflated catheter elicits a reflex contraction of the pelvic floor and anal sphincter that can be felt by inserting a finger into the rectum. A similar reflex contraction of the pelvic floor occurs in response to squeezing the glans penis. The basis for this reflex appears to depend on the similarity in embyronic origin of the bladder and anal sphincters. This test is useful in determining the degree and nature of the neurological deficit following cord injury.

Voluntary voiding in the absence of spontaneous detrusor contraction can be initiated by increasing the intra-abdominal and intravesical pressure by straining against a closed glottis. If, when bladder contractions occur, the external sphincter is contracted, the bladder contractions will subside in a matter of seconds, thus ameliorating the desire to void. As bladder filling continues, the detrusor pressure spikes become more frequent and stronger, and they are more difficult to inhibit until the urge to void is irresistible (Fig. 14–4).

If voiding is appropriate in response to the desire to void that accompanies bladder contraction, voluntary contractions of the pelvic floor are inhibited. Relaxation of the external urinary sphincter and strong micturition contractions of the detrusor allow the bladder to start to empty. As the bladder muscle contracts and tension increases around the incompressible urine content, the bladder shape changes in a way that may be likened to converting the form of the bladder from that of a narrow-necked Florence flask to more closely simulate a wide-mouthed Erlenmeyer flask. The net effect is to open the bladder neck and permit voiding. There is no distinct internal sphincter other than the detrusor muscle of the bladder neck. This mechanism of opening the internal sphincter also explains incontinence resulting from overfilling of the bladder.

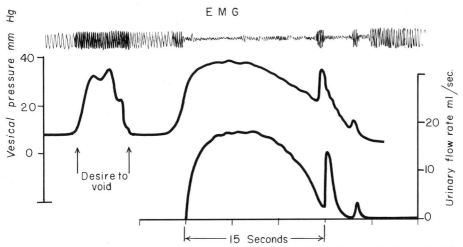

Figure 14–4 Bladder (vesical) pressure (mm Hg), urinary flow (ml/sec) and electrical activity (EMG) of the external urinary sphincter during gradual bladder distention to a volume sufficient to elicit spontaneous bladder contractions and desire to void. Voiding begins when the external sphincter is voluntarily relaxed, as indicated by a reduction in EMG electrical activity of the sphincteric muscles. (Adapted from Boyarsky, S.: The Neurogenic Bladder (S. Boyarsky, ed.). Williams and Wilkins, Baltimore, 1967.)

Returning to the events of the cystometrogram, if the bladder has been effectively denervated (as during spinal shock after acute transection of the spinal cord, by extensive damage to the sacral area of the cord, by destruction of the pelvic nerves or by deep anesthesia), flaccid paralysis of the bladder results. Increased filling will then result in progressively increased bladder pressure as the limits of elasticity of the bladder wall are reached. This phase is called segment II of the cystometrogram (Fig. 14-3). This segment is the most likely section to show the hysteresis effect mentioned earlier, so that if the bladder is filled once, then emptied and refilled a second time, a striking decrease in the pressure is observed in comparison to the pressure resulting from the first filling. This situation is especially important during filling to relatively large volumes and remains an ever-present source of error in both diagnostic and experimental studies.

A discussion of the mechanics of micturition would be incomplete without describing the mechanisms that limit vesicoureteral reflux. The limited nature of our understanding of these important mechanisms is documented by the number of operative procedures that have been used to correct the occurrence of reflux. In the normal ureter, a bolus of urine is transported in a smooth, unidirectional process from the renal pelvis to the bladder. The rate of ureteral contractions appears to be related to the intrinsic contractile response of ureteral muscle. Studies have shown that the ureteral smooth muscle behaves as a unitary type whose most excitable portion is located in the renal pelvis or proximal ureter.[21] The ureter responds to stretch resulting from a bolus of urine with a contraction that spreads distally. The mechanical wave of contraction is preceded by an action potential that travels from the renal pelvis to the bladder but does not enter the intravesical portion of the ureter.[14] Pressures have been measured, and that in the pelvis is relatively low (of the order of 2 to 3 mm. Hg), while the pressure in the remainder of the ureter can be as high as 80 mm. Hg.[14] This pressure in the lower ureter is considerably higher than that in the bladder during normal voiding.

At least three factors prevent reflux of urine from the bladder into the ureter. First, it can be verified in experimental animals that a peristaltic contraction in the ureter can be induced by increasing the bladder pressure. A second mechanism is the anatomical arrangement of the muscle fibers that make up the longitudinal muscle of the lower ureter. These fibers insert into the bladder neck, trigone and proximal urethra, and contractions of the bladder elongate and flatten the lower portion of the ureters, thus reducing the possibility of urinary reflux.[19, 22] Finally, the ureters pass through the bladder wall in a diagonal direction. When the detrusor muscle contracts, it compresses this portion of the ureter and reflux is prevented. It has been suggested that the dual innervation of the bladder and ureters is important in preventing reflux, but current evidence suggests that active, neurologically mediated contraction of the distal ureter is not an important factor in this connection.

The account of voiding presented previously and its interrelationships to cystometrograms still leave open several questions of clinical significance. First, it would be very interesting to understand the neural mechanisms that have led to the characterization of the micturition reflex as the longest phasic reflex in the body. The neurophysiological basis for the prolongation of this reflex is poorly understood.

The pressure, flow and sphincteric electrical activities during voiding in normal subjects are summarized in Fig. 14-4. Pressure in the bladder rises before the muscle action potentials in external urinary sphincter disappear; when the contraction of the external sphincters is voluntarily stopped or relaxed, urine flow starts and continues as long as the bladder wall contracts. Complete emptying of the bladder is accomplished by several forceful contractions of the bladder at the end, and flow ceases.

Innervation of the Bladder

Peripheral Innervation

The bladder has both sensory and motor innervation. Several types of receptors have been described in the bladder wall, ranging from highly organized structures such as pacinian corpuscles to free nerve endings. Evidence is not available to assign functional roles to any particular type of sensory ending, but some observations suggest that several types of endings may arise from one

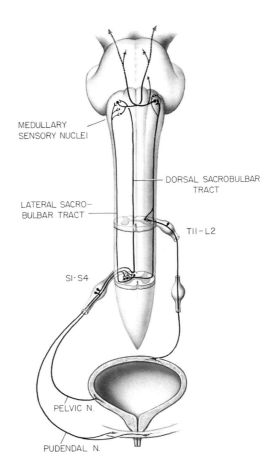

Figure 14—5 Schematic representation of the sensory innervation of the bladder and external sphincter.

MEDULLARY SENSORY NUCLEI

DORSAL SACROBULBAR TRACT

LATERAL SACRO—BULBAR TRACT

TII–L2

SI–S4

PELVIC N.

PUDENDAL N.

sensory neuron, hence producing no clear correlation between structure and function.

The sensory fibers from the bladder and urethra follow one of three pathways (Fig. 14–1). Sensory fibers from the muscle of the external sphincter pass to the first, second and third sacral segments of the spinal cord via the pudendal nerves. These nerves also carry the efferent limb of a stretch or myotatic reflex that serves the external sphincters. The sensory fibers of the bladder pass to the spinal cord via the pelvic nerves (nervi erigentes), and these serve as the afferent limb of the micturition reflex. These fibers traverse the dorsal root ganglia of S2, S3 and S4 and connect either directly or through interneurons with the preganglionic parasympathetic motor neurons in the intermediate gray matter of the sacral cord to complete the neural arc of the micturition reflex. Some sensory fibers decussate within the spinal cord and synapse with middle-sized cells along the lateral margins of the base of the dorsal horns, giving rise to the ascending sacrobulbar tract. In addition, some sensory fibers terminate in the dorsal horn cells to subserve the sensations of

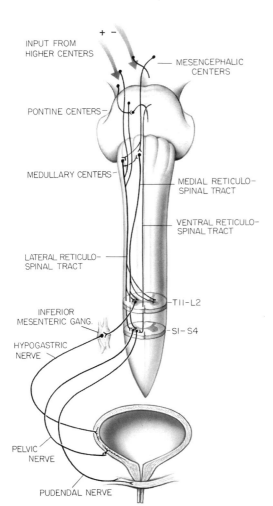

Figure 14–6 Schematic representation of the motor innervation of the bladder and external sphincter.

pain and temperature, as well as continuing directly up the cord in the dorsal columns. It is apparent from a functional standpoint that the sacral micturition centers are organized so that at least some sensory neurons must synapse with inhibitory interneurons that fire on the ventral horn cells that supply the external sphincter.

Sensory fibers from the bladder also pass to the central nervous system via the sympathetic fibers of the hypogastric nerves to synapse in the spinal segments T11-12, L1-2. The role of these sensory axons in normal micturition is not clear, but they may explain the ability of the patient with lumbar or sacral spinal cord transection to experience the sensation of bladder fullness and discomfort (Fig. 14-5).

The motor innervation of the bladder wall is by both sympathetic and parasympathetic nerves. Preganglionic parasympathetic fibers arise from cell bodies in the lateral areas of the intermediate gray matter of the sacral cord and pass via S2, S3 and S4 roots to the bladder through the pelvic nerves (nervi erigentes) to synapse with postganglionic neurons in the bladder or vesical plexus (Fig. 14-6). Postganglionic cholinergic axons arise in these ganglia and pass directly to innervate the muscle fibers. Recent evidence suggests that each fiber is innervated by a postganglion axon; however, one axon may supply several fibers.

The sympathetic preganglionic fibers arise in nerve cells in the intermediolateral gray matter of the lower thoracic and upper lumbar cord and synapse in the inferior mesenteric ganglia or in the pelvic plexus. The postganglionic adrenergic fibers then pass via the hypogastric nerves to the bladder and pelvic organs.

Adrenergic postganglionic sympathetic motor fibers appear to be mingled with the postganglionic parasympathetic fibers supplying the bladder muscle. The parasympathetic nerves produce contraction of the bladder wall. The role of the sympathetic innervation is still in doubt. The best explanation is that it inhibits bladder muscle contraction, thus preventing bladder emptying during orgasm and ejaculation.[6]

Central Neurological Connections

ASCENDING AND DESCENDING PATHWAYS.   Sensory fibers entering the cord by way of the pelvic nerves ascend via two pathways. The first group of fibers are extensions of dorsal root neurons that course upward in the medial superficial layer of the dorsal columns. It is thought that impulses related to passive distension are conducted via this route to terminate in the medulla.[12]

A second set of ascending fibers is composed of the axons of second order neurons located in the intermediolateral nucleus of the sacral cord. The fibers decussate almost completely in man and travel rostrally in the superficial layers of the dorsal half of the lateral column of the lumbar cord. They shift ventrally above the midthoracic level to lie in the ventral half of the lateral columns. In the rostral cervical segments, they lie in the dorsal cord and terminate in the medulla. These fibers have been called the "sacrobulbar tract."

There appear to be at least three important systems of descending fibers: lateral, ventral and medial reticulospinal tracts. The lateral tract originates in the mesencephalon, pons and medulla and fuses to form a lateral reticulospinal tract in the lower cord. These fibers are situated in the superficial layers of the dorsolateral column. They are facilitatory to both the micturition reflex and the external sphincter, and they terminate on the preganglionic parasympathetic neurons transversing the pelvic nerves and the somatic motor neurons of the sacral segments.

The ventroreticulospinal tracts originate in the medial reticular formation of the medulla, close to the hypoglossal nucleus. They are located in the ventral columns of the upper cervical cord but shift dorsally below the midthoracic level and fuse with the lateral reticulospinal tract. These tracts terminate on the same neurons as the lateral reticulospinal tract but appear to be inhibitory rather than facilitatory to both types of sacral motor neurons. A third group of fibers (medial reticular spinal tract), originating in the reticular formation of the pons, conveys tonic impulses to the ventral horn cells of the external sphincter. These fibers are located in the ventral columns of the cord.

ROLE OF HIGHER CENTERS.   The influence of higher neural centers on the sacral micturition reflex has been documented in both clinical and laboratory studies. The importance of such centers is recognized, but their role in normal bladder function is not completely known. This situation appears to have arisen from the failure of some investigators to control the effect of a number of variables on bladder function. For example, many laboratory studies fail to report the degree of bladder filling, the previous history of bladder filling, whether the animals were cage-trained or housebroken and even the degree and type of anesthesia employed. With these reservations in mind, it can be concluded that bladder function is represented at several levels of the brain stem reticular formation by both facilitatory and inhibitory neuron pools. There is typically an overlap between areas, yet there is enough separation to conclude that they are reciprocally acting centers in the medulla, anterior pons, mesencephalon and possibly the hypothalamus.

The role of medullary centers is not completely resolved. Ruch and Tang[17] have reported that, in anesthetized cats, bladder contractions cannot be elicited in an animal with an inferior collicular transection and hence an intact medulla and spinal cord. Kuru,[12] on the other hand, has reported both sensory and motor nuclei in the medulla. One group of fibers ascending in the anterolateral column terminates in a nucleus just lateral to the dorsal sensory nucleus of the vagus and represents the most anterior extension of the gracile nucleus. Kuru has termed this nucleus the "paraalar nucleus" because of its close relationship to the ala cinerea. This nucleus is also supplied by fibers transversing the dorsal columns of the spinal cord.

A second group of fibers ascending via the ventrolateral columns bends medially from the external arcuate fibers, passes between the trigeminal and cuneate nuclei and terminates in a nucleus just lateral to the solitary fascicle. Kuru[12] has termed this the "juxtasolitary nucleus." Finally, a third group of fibers of the sacrobulbar tract terminates in the subtrigeminal region of the lateral reticular nucleus.

In addition to the nuclei already mentioned, stimulation experiments have revealed both "vesicofascilitatory" and "vesicoinhibitory" centers in the medullary reticular formation. Terming these centers facilitatory or inhibitory seems more appropriate, if they are viewed as influencing the excitability of the spinal reflex arc responsible for micturition. The facilitatory center is located in the ventrolateral reticular formation and the inhibitory area in the dorsomedial reticular formation. The vesicofacilitatory center sends its fibers to the sacral micturition center via the lateral reticulospinal tract, while the inhibitory area connects via the ventral reticulospinal tracts. Both of these medullary centers receive fibers from mesencephalic and pontine levels of the brain stem.

The observation of Ruch and others[18, 23] have confirmed that the anterior pons contains a strongly facilitatory micturition center. In addition, both vesicoinhibitory and sphincteric facilitatory areas occur in the anterior pons. The centers are known to connect both with the medullary centers and directly with the intermediolateral somatic motor nuclei of the sacral cord via the ventroreticulospinal tract. A similar situation exists in the mesencephalon, where the reticular formation contains both facilitatory and inhibitory centers that connect to pontine and medullary centers, as well as fibers that synapse in thalamic nuclei. These interconnections are presented graphically in Figures 14–5 and 14-6.

REFERENCES

1. Bard, P.: The hypothalamus and sexual behavior. Res. Publ. Assoc. Res. Nervous Mental Diseases, 20:551-579, 1940.
2. Beach, F. A.: Effects of cortical lesions upon the copulatory behavior of male rats. J. Comp. Psychol., 29:193-244, 1940.
3. Beach, F. A.: Effects of injury to the cerebral cortex upon the sexually receptive behavior in the female rat. Psychosomatic Med., 6:40-55, 1944.
4. Burns, R. K.: Role of hormones in the differentiation of sex. In: William C. Young (ed.): *Sex and Internal Secretions,* 3rd edition, Vol. 1, pp. 76-160. Williams and Wilkins, Baltimore, 1961.
5. Davidson, J. M.: Activation of the male rats' sexual behavior by intracerebral implantation of androgen. Endocrinol. 79:783-794, 1966.
6. Edvardsen, P.: Nervous control of urinary bladder in cats. IV. Effects of autonomic blocking agents on responses to peripheral nerve stimulation. Acta Physiol. Scand., 72:234-247, 1968.
7. Fisher, A. E.: Maternal and sexual behaviour induced by intracranial chemical stimulation. Science, 124:228-229, 1956.
8. Gowen, J. W.: Cytologic and genetic basis of sex. In: William C. Young (ed.): *Sex and Internal Secretions,* 3rd edition, Vol. 1, pp. 3-75. Williams and Wilkins, Baltimore, 1961.
9. Hall, R., Anderson, J., and Smart, G.-A.: *Clinical Endocrinology.* Philadelphia, J. B. Lippincott Co., 1969.
10. Harris, G. W., Michael, R. P., and Scott, P. P.: Neurological site of stilbestrol in eliciting sexual behavior. Ciba Foundation Symposium on Neurological Basis of Behaviour. Boston, Little, Brown and Co., 1958.
11. Herman, M.: Role of somesthetic stimuli in the development of sexual excitement in man. Arch. Neurol. Psychiat., 64:42-56, 1950.
12. Kuru, M.: Nervous control of micturition. Physiol. Rev., 45:425-494, 1965.
13. Lisk, R. D.: Diencephalic placement of estradiol and sexual receptivity in the female rat. Am. J. Physiol., 203:493-496, 1962.
14. Mason, R. C.: Unpublished data.
15. Newman, H. F., Northrup, J. D., and Devlin, J.: Mechanism of human penile erection. Invest. Urol. 1:350-353, 1963-64.
16. Remington, V. W., and Alexander, R. S.: Stretch behavior of the bladder as an approach to vascular distensibility. Am. J. Physiol., 181:240-248, 1955.

17. Ruch, T. C., and Tang, P. C.: The higher control of the bladder. In: Saul Boyarsky (ed.): *The Neurogenic Bladder,* pp. 34-45. Williams and Wilkins, Baltimore, 1967.
18. Scott, F. B., Quesada, E. M., and Cardus, D.: The use of combined urofluorometry, cystometry and electromyography in evaluation of neurogenic bladder dysfunction. In: Saul Boyarsky (ed.): *The Neurogenic Bladder,* pp. 106–114. Williams and Wilkins, Baltimore, 1967.
19. Tanagho, E. A., and Pugh, R. C. B.: The anatomy and function of the ureterovesical junction. Brit. J. Urol., *38*:151-165, 1963.
20. Veenema, R. J., Carpenter, F. G., and Root, W. S.: Residual urine, an important factor in interpretation of cystometrograms. An experimental study. J. Urol., *68*:237-241, 1952.
21. Weiss, R. M., Wagner, M. L., and Hoffman, B. F.: Localization of the pacemaker for peristalsis in the intact canine ureter. Invest. Neurol., 5:42-48,1967.
22. Woodburne, R. T.: Anatomy of the bladder. In: Saul Boyarsky (ed.): *The Neurogenic Bladder,* pp. 3-17. Williams and Wilkins, Baltimore, 1967.
23. Zinner, N. R., and Ritter, R. C.: Bladder physiology—a review with emphasis on hydrodynamic principles. In: Saul Boyarsky (ed.): *The Neurogenic Bladder,* pp. 18–31. Williams and Wilkins, Baltimore, 1967.

Chapter 15

AUTONOMIC FUNCTION IN THE ISOLATED SPINAL CORD

by John M. Miller, III, M.D.

INTRODUCTION

Spinal Man

Sir Charles Sherrington has said, "The greatest motor organ—the skeletal musculature—is at the command of the sense organs. For each individual creature, the material universe is thus separated into two parts, the part that is 'me' and the part that is 'not me.' By high spinal transection the splendid motor machinery of the vertebrate is separated from all the universe except that fraction of the 'material me.' "[22] The consequences of removing the voluntary control from large portions of the skeletal musculature are devastating, but it is remarkable how much of the homeostatic mechanisms is operative at spinal level alone. The tetraplegic patient is capable of grossly maintaining the more basic vital functions such as the circulation, alimentation, defecation, micturition and sexual reproduction through spinal reflexes without any contribution from higher nervous centers. Moreover, there is evidence that these functions may improve with the passage of time and with training, as seen clinically in the development of postural tolerance, improved temperature control and bowel and bladder training.

The functional significance of these spinal autonomic reflexes in intact vertebrates is unclear because they are modified and regulated by medullary or higher centers within the central nervous system. In the patient with spinal cord transection, we deal less with an "abnormal physiology" than with an

265

"altered physiology" and are dependent on the development and training of more primitive spinal reflexes that are now isolated and freed of higher control.

In this chapter we will discuss the responses of patients with a fully viable, functional spinal cord, completely severed from the brain at various levels, with the intrinsic function described below and termed "spinal man." We will not deal with spinal shock nor with incomplete cord lesions.

The spinal skeletal muscle reflexes are well presented in the summaries of Sherrington,[23] and these are not treated here. The functional significance of the residual motor capacities at various levels of cord transection have likewise been adequately described by Long and others[17] and are also not treated in this chapter except for the postural adjustments involved in these functions.

In this chapter, "tetraplegic" will refer to any complete lesion above T1, and all lower lesions will be referred to as "paraplegia" with a qualifying level; this is a useful distinction in the study of autonomic function because of the emergence of all the sympathetic nerve fibers below the C8-T1 level.

The Spinal Autonomic Nerves

Because of the significance of the level of the lesion in the autonomic responses in spinal man, a brief review of the peripheral portions of the two sections of the autonomic nervous system will be presented. Both the sympathetic (or thoracolumbar) system and the parasympathetic (or craniosacral) system share the common characteristic that all fibers emanating from the central nervous system (preganglionic fibers) synapse outside the central nervous system in a ganglion with one or more postganglionic fibers before reaching their end-organ. Each preganglionic fiber may branch many times; this results in the phenomenon of "spread" of an autonomic outflow. In the sympathetic system, the ratio of preganglionic fibers to postganglionic fibers may be as high as 1 to 32; in the parasympathetic, this ratio is usually only 1 to 2. The high ratios are in those nerves involving diffuse autonomic responses, and the low ratios in those involving fairly discrete organ responses.

SYMPATHETIC SYSTEM. For man, the spinal sympathetic preganglionic efferent fibers descend through the lateral column of the cervical cord and pass with the ventral roots of the spinal nerves from T1 to L2 levels. After leaving the spinal canal, these preganglionic fibers separate from the spinal nerve via the myelinated white rami communicantes and pass into the vertebral ganglia of the sympathetic chain. Here some of the preganglionic fibers synapse with segmental postganglionic fibers. Others branch and ascend or descend to other ganglia of the sympathetic chain, or pass through the paravertebral ganglia, and with the splanchnic nerves go to more remote sympathetic ganglia. Although the white rami are confined to the T1-L2 segments, *all* spinal nerves have associated vertebral ganglia of the sympathetic chain which supply the corresponding segments. Because of the multiple branching of many preganglionic fibers ascending and descending the sympathetic chain, discrete segmental responses are uncommon, although a segmental pattern may be seen to "spread" up and down much of the sympathetic chain.

Postganglionic fibers to the *head*, *limbs* and *body wall* accompany the corre-

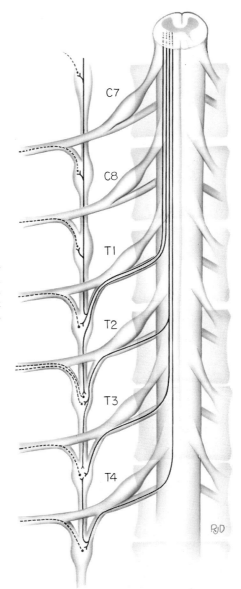

Figure 15–1 A schematic diagram of the lower cervical and upper thoracic spinal cord showing: Gray ramus communicans, white ramus communicans, sympathetic ganglia, ventral root of spinal nerves, dorsal root of spinal nerves, sympathetic tract, and branching in a ganglion.

sponding spinal nerve to this segment and innervate the blood vessels, sweat glands, hair follicles, and so on. They regain the spinal nerve via unmyelinated fibers which leave the paravertebral ganglion via the gray rami communicandi. Postganglionic fibers to the *abdominal* and *thoracic viscera* leave the prevertebral ganglia and follow a blood vessel in a perivascular plexus to the appropriate gland or organ. Some preganglionic fibers end directly in the adrenal medulla, a gland of similar embryonic origin to the sympathetic chain in which the chromaffin cells are in fact adapted postganglionic fibers.

Transection of the spinal cord above T1 abolishes all suprasegmental control over the sympathetic nervous system, and all subsequent sympathetic action must function under the control of an autonomous cord. However, transection below L2 leaves the sympathetic system intact, even though the somatic functions below that level are impaired. At the intervening levels of spinal cord transection (T1-L2), the pattern of spread along the sympathetic chain makes segmental localization of sympathetic outflow imprecise.

PARASYMPATHETIC SYSTEM. The *cranial* portion of the parasympathetic nervous system is intact at any level of cord transection. Of the four brain centers for parasympathetic outflow, two have special significance after cord transection. The *hypothalamic* outflow to the neurohypophysis (pituitary gland) and the *medullary* outflow, through the vagus (cranial nerve X), innervates the *heart, bronchial tree* and the *alimentary tract* down to the splenic flexure of the colon. Although the autonomic nervous system is often thought of as having two reciprocal components, alterations in the "tone" of the vagus alone, without a sympathetic component, can alter heart rate, peristaltic activity and respiratory responses. Moreover, sympathetic autonomy exists at the spinal level within the isolated cord segments. These factors, together with the anatomical connections between the two systems, especially between the vagus and the superior cervical ganglia, make isolated sympathetic-parasympathetic activities difficult to assess.

The sacral portion of the parasympathetic system emerges from the ventral roots of S3-4, with inconstant fibers from S2 and S5, and leave the spinal nerves as the pelvic nerves in lower animals. In man, they accompany the corresponding spinal nerves to synapse with postganglionic fibers in plexi in the walls of the *rectum* and *bladder*, thus innervating these organs and the blood vessels of the genitalia.

CARDIOVASCULAR RESPONSES

In intact man, adjustments occur within the vascular system with changes in posture to insure a nearly constant blood pressure. These changes, initiated through baroreceptors in the high pressure (arterial) and low pressure (venous) systems and mediated via the autonomic nervous system, include changes in heart rate, cardiac output and adjustments of blood flow through the visceral and peripheral vascular beds.[15] In the spinal patient, there may be a separation of the baroreceptors from the neural effector mechanisms, causing blood pressure regulation and regional circulation to be abnormal.

Postural Adjustments in the Spinal Man

The responses of the spinal patient to postural change are influenced by several factors:
1. The length of time after the initial injury.
2. The level of the cord transection.
3. The way the patient has been managed from the time of injury. Immediately after spinal injury, patients often develop "spinal shock," during which all neural reflexes dependent on the spinal cord are absent. The rate of return of spinal reflexes varies, but is usually complete in 2 to 6 weeks.

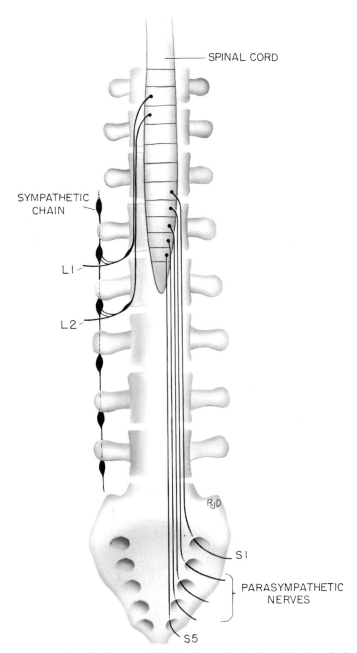

SPINAL CORD

SYMPATHETIC CHAIN

L1

L2

RJD

S1

PARASYMPATHETIC NERVES

S5

Figure 15 – 2   A schematic diagram of the lumbosacral spinal cord showing the last two (L1-L2) sympathetic efferent nerves passing to the sympathetic chain from the somatic nerves. The parasympathetic nerves are shown arising from the spinal segments S1-S5.

A lesion at the L3 spinal cord level would eliminate all of the somatic motor and sensory fibers below the lesion as well as all of the parasympathetic nerves, but the whole of the sympathetic innervation would remain intact.

Level of the Lesion

Most patients with chronic spinal lesions at C7 or above experience hypotension, tachycardia and loss of consciousness within two minutes of being tilted to 60°. In contrast, patients with lesions at or below T6 respond to tilting much as do normal subjects who have been at bed rest for similar periods.[13] Patients with lesions between C7 and T6 show intermediate responses.

The fall in blood pressure is due to failure of the compensatory cardiovascular mechanisms. Effective vasoconstriction (arterial and venous) does not occur, allowing a peripheral pooling of blood, a decreased venous return and a lower cardiac output. Cardioacceleration normally is a result of both a reduction of vagal tone and an activation of sympathetic cardioaccelerator stimulation. Without the sympathetic activation heart rate responds only to the vagal reduction and rises to an appropriate maximal tachycardia of 120 beats per minute. This is inadequate compensation and the cardiac output falls because of inadequate venous return.

Despite fixed lesions, spinal patients develop improved tolerance to tilting with time, especially when they are tilted frequently. The mechanism of this improvement is not known, but several factors seem to contribute. Reflexes arising in the isolated spinal cord may be developed. There is evidence that baroreceptors within the cord and changes in arterial pO_2 and pCO_2, such as occur with severe hypotension, can stimulate reflex vasomotor constriction at a cord level. Urinary excretion of norepinephrine is higher in quadriplegics who do not faint when tilted.[14, 27] Increased sensitivity of vascular beds to levels of circulating catecholamine may also occur. The blood volume of spinal patients undergoing an active rehabilitation program for two or three months is greater than normal, and this may help to maintain cardiac output during postural change.[16] The mechanism of the increased blood volume is not clear. Exercise, in normal man, causes an increased blood volume, and the intensity of exercise in the rehabilitation program may contribute. Many spinal patients with high lesions have chronically high circulating levels of plasma cortisol, ADH and aldosterone, particularly if they are repeatedly tilted, all of which would help in maintaining an expanded blood volume.[27]

Interpretation of changes in patients undergoing rehabilitation is complicated by several factors occurring at the same time. In addition to the physiological readjustment that occurs, the patients are usually started on an active program of tilting and exercise to counteract the effects of chronic bed rest and inactivity. Also, resumption of a normal diet helps to reverse the metabolic effects of trauma deprivation. The several effects of these complicating aspects of any chronic illness are discussed in Chapter 12, but no effective separation can be made of each in a given patient.

RESPONSES OF SPINAL PATIENTS TO STRESS

Recovery From Acute Blood Loss

Intact animals respond to blood loss of up to one-third their total blood volume with transient hypotension, but within a few minutes the blood pressure is restored to resting levels by an increase in peripheral vascular resistance. This response is mediated by the sympathetic adrenergic nervous system and is associated with higher circulating levels of catecholamine. Animals with chronic high spinal lesions respond to comparable blood loss with a similar although slower compensation.[5] In the spinal animals, as in normal ones, there is vaso-constriction in the periphery which can be abolished by cutting the peripheral nerves or the ventral nerve roots (motor and sympathetic) but not the dorsal (sensory) spinal nerve roots. Blood levels of norepinephrine rise, even in the adrenalectomized animal, presumably by release of the catecholamine from other stores. This neurogenically mediated vasoconstriction appears to arise directly from the isolated spinal cord, but it is not known whether it is initiated by pressure-sensitive structures within the cord or as a response to some other manifestation of the hypotension such as anoxia.

Responses to Hypoxia

The electrical activity of the inferior cardiac nerve, a branch of the sympa-thetic adrenergic nervous system, is used as an index of sympathetic nerve activity of the spinal cord.[1] In intact animals, this nerve exhibits a background of electrical activity with bursts of increased activity that occur between the peaks of aortic pulse pressure. The electrical activity is inhibited when the blood pressure is raised, and increased when it is lowered. In spinal animals, this electrical activity persists even after transection of the cervical cord. This would indicate that the activity originates within the cord rather than in the higher central nervous system, and reflects intrinsic sympathetic activity.

When these animals were made hypoxic by breathing pure nitrogen, the electrical activity increased; it was decreased by breathing 90 per cent O_2. This suggests that at least in animals the isolated spinal cord can respond to hypoxia by increased sympathetic nerve activity, which in turn may play a part in increasing peripheral vasomotor tone in response to hypotension.

Response to Hypercapnia

The direct local effect of CO_2 on blood vessels is to cause dilation, but in intact man breathing CO_2 causes an increase in blood pressure owing to a rise in cardiac output and an increase in peripheral resistance. The cardiac and peripheral vascular effects are mediated by the central nervous system and by the sympathetic nervous system. Thus, there is a competing peripheral and central action of CO_2, the local dilating effects occurring, for example, in exercising muscles while the central neurogenic effect overrides the local effect to maintain systemic blood pressure.

In spinal patients with lesions below T6 and who breathe 5 per cent CO_2 in air, the responses are similar to normal patients, with an increased peripheral resistance and a rise in cardiac output with a slight rise in systemic blood pressure.[19] Patients with higher cord transections (above T2) do not respond with an increased cardiac output, but do develop increased peripheral resis-tance and a moderate to severe hypertension. In tetraplegic patients, the hypotension of passive tilting can be abolished or retarded by breathing 5 per cent CO_2 in air.[10] This peripheral constriction of both the arteriolar and venous beds must be initiated by a direct action of the CO_2 on the spinal cord itself or at the sympathetic ganglia.

Breathing 5 per cent CO_2 increases the circulating levels of norepinephrine in intact man, and if present in the spinal patients, this could contribute to enhancing peripheral vasoconstriction. The increased respiratory rate and tidal volume during hypercapnia occur in all spinal patients and, as in normal patients, is due to a central stimulating effect mediated through the phrenic nerves.

Paradoxical Responses

Many changes in blood pressure and pulse rate observed in normal man do not occur, or have a paradoxical effect, in tetraplegics.[6] In intact man mild to moderate exercise causes an increase in the blood pressure and pulse rate, but in tetraplegics exercises do not raise the blood pressure, although the heart rate is increased. Eating, drinking, defecation (or rectal stimulation) and bladder emptying all cause slight elevation of the blood pressure and fall in the pulse rate in normal man; the reverse is true in tetraplegics.

One of the most striking examples of a paradoxical response is the response to Procaine block of the carotid nerves (cranial nerves IX and X) bilaterally. In normal man the response to this procedure is an immediate tachycardia, with an increase in the cardiac output, and hypertension. This may be followed by a transient compensatory fall in blood pressure, but is followed in turn by another rise in blood pressure owing to the increased peripheral resistance, even though the cardiac output returns to normal. Carotid nerve block in the tetraplegic patient causes an immediate decrease in cardiac output and gradual fall in the blood pressure.[18] It is likely that in the normal subject block of the cardiac depressor nerve (vagus) leads to a pressor response in the vasomotor center. The sympathetic effectors causing the increased peripheral resistance require the integrity of the cervical spinal cord to function; thus in the tetraplegic patient, no such response is possible.

AUTONOMIC HYPERREFLEXIA

Much of the physiological study of the autonomic cardiovascular responses in spinal patients has been stimulated by the occurrence of a clinical syndrome termed "autonomic hyperreflexia."[7] In many patients with spinal lesions, distension of the bladder or bowel causes flushing of the face, sweating of the forehead, constriction of the pupils of the eyes, nasal congestion and a feeling of oppression in the chest. Clinical examination shows bradycardia and an elevation of blood pressure. A similar syndrome can be produced by other stimuli, including parturition, or even a mild stimulus such as squeezing the calf.

The nature and the degree of the cardiovascular response seem to depend on the level of cord transection and the time interval from the initial injury.

Blood Pressure

Bladder distention causes a rise in blood pressure in patients with a spinal lesion above T6, but hardly at all in patients with lower lesions. The peaks of the blood pressure elevation correspond to the highest bladder pressures associated with rhythmic detrusor contractions.[7] This blood pressure elevation does not occur in the period of spinal shock, but after the patient has regained some tolerance to tilting.[18] In tetraplegic patients during obstetrical deliveries, the hypertension may be so severe during the second stage of labor as to warrant instrumental delivery or cesarian section to terminate pregnancy.[21]

In subjects with very low lesions (around L2) but with intact cord below, the blood pressure may fall when the bladder is distended, even though there is an associated vasoconstriction in the toes and calf muscles.

Peripheral Arterial Responses

In the patient with a T6 or higher lesion, distention of the bladder causes a constriction in calf muscle blood vessels, synchronous with each detrusor contraction of the bladder. When the bladder pressure is high or the detrusor contractions are close together, the calf blood flow may be continuously reduced. Simultaneously the forearm muscle blood flow increases up to double resting levels. This rise of forearm flow is much greater than would be expected from the greater perfusion caused by the increased blood pressure, and it indicates active vasodilation of the vessels. The blood vessels in the arm, innervated as they are by sympathetic cholinergic vasodilator nerves leaving the cord above the level of the transection, have their central sympathetic connections intact.

In patients with lesions at or above T1, bladder distention also causes a pronounced fall in calf blood flow and rise in forearm blood flow. The mechanism of the increased forearm flow in these cases comes from the isolated cord. It is possible that the reflex is initiated by baroreceptors in the proximal great veins and mediated directly to and from the cord.[11] In one case report, of a patient with a T6 level lesion on the left and T10 level on the right, both the calf and forearm blood flow increased on the right where the suprasegmental sympathetic innervation was almost complete; however, the calf blood flow fell on the left, the forearm blood flow rose and the patient remained normotensive. On the right side, the calf was supplied with isolated cord sympathetic innervation. In subjects with low lesions (T10-L4), the calf blood flow falls in response to bladder distention the same as it does in higher lesions, but no hypertension occurs.

Skin blood flow in the *feet* and *toes* is reduced with bladder distention in cord transections at any level, but the blood flow to the skin of the *fingers* is variable. In high cord transections there is an initial moderate rise in finger blood flow for about 10 minutes, followed by marked decrease in flow. Presumably the initial increase is due to the mechanical effect of increased blood pressure and perfusion pressure, but the fall in flow is a response to actively induced vasoconstriction effected by spread of sympathetic activity generated at cord level. The hand blood flow is innervated in part by the same sympathetic segments (T3-T9) that supply the blood vessels of the splanchnic bed (T5-T11) and may reflect vasoconstriction in that bed as well.

The skin of the face actively vasodilates as the blood pressure rises; this is a function of both the intact carotid sinus mechanism and the parasympathetic innervation to this area. It occurs only if there is a rise in the blood pressure, as there is in patients with lesions above T6.

The Heart

In patients with lesions below T10 the heart rate and cardiac output do not change with bladder distention, even if the blood pressure rises or falls slightly. In subjects with higher lesions (above T6), the heart rate *decreases* because the intact sinoaortic pressure sensors initiate increased vagal tone.[18] The *cardiac output* remains unchanged even when severe hypertension occurs, but the stroke volume may increase if bradycardia occurs. The hypertension of autonomic hyperreflexia is almost purely a function of increased peripheral resistance and shift of the splanchnic blood into the systemic circulation, rather than a change in the cardiac output.

Cardiac arrhythmias and fluoroscopic evidence of right ventricular enlargement have been described in autonomic hyperreflexia, particularly during obstetrical labor.[12] The arrhythmias include ventricular premature contractions, sinus tachycardia and the Wenckebach phenomenon. These abnormalities may be ascribed to the physiological stress of a bradycardia in the face of an increased "forward load" from the increased peripheral resistance, as well as enhanced venous return.

The Veins

The veins contain at least four-fifths of the total blood volume and are under active sympathetic innervation; change in venous tone is important to the distribution of the circulating blood volume. In patients with high cord transections with autonomic hyperreflexia, there is a rise in venous pressure of the antecubital vein. This rise is associated with right ventricular dilatation and could reflect either back pressure from the heart or increased forearm blood flow. However, the heart rate and the forearm blood flow remain steady after the onset of the hypertension, while the venous pressure continues to rise.[7]

In summary, distention of the bladder or other viscera in a subject with spinal cord transection above T6 results in a generalized spread of sympathetic activity, causing constriction of the blood vessels in the lower extremities and in the blood reservoirs of the splanchnic bed as well. In patients with lesions below T6 vasodilation in the upper extremities, head and neck prevents a rise in blood pressure, but in patients with higher lesions the hypertension often occurs.

THE REGULATION OF BODY TEMPERATURE IN SPINAL MAN

Thermoregulation in normal man is reviewed in Chapter 7. Spinal man has difficulty in regulating his temperature in a changing environment and the responses to thermal stress vary according to several factors:

1. The time after injury.
2. The level of the cord transection.
3. The relationship between deep and superficial temperature change.

Both spinal animals and spinal man regulate the body temperature very poorly in the days immediately after injury. In animal studies some thermoregulating stability recovers within 7 to 10 days,[25] but detailed studies in man have not been done.

The ability of chronic spinal patients to withstand changes in temperature depends on the level of their lesions. Guttman[14] has concluded that T8 is the highest lesion with which a patient can maintain rectal temperature at 37°C in an ambient temperature ranging from 18 to 40°C. Patients with higher lesions are poikilothermic in response to cooling or heating. In laboratory studies, patients with *cervical* cord transections do not shiver or increase their heat production until their central temperatures (measured at the ear drum or under the tongue) falls to approximately 35.6°C when the sentient skin is kept warm (i.e., above 34°C).[9] Exposure of the sentient skin to an ambient temperature of 22 to 24°C did not modify the response to central cooling. It is not known whether exposure to lower ambient temperature would enhance the response.

In patients with lesions from T2 to L1, in whom the sentient skin was kept warm (above 34°C) central cooling did not initiate shivering until the ear temperature fell to approximately 35.6°C, as in the tetraplegics.[8] However, cooling the sentient skin in conjunction with a falling central temperature caused shivering sooner. Skin response is dependent on the area of innervated skin and the amount and rate of cooling. Patients with lesions at T10 or below will shiver by skin cooling alone without a fall in deep temperature. Similar studies have not been performed with heat, but results of such studies would be expected to parallel those obtained in the cold.

Rudimentary Thermal Responses at Cord Level

In spinal patients shivering occurs only in muscles innervated above the level of the lesion.[22] There is, however, evidence for rudimentary thermoregulation at cord level. Direct cooling of the spinal cord of intact unanesthetized dogs caused shivering when the spinal cord was cooled by 3.6°C. The shivering became more vigorous as the cord was cooled further despite no apparent change in central body temperature.[24]

Spinal man also has primitive thermoregulatory responses in the areas innervated by the isolated spinal cord.[20] When exposed to an ambient temperature of 30°C, there was a gradual rise in rectal and sublingual temperature and sparse sweating, and vasodilation in the skin occurred below the level of the lesion within 10 minutes. The onset of sweating was sluggish and only about 20 per cent of the sweat glands were activated. The sweating rapidly decreased when the ambient temperature returned to neutral. Vasodilation in the skin followed the onset of sweating by about 10 minutes and occurred only after the central temperature was elevated; it is possible that the elevated skin temperature itself accounted in part for the vasodilation rather than this being the result of a true spinal reflex. The possibility of training this primitive thermoregulatory response at spinal level has not been adequately explored.

OTHER VISCERAL RESPONSES IN THE ISOLATED SPINAL CORD

The visceral autonomic reflexes, except for micturition and sexual function, in spinal man have not been extensively studied. In addition, reference will be made in this section to the pulmonary function, alimentation and defecation of spinal man where information is available to explain the functional result of spinal cord transection.

Pulmonary Function

In man, the efferent nerves to skeletal muscles involved in respiration originate from many segments along the length of the spinal cord. The phrenic nerves to the diaphragm originate at C2 to C4; the thoracic nerves to the intercostal muscles from T1 to T6; and nerves to the abdominal muscles from T7 to L1. The principal efferent neural fibers pass along cranial nerves IX and X, principally from the chemoreceptors in the aortic and carotid bodies, but also from stretch receptors in the lung, aortic arch and large veins. In quiet, normal breathing the principal regulation of respiration is at a suprasegmental, supraspinal level. In spinal man, the cranial nerve portions are intact and the medullary respiratory centers function normally, the impairment of the effector muscles being determined by the level of the lesion. In patients with lesions above C7, the entire tidal volume is a result of diaphragmatic activity alone, in contrast to normal individuals in whom expansion of the rib cage accounts for most of the tidal volume.[2] Gastric pressures have been measured and found to increase to three times the normal level during inspiration. The calculated work done in moving the abdominal viscera (pressure × volume) is thus nine times that of intact subjects. The increased work of displacing the abdominal viscera by the diaphragm makes even quiet breathing in tetraplegic patients more laborious than normal.[2] In subjects with lower lesions, the accessory muscles of respiration, especially the intercostals, assume greater amounts of the work load of breathing.

There is a decreased respiratory sensitivity to low arterial pO_2 in tetraplegics with chronic hypoventilation, but this is decreased sensitivity of the pO_2 chemoreceptors rather than alteration in spinal cord function. In both paraplegics and tetraplegics with normal resting pO_2 and pCO_2 the ventilation response to hypercapnea is unimpaired.

Alimentation

In spinal man the cranial portion of the parasympathetic outflow is intact and supplies the entire alimentary tract to the splenic flexure of the colon. Below that level, the bowel receives parasympathetic innervation from the second to fifth sacral cord segments. The precise relationship between the sympathetic-parasympathetic reciprocal relationship in the gut and its related glands is not clear in intact man and has not been adequately studied in spinal cord transection. The peristaltic activity and the propagation of digestive products through the gut is an intrinsic function of the gut itself, dependent on the autonomic plexi in the bowel wall and not, in chronic preparations, related to any central nervous system connections. Thus in spinal man, at any level, the digestion, absorption and elimination of foodstuffs proceeds in a nearly normal fashion. During the period of spinal shock both paralytic ileus and hypermotility of the bowel have been reported and in dogs liquid, mucus-ridden stools may persist for many months after cord transection. These phenomena have been attributed to unopposed vagal secretory activity. In tetraplegic man, gastric hyperacidity and a high incidence of upper gastrointestinal hemorrhage from duodenal ulcer have been described and have been attributed to unopposed vagal action, but they could be rather a response to stress.

Cachexia is often associated with high spinal cord injury, but there is no evidence for malabsorption or a primary disorder of the gastrointestinal tract, so the weight loss is probably due to inadequate food intake. One theory of the regulation of hunger and satiety is that the heat generated from the specific dynamic action of ingested foods is detected by thermoregulators in the hypothalamus, and this controls, or contributes to, the sensation of hunger and its satisfaction. Although this theory does not postulate the integrity of the spinal cord, it is possible that the failure of thermoregulation is a contributing factor to the poor appetite of tetraplegics.

Defecation

The reflex component of defecation involves only the sacral portion of the spinal cord and the peripheral nerves to this segment. Defecation will occur in spinal animals and man when the sacral cord segments have been destroyed, but is less forceful and less complete than in normals. The principal stimulus to defecation is the distention of the rectum. The parasympathetic innervation to the internal sphincter is inhibitory, and on distention of the rectum release of the sphincter occurs and evacuation follows. The voluntary (skeletal muscle) contribution to defecation consists only of closing the external sphincter to *inhibit* reflex emptying of the bowel, or the contraction of the diaphragm and abdominal muscles with a closed glottis (Valsalva maneuver) to increase the intra-abdominal pressure to initiate or facilitate defecation. Neither is possible in the spinal patient. There is probably no sympathetic contribution to normal defecation.

Electromyographic studies have shown that the basic electrical rhythm of the internal anal sphincter is no different in the spinal patient than the normal.[26] There is a continuous pulsatile activity in the annular muscles of the internal sphincter which is inhibited by mechanical distention of the rectum.

Patients with sacral cord and cauda equina lesions may regain some of their sphincter tone and have peristaltic movements to provide an incomplete evacuation; this, supported by animal experiments, suggests that defecation is in part controlled by peripheral nervous plexi on the bowel wall, independent of the spinal cord.

Micturition

Micturition in intact man is complex and the neurophysiological mechanism is poorly understood. The major events in active voiding, even in intact man, are integrated at spinal level; supraspinal influences are inhibitory or facilitory. We will deal here only with the spinal portion of the voiding reflex. For details of higher integration the reader is referred to Chapter 14.

The "tone" of the bladder wall is intrinsic and not dependent on spinal reflexes; the usual intravesical pressure is 10 cm H_2O, regardless of the volume of liquid contained therein, and with slow filling from the ureters, this pressure remains constant. Afferent stimuli from the bladder wall pass along the pelvic nerves to the sacral cord to the central nervous system. Efferent fibers to the detrusor muscle (which also comprises the internal sphincter) emerge with the S3-4 pelvic nerves and constitute the parasympathetic nerve supply to the bladder. The sympathetic nerve supply to the bladder passes from the lower thoracic and upper lumbar spinal segments and reaches the bladder neck via the hypogastric nerves. This sympathetic supply plays no part in normal micturition, but functions only to close the bladder neck at ejaculation to prevent retrograde flow of semen. The internal sphincter is not truly an annular sphincter, but an extension of the detrusor muscle. In voiding there is opening of the internal sphincter as part of the contraction of the detrusor muscle.

In the simplest voiding pattern, stretch receptors in the bladder wall transmit impulses to the spinal cord and initiate a parasympathetic discharge, which stimulates a detrusor contraction, increasing the intravesical pressure and opening the internal sphincter. The external sphincter is skeletal muscle and under voluntary control. Normally it is in a state of constant activity, except for a few seconds before micturition and throughout voiding.

In spinal man with lesions above S2, the above voiding pattern is present in a primitive way. In the absence of the cortical facilitory influence in normal voluntary voiding, the emptying may be less complete, particularly if the bladder wall may have been damaged by distention or infection. This reflex is dependent upon the integrity of the pelvic nerves; these leave the cord in the cauda equina, and the characteristics of the bladder in cauda equina lesions are quite different. Bors[3] distinguishes between "upper motor neuron" bladder and "lower motor neuron" bladder. In the "upper motor neuron," voiding contractions are seen on cystometrogram. The cystogram is symmetrical; cold stimuli such as ice water in the bladder produce strong detrusor contractions; and autonomic reflex emptying can usually be accomplished by training. In the "lower motor neuron" bladder, no effective detrusor contractions are seen on the cystometrogram; the cystogram is asymmetric; there are no cold water contractions of the detrusor; and bladder emptying is accomplished only by manual expression of the urine.

The upper motor neuron pattern of autonomic reflex bladder emptying improves as the level of the cord transection becomes progressively higher. The most efficient emptying usually occurs in cervical cord transection but the neuroanatomical explanation for this is not clear. Possibly the sympathetic autonomic nervous system inhibits normal voiding, except in the isolated spinal cord with the cervical connection severed.

Sexual Function

The basic reflexes for sexual activity are located in the sacral portion of the spinal cord. In the frog with extirpation of the entire spinal cord except for the sacral 3rd and 4th segments, tactile stimulation of the genitalia causes the animal to assume the copulatory position throughout the mating season. In spinal dogs and cats (cervical lesions), manipulation of the genitalia usually causes sexual arousal manifested by appropriate movement of the hind limbs and tail, ejaculation and orgasm. In man both the facilitory and inhibitory cortical influences are of great importance in sexual function, but nevertheless the retention of sexual function after cord transection exists to a surprising degree. During spinal shock, none of these reflexes are present, although general vasodilation may lead to persistent priapism in the male. Like sweating, micturition and vasoconstriction, the sexual autonomic reflexes return somewhat later than the skeletal muscle spinal reflexes upon the subsiding of spinal shock.

There are more male than female paraplegics; consequently, more data is available for men. Erection in the male is caused by local vasodilation. Parasympathetic fibers emerging from S3-4 descend via the cauda equina and pelvic nerves to dilate the arteries supplying the venous sinuses (corpora) along the shaft of the penis. Erection is maintained as long as these sinuses are distended with blood. In intact man, cortical facilitation in response to visual stimuli or erotic thoughts can initiate erection, but the maintenance of a complete erection depends on the integrity of the somatic afferent fibers from the tactile receptors in the skin of the penis, principally the glans, which reach the cord via the pudendal nerves and cauda equina.

Ejaculation and orgasm are sympathetic functions and employ the same somatic afferents of the internal pudendal nerve. The efferents leave from the lower sympathetic chain and form the hypogastric nerves. Patients with cauda equina lesions are unable to achieve or maintain erections by stimulation of the penis, because this part of the reflex pathway has been disrupted. They may achieve an incomplete erection from cortical stimulation, however. In these patients, the entire sympathetic system is intact, and the incomplete erection is produced by increasing the sympathetic constrictor tone to the penile arteries.

In spinal man the ability to achieve and maintain an erection varies with the level of the lesion.[4] Erections occur in 80 per cent of patients with cervical cord lesion. Of these, 33 per cent can maintain the erection long enough to carry out successful coitus. Only about 5 per cent actually ejaculate, but many report a pleasant feeling associated with orgasm and sustain flexor spasms of the legs at that time. Fewer patients with lower thoracic lesions have erections, and only about 15 per cent can successfully complete intercourse. Patients with lumbar cord lesions (not cauda equina lesions) have a much lower incidence of erection. If erection can be achieved, however, they are more likely to be able to ejaculate, presumably because of the more complete sympathetic innervation.

When cord transection occurs in childhood, pubertal changes and the development of secondary sexual characteristics occur at the normal times. However, there is often infertility and tubular testicular atrophy, especially in patients with lesions higher than T10.[4] These observations indicate that infertility may be related to the failure of thermal regulation of the testicular temperature, as there is evidence that the production of mature spermatozoa is sensitive to high temperatures. There is no correlation between this type of testicular atrophy and sexual performance, 17-keto steroid excretions or sex desire.

The lack of sensation from the genitalia, the difficulty in finding a partner, and the inconvenience of removing indwelling catheters contribute to the decrease in libido and erotic fantasies reported in the paraplegic male, but phantom orgasms in dreams are reported.

The female who sustains a cord transection in childhood achieves menarche at the usual age and the menstrual periods and ovulation continue unabated until menopause. The ovaries are not thermally sensitive and function normally. Primates with cord transection in adult life are reported to menstruate spontaneously after the injury and continue regularly thereafter. The human female may have a period of amenorrhea or irregular menses after cord transection. In general, the menses and ovulation, with inherently implied fertility, are not disturbed by cord transection at any level. As in the male, sexual arousal depends on the integrity of the sacral cord and its peripheral connections. Because of the passive role of the female in intercourse, successful marital adjustment is common. When the cord is intact below the lesion, appropriate movements, secretion of vaginal lubricants and, occasionally, a modified form of orgasm all may occur.

Libido decreases in females following cord transection, but pregnancy occurs in patients with all levels of cord transection, and gestation, parturition and lactation occur normally. There appears to be a higher incidence of prematurity and spontaneous abortion, but sufficient numbers are not available for statistical analysis.

In the pregnant paraplegic, the absence of pain often makes it difficult for the patient to know that labor has begun. In lesions above T10, assistance may be required in the second stage of labor to make up for the absent abdominals in "bearing down." In patients with lesions above T6, autonomic hyperreflexia is a hazard during labor and can be confused with eclampsia. If the hypertension is severe, labor must be terminated by instrumental vaginal delivery, or cesarian section.[21]

CONCLUSION

The hypothesis of this chapter is that following spinal cord transection in man, the autonomic responses innervated by the isolated cord function like those in a phylogenetically more primitive species. Understanding the extent to which the basic spinal cord physiology can be utilized and adapted is essential to the continuing care of spinal man.

REFERENCES

1. Alexander, R. S.: The effects of blood flow and anoxia on spinal cardiovascular centers. Am. J. Physiol., *143*:698–708, 1945.
2. Bergofsky, E. H.: Quantitation of the function of respiratory muscles in normal individuals and quadriplegic patients. Arch. Phys. Med. Rehabil., *45*:575–580, 1964.
3. Bors, E.: Neurogenic bladder. Urological Survey, 7:177–250, 1957.

4. Bors, E., Engle, T. T., Rosenquist, R. C. and Holliger, V. H.: Fertility in Paraplegic Males: a Preliminary Report of Endocrine Studies. J. Clin. Endocr., *10*:381-388, 1950.
5. Brooks, C. M.: The reaction of chronic spinal animals to hemorrhage. Am. J. Physiol., *114*:30-39, 1935.
6. Cole, T. M., Kottke, F. J., Olson, M., Stradal, L. and Niederloh, J.: Alterations of cardiovascular control in high spinal myelomalacia. Arch. Phys. Med. Rehabil., *48*:359-368, 1967.
7. Cunningham, D. J. C., Guttmann, L., Whitteridge, D. and Wyndham, C. H.: Cardiovascular responses to bladder distention in paraplegic patients. J. Physiol. (London), *121*:581-592, 1953.
8. Downey, J. A., Chiodi, H. P. and Darling, R. C.: Central temperature regulation in the spinal man. Appl. Physiol., *22*:91-94, 1967.
9. Downey, J. A., Chiodi, H. P., Darling, R. C. and Sarno, J. A.: Oxygen consumption related to body temperature change in quadriplegic subjects (abstract). Physiologist, *8*:155, 1965.
10. Downey, J. A., Chiodi, H. P. and Miller, J. M.: The effect of inhalation of 5 per cent carbon dioxide in air on postural hypotension in quadriplegia. Arch. Phys. Med. Rehabil., *47*:422-426, 1966.
11. Gilliatt, R. W., Guttmann, L. and Whitteridge, D.: Inspiratory vaso-constriction in patients after spinal injuries. J. Physiol., *107*:67-75, 1948.
12. Guttmann, L., Frankel, H. L. and Paeslack, V.: Cardiac irregularities during labour in paraplegic women. Paraplegia, *3*:144-151, 1965.
13. Guttmann, L., Munro, A. F., Robinson, R. and Walsh, J. J.: Effect of tilting on the cardiovascular responses and plasma catecholamine levels in spinal man. Paraplegia, *1*:4-18, 1963.
14. Guttmann, L., Silver, J. and Wyndham, C. H.: Thermoregulation in spinal man. J. Physiol. (London), *142*:406-419, 1958.
15. Heymans, C. and Neil, E.: *Reflexogenic Areas of the Cardiovascular System.* London, Churchill, 1958.
16. LaBan, M. M., Johnson, H. E. and Verdon, T. A. Jr.: Blood volume following spinal cord injury. Arch. Phys. Med. Rehabil., *50*:439-441, 447, 1969.
17. Long, C. and Lawton, E. B.: Functional significance of spinal cord lesion level. Arch. Phys. Med. Rehabil., *36*:249-255, 1955.
18. Mertens, H. G., Harms, S., Harms, H. and Jungmann, H.: The regulation of the circulation in patients with cervical cord transection. Deut. Med. Wochschr., *85*:180-185, 1960. English edition: German Medical Monthly, *5*:189-192, 1960.
19. Miller, J. M., Downey, J. A. and Darling, R. C.: The cardiovascular effects of breathing 5 per cent carbon dioxide. Arch. Phys. Med. Rehabil., *50*:442-447, 1969.
20. Randall, W. C., Wurster, R. D. and Lewin, R. J.: Responses of patients with high spinal transection to high ambient temperatures. J. Appl. Physiol., *21*:985-993, 1966.
21. Robertson, D. N. S. and Guttmann, L.: The paraplegic patient in pregnancy and labour. Proc. Roy. Soc. Med., *56*:381-387, 1963.
22. Sherrington, C. S.: Notes on temperature after spinal transection, with some observations on shivering. J. Physiol. (London), *58*:405-424, 1924.
23. Sherrington, C. S.: The spinal cord. *In:* Schäfer, E. A. (ed.): *Text Book of Physiology.* Edinburgh, Y.J. Pentland, 1900, V.2, pp. 849-856.
24. Simon, E., Rautenberg, W. and Jessen, C.: Initiation of shivering in unanaesthetized dogs by local cooling within the vertebral canal. Experientia, *21*:476-477, 1965.
25. Thauer, R.: Der nervöse Mechanismus der chemischen Temperaturregulation des Warmbluters. Naturwissenschaften, *51*:73-80, 1964.
26. Ustach, T. J., Tobon, F., Hambrecht, T., Bass, D. D. and Shuster, M. M.: Electrophysiological aspects of human sphincter function. J. Clin. Invest., *49*:41-48, 1970.
27. Vallbona, C., Lipscomb, H. S. and Carter, R. E.: Endocrine responses to orthostatic hypotension in quadriplegia. Arch. Phys. Med. Rehabil., *47*:412-421, 1966.

Chapter 16

EFFECT OF FORCE ON SKELETAL TISSUES

by C. Andrew L. Bassett, M.D., Sc.D. (med.)

INTRODUCTION

It generally is recognized that increased use leads to hypertrophy and disuse to atrophy. Furthermore, there seems to be an innate relationship between form and function. These facts rule the life of the athlete and shape the therapeutic plans of the physician. Until the nineteenth century, however, little was known about the mechanisms behind form and function, hypertrophy and increased use, atrophy and disuse. The first glimmer of understanding was provided when Swiss and German efforts linked engineering principles and anatomy. These early efforts to explain the way in which physical forces might shape the skeleton, after initial form is determined genetically, have stood the test of time and provide the basis for many of our current concepts. More recently, increasing attention has been devoted to effects of physical forces on the behavior of connective tissue cells and on responses of extracellular matrices of skeletal tissues. In fact, the interaction between these cells and their structural, extracellular by-products now seems to be the foundation of control mechanisms relating physical force, orientation and mass. It is important, therefore, that the reader have a working knowledge of the properties of the two major structural, extracellular by-products of connective tissue cells, collagen and mucopolysaccharide. Since an extensive discussion of these macromolecular biopolymers is outside the scope of this chapter, the reader is referred to an excellent review entitled *Physiology of Connective Tissue* by M. Chvapil (1967) for specific details.

Collagen is the primary structural component of both mineralized and non-mineralized connective tissues and it will serve as a central focus in several sections of this chapter. Recently the electromechanical behavior of this fibrous (crystalline) protein has been the subject of increasing attention, and it has been proposed that the electromechanical properties of collagen are intimately involved in controlling the activity of connective tissue cells. Furthermore, since bone—a mineralized, collagenous tissue—has been studied very intensively, it will serve as the supporting framework for the chapter.

MECHANICAL FORCES AND BONE ARCHITECTURE

The relationship between the form a bone assumes and its function has been the subject of continuing study since 1867. Before the results of those studies are considered, however, it is important to grasp the broader meaning of the word "form." The most comprehensive view of this subject is to be found in a magnificent two-volume work entitled *On Growth and Form* by d'Arcy W. Thompson (1943). For those who wish to bask in the pure joy of discovery, Thompson describes in clear biological, mathematical and mechanical terms the molding forces that have shaped such diverse creatures as the periwinkle, the dinosaur and the mammals. In a rewarding little book entitled simply *Bones*, a disciple of Thompson, P.D.F. Murray (1936), reviewed, specifically, mechanical factors responsible for the organization of bone. With the information at hand in 1936, he traced hierarchical ordering of subunits that results in the ultimate shape of a bone. More recently Weiss (1965) has described the ramifications of the term "form" in these words,

Form, in contradistinction to random shape, contains parts or elements in a definite, characteristically recurrent array in space. Thus form is the result of the orderly manner in which those elements are combined and arranged. Static form is but the outcome of formative dynamics. . . .

Since the elements of living systems come in a hierarchy of different orders of magnitude and complexity—organs, cells, organelles, macromolecular complexes, macromolecules—the population of elements whose ordered array defines form is heterogeneous and composite. Form of a higher order of complexity accordingly can emerge from the ordered assembly of simpler formed elements of mutual fit. This compounding of higher order proceeds stepwise.

So it is in bone, in which ordered tropocollagen units form ordered fibrils in the presence of highly structured macromolecules of protein-polysaccharide. The fibrils in turn become calcified in a strictly ordered pattern; they are then formed into parallel fiber bundles and lamellae to form the osteons and trabeculae that finally constitute a bone. (An osteon can be defined as the volume of bone, generally cylindrical in shape, enclosing a central haversian canal from its point of origin to its point of division or connection with a Volkmann canal.) Throughout the hierarchy of this organization, the spiral pattern, inherent in the helix of the collagen macromolecule, is repeated in the collagen bundles in lamellae and in the osteons of a long bone. Although it is clear that highly ordered form can result from a systematic assembly of structural subunits, it is not yet known precisely how forces direct this construction process. If one excludes recrystallization and "stress working" (molecular reordering as a result of stress), the cell is primarily responsible for the production and assembly of the extracellular inanimate subunits. In simple terms we can ask, "How does the cell 'know' when, where, how, and in what orientation to produce bone elements whose form and mass are balanced economically with strength and weight?"

Wolff's Law

In 1867, Culmann, a Swiss engineer who had observed that the trabecular structure of the femoral neck resembled that of a Fairbain crane, collaborated with Meyer to put forth a theory that bone trabeculae are oriented along trajectories arising from compression and tension. Popularized and modified by Wolff between 1870 and 1892, this basic concept now is commonly referred to as Wolff's Law (1892). In its most elementary form this law states that a bone becomes adapted during its growth to functional forces acting upon it. Numerous modifications to the law have been proposed since the 1890s. One of these, introduced by Thoma in 1907, drew attention not only to the quantity of the force, but also to the length of time it acted, thereby implying the importance of cyclic or dynamic loading in the living animal. Jansen (1920) was the first to propose that effects of compression and tension were different and rejected the role of tension in bone formation. He restated Wolff's Law in the following terms: "The form of a bone being given, bone elements place or displace themselves in the direction of functional pressure."

Despite Jansen's views, a dichotomy still seems to exist in interpretations of the effects of compressive and tensile forces on bone formation. For example, many articles and textbooks dealing with fracture care express the opinion, almost universally accepted by clinical orthopedics, that compression leads to bone resorption. Yet it has been demonstrated that *static* compression both in cancellous bone, up to 4000 lbs per sq in, and in cortical bone, from 6000 to 12,000 lbs per sq in, does not result in resorption. In the application of orthodontic forces, which are miniscule when compared with the figures cited immediately above, bone is known to be deposited on the tensile side of the tooth and removed on the "compressive" side. Furthermore, both osteoblastic and osteoclastic activities coexist within a few micra of one another in primary healing of fractures, in reorganizing bone grafts and in the tuberous insertions of muscles, a site where tensile forces are believed to predominate.

Much of the early dilemma in deciding whether a compressive or a tensile force stimulated osteogenesis or osteoclasis now can be resolved by recognizing that few forces are "pure" and that it is the *net* force that is important. Consider, for example, the situation in bowed weight-bearing long bones of large mammals, which generally are loaded in bending. If such a mechanical system is considered solely on the basis of in vitro testing, the concave side of the bone is under compression, while the convex side is under tension. This situation probably does not exist in a normally bowed bone in the living animal. In Frost's opinion (1964), the role of tension loading in bones has been exaggerated in biomechanical thinking. This should not be interpreted to mean that tension loading does not exist. It obviously does at muscle attachments, including the large ones at the trochanters, at various tuberosities and at the broad fleshy origins of many muscles. But it is doubtful that significant tension loads are generated in the shafts of long bones by bending, the reason being that in these bones the compression loads seem to outweigh the bending loads by more than three to one.

Unfortunately, most analyses of stress-strain patterns in whole bone have been derived from static or dynamic in vitro testing and in the absence of active musculature. When an attempt is made to correlate data arising from such studies with indices of living bone remodeling (the summation of osteoclastic and osteoblastic activity), much confusion may result. It remains to be proved whether convexity in the living animal is always, intermittently or never characterized by *net* tensile forces. Certainly, one would predict that if bowing were great and a large load were applied rapidly, the convex surface of a tubular bone would be under *net* tension. Under these conditions, if osteogenesis is stimulated by compression and destruction by tension, the concave cortex would become thicker and the convex would be thinner. This correlation can be observed in a variety of clinical problems which produce significant bowing of the weight-bearing long bones.

One of the best current interpretations of the effects of compression on the one hand and tension on the other was made by Enlow (1968):

> ...bone is a most sensitive and labile tissue.... It is believed that there is a threshold level within which both pressure and tension function to stimulate osteogenesis. If this level is exceeded, both pressure and tension serve to induce resorption.

This statement probably can be improved by expanding it to include the concepts of static forces as opposed to dynamic forces, because load levels, loading rates, stress concentrations are all important. Furthermore, it must be remembered that the mechanical behavior of bone is determined both by its elastic and viscoelastic properties. It is likely that bone is at least a two-phase material (fiberglass is a common example) and possibly a three-phase material. Bone has been compared to prestressed concrete, its collagen fibrils being in a state of tension (even in an unloaded bone) and its apatite in a state of compression. Any elastic system loaded in tension develops compressive forces at right angles to the axis of loading. This factor may assume a dominant role in interpreting osteogenesis in orthodontic movement, in suture growth, in healing of isolated cortical defects and in any attempt to link the compacting forces of an in vitro bone forming system (Bassett, 1962, 1964) with osteogenesis in vivo. Of one thing we can be confident: when we grasp the full picture, we shall likely find that Nature responds consistently to basic principles. For those interested in a more comprehensive, modern view of Wolff's Law, the writings of Enlow (1968), Frost (1964), Johnson (1966) and Trueta (1968) are recommended.

It will be noted in the foregoing discussion of Wolff's Law that the major emphasis in the past has been placed on alignment of trabeculae and other osseous structures along axes of stress. Orientation and form, however, are not the sole effects of mechanical stimuli in bone, for as Paget wrote in 1853, "Nature strives for safety before symmetry." As knowledge of bone physiology and disease has grown, Galileo's observation relating bone mass and the forces acting on it has become increasingly important. In fact, it seems appropriate to expand Jansen's (1920) rephrasing of Wolff's Law to state, "The form of a bone being given, the bone elements place or displace themselves in the direction of functional forces and increase or decrease their mass to reflect the amount of the functional forces" (Bassett, 1968). In the next two sections, we will summarize information relevant to the second portion of this restatement of Wolff's Law, namely that "[bone elements] increase or decrease their mass to reflect the amount of functional force."

Osteopenia as a Result of Bed Rest, Disuse and Weightlessness

In the past several decades, investigators have become increasingly aware that bone mass is determined to a significant degree by mechanical stimuli. When these stimuli are reduced by prolonged recumbency, immobilization, flaccid paralysis or weightlessness, bone atrophy ensues. As a result, the individual develops hypercalciuria and a negative calcium balance. Skeletal loss is nearly directly proportional to total negative calcium balance, and the alterations in physical parameters of atrophied bone are due mainly to the decrease in bone mass. When bone resorption is sufficiently advanced, reduction of bone mass can be detected radiographically. Depending upon the method used, changes in mass from 2 per cent upward are measurable by photon scanning, step wedge densitometry and by standard x-rays for losses in excess of 25 per cent. Unfortunately, the terms "demineralized" and "decalcified" have gained wide acceptance in clinical use, where they usually are synonymous with diminished radiographic density. It is argued that since the x-ray beam detects mainly calcium in bone, increased penetrance is secondary to loss of mineral. Such an interpretation ignores the basic mechanism of bone resorption, in which both the organic and inorganic fractions are lost almost simultaneously except occasionally during perilacunar resorption by osteocytes (calciolysis). It would appear, therefore, that a term such as "deossified" would be more appropriate to describe osteopenic (osteoporotic) bone.

The first studies linking bed rest and increased urinary calcium excretion were made in 1929. Since then, a number of investigations have confirmed and expanded the original observations. These have been reviewed recently by Birge and Whedon (1968) and by Issekutz, et al. (1966). Most of the studies demonstrate clearly that bed rest, either enforced by disease or in normal volunteers, results in a rapid decrease in bone mass. This loss has been followed recently by means of x-ray densitometry of the os calcis and has been documented to be significant within two weeks. Generally, bed rest studies also have sought information on the effects of exercise and weight bearing in ameliorating the increased urinary calcium excretion associated with bone loss. Results of weight bearing have been more satisfactory than of exercise alone. For example, 3 hours of quiet standing per day was found to induce a slow decline of the elevated calcium excretion. Some investigators have concluded that hypercalciuria secondary to prolonged recumbency is due to absence of longitudinal pressure (weight bearing) on the bones, rather than to physical inactivity during rest. In fact, in one study subjects did not decrease urinary calcium output even with 4 hours of vigorous exercise per day, if it was performed in the supine position. This interpretation of the importance of weight bearing is buttressed by the finding that dynamic axial compression (up to 100 pounds, achieved by means of springs with the subject still in bed) will produce results that mimic weight bearing. In a similar vein, the use of an oscillating bed decreases negative calcium balance in recumbent subjects without planned exercise regimes. A program of axial compression exercise using springs, similar to the one described above, has been adopted by the National Aeronautics and Space Administration (NASA) for the astronauts and, despite other variables, may have reduced both loss of bone mass and negative calcium balance. For those who are interested in gaining a more complete picture of this subject, the reviews by Birge and Whedon (1968) and by Hattner and McMillan (1968) are recommended.

The effects of prolonged bed rest on the whole skeleton are reproduced by immobilization in plaster casts that incorporate most of the body, by extensive poliomyelitis and other amyotonic diseases, by weightlessness or by buoyancy. Furthermore, local osteopenia can be induced by a variety of techniques. Long bones supported by casts or by rigid plates and screws, extremities subjected to nerve or tendon section and bone grafts placed in non-functional sites all contribute to bone atrophy.

A loss of bone mass, as measured by increased urinary calcium excretion, has been documented in patients with poliomyelitis and may give rise to urolithiasis as a result of prolonged hypercalciuria. Interestingly, weight bearing fails to correct the increased negative calcium balance in patients with extensive poliomyelitic paralysis. This observation suggests that the role of muscle activity in reversing disuse atrophy of bone is not yet fully understood.

The few data that are available on the effects of weightlessness arise from the NASA Gemini IV, V and VII missions. These lead to the conclusion that prolonged space flight will cause a significant reduction in bone mass. The extent of this problem has not yet been defined and is dependent upon more concrete information, which, unfortunately, can be gained only from orbital or interplanetary flight. Attempts to simulate the weightless state on earth have been limited largely to studies of the effect of buoyancy on the skeleton. There is a conspicuous loss of bone mass in major weight-bearing bones of beagles placed in a water buoyant environment for 32 days. A return to active weight bearing reverses the changes. At this point it should be noted that animals raised in increased gravitational fields demonstrate changes in bone shape and a larger bone mass. Similar findings resulted when the weight of immature animals was increased acutely by artificial means and when quadriped animals were forced to adopt permanently a bipedal mode of ambulation. Furthermore, recent studies have demonstrated that bone hypertrophies in normal rats subjected to exercise.

In studies of more localized bone atrophy many experimental models have been used. Disuse osteoporosis has been induced by plaster immobilization of limbs, by nerve section and by tendon section. Most of the investigations have produced variable effects on osteogenesis, but a marked increase in osteoclastic activity. It still is not clear whether vascular changes are primarily responsible for the bone resorption or secondarily associated with it. Interestingly, combination of parathyroidectomy and thyroidectomy with immobilization has been reported to prevent disuse osteoporosis.

Investigators in Switzerland have suggested that excessively rigid internal fixation of fractures causes osteoporosis and architectural disorganization in the supported segment by reducing the normal mechanical stimuli. Recently it was found that application of two compression fracture plates at right angles will reduce strain levels in the canine femur by a mean of 45 per cent. Reduction of mechanical stimuli in autogenous, cortical bone grafts, transplanted to non-functional sites in soft tissues, also may be responsible for the initial osteoporosis and subsequent resorption of these grafts. If bone transplants are spring loaded and placed in soft tissues, however, extensive remodeling occurs. Resorption appears characteristically on the convex side of the bone and formation on the concave; this produces a drift in the axis of the bowed graft toward the axis of the load. This behavior, and that of cortical bone grafts placed across actively growing epiphyses, demonstrates, as proposed earlier in this chapter, that cyclic, *net* tensile forces probably result in osteoclasia.

These observations on fracture fixation and bone grafting in animals indicate that cells invading and within bone are extremely sensitive to changes in mechanical stimuli. Similar findings have been documented in tissue culture studies. Recently the rate of P^{32} release into the medium by bone samples was found to be dependent upon the amount of mechanical stress focused on the explant. Furthermore, in vitro studies conducted 10 years ago in this laboratory demonstrated that mechanical forces controlled, in part, the differentiation of bone or fibrous tissue from mesenchymal cells.

A discussion of postmenopausal, senile and steroid-induced osteoporosis is outside the scope of this chapter. On the other hand, from the evidence currently available it is likely that disuse must be considered a major etiologic factor in both postmenopausal and senile types. Skeletal atrophy may result from the simultaneous action of several different factors. For example, prolonged negative calcium balance (whether from inadequate intake or absorption or from excessive excretion) can cause osteoporosis. The changing pattern of physical activity in aging individuals who "hurt" undoubtedly has an additive effect on bone atrophy and must be considered in an evaluation of the total picture. Certainly immobilization of patients with osteoporosis is not to be recommended; on the contrary, every effort must be made to improve skeletal loading patterns and muscle tone.

Fatigue (Stress) Fractures

In the discussion of Wolff's Law, Enlow's view of the role of compression and tension on bone was emphasized. From his interpretation and from other data cited earlier, it seems likely that the rate and magnitude of loading are critical to maintaining or increasing bone mass. Furthermore, intermittent compression and tension operate within threshold levels to stimulate osteogenesis. If these levels are exceeded or if a continuous, *net* tensile force exists, resorption may result. This concept is *central* to an understanding of fatigue fractures and other situations characterized by bone resorption in regions of excessive loading (e.g., osteoarthritic "cysts").

Although it has long been recognized that fatigue (stress, march) fractures may occur when bone is subjected to repeated, excessive mechanical demands, it was not until 1963 that Lent Johnson and his co-workers documented the sequence of pathologic events. From their studies of the histogenesis of the lesion, it is evident that deossification, microfracture and osteocyte death do not precede fracture. Prior to resorption of bone, clearly defined changes in organization were observed in the collagen bundles; osteoclasis followed. The disorganization seems to be generated by the continued, elevated stress in the bone and by the resultant elastic deformation and recoil. Characteristically lesions were located in unosteonized regions of the cortex; development of lesions was followed by a healing phase in which both endosteal and periosteal callus buttressed the region of resorption. The reader is referred to Morris and Blickenstaff (1967) for a more complete presentation of this problem.

From the foregoing discussion, it is evident that there is a direct relationship between mechanical stress and the mass and orientation of bony structures. Both the amount and direction of the stress apparently are reflected in the activity of bone cells. Since the cells of bone are primarily responsible for the elaboration and destruction of extracellular osseous matrix, it is essential to determine the mechanisms by which stress affects the behavior of these osseous and preosseous cells. Current concepts of the mechanism will be considered later.

MECHANICAL FORCES AND CARTILAGE

At the outset of this discussion, it was noted that collagen is the common structural element of the connective tissue. This fibrous protein is the major organic fraction of bone and accounts for 20 per cent of its total dry, fat-free weight. Cartilage exists in several forms, each of which has a larger content of collagen than does bone. For example, dry, ash-free hyalin cartilage, such as covers the articular surfaces of joints, contains 50 per cent collagen, as does the nucleus pulposus. The fibers of each type of cartilage have a characteristic orientation that most frequently reflects the stress patterns. In hyalin cartilage, the collagen fibers are arranged in von Benninghoff's arcades. Those at the joint surfaces are aligned parallel to the underlying bony contours and, thereby, resist lateral expansion of the cartilage during loading. Collagen in this superficial layer is subjected primarily to tensile forces. Deeper in the cartilage, collagen bundles are perpendicular to the bony surfaces, are arranged in columns and are loaded mainly in compression. It is believed that highly charged, protein-polysaccharide molecules may be linked in some manner to the collagen fibers. These molecules would serve, together with the incompressible extracellular fluid, to stabilize the structure against major deformation during cyclic compression.

Articular Cartilage

It is evident from a variety of sources that mechanical forces control not only the histogenesis of cartilage but also its maintenance. Just as in bone and other connective tissues, the cells of cartilage synthesize the complex macromolecules of the extracellular matrix. Furthermore, it is conceivable that these cells are responsible in part for the alignment of collagen fibers in the tissue. It is important, therefore, to document how mechanical forces affect cartilage.

Although the histogenesis of cartilage was studied extensively in vitro during the period from 1920 to 1940, little specific information concerning the role of dynamic or static stresses on development was available until recently. In the past four years, however, much has been accomplished to demonstrate the importance of mechanical forces on the development of cartilage. The elegant studies by Drachman and Sokoloff (1966) show clearly that spontaneous movements by the embryo during its development are essential to the primary formation of joint cavities and their associated ligaments. Muscle paralysis was induced in growing chick embryos by two neuromuscular blocking agents, decamethonium bromide and type A botulinum toxin, and by spinal cord extirpation. All three methods of paralysis resulted in a failure of the joint cavity to form and in poorly sculptured articular surfaces. When cavitation failed to occur, the interzone of the paralyzed joints was filled first by a fibrous or cartilaginous tissue.

Organ culture experiments also point directly to the essential nature of mechanical stimuli in the evocation of cartilage (Hall, 1968). Hall repeated the interesting experiments of Glucksmann that had been interpreted to show that mechanical factors determined whether cartilage or bone would develop in a tissue capable of forming both. The results of Hall's studies demonstrate that germinal cells of avian membrane bones may be induced to form cartilage by movement. Hall did not observe cartilage formation when static compression was applied by means of Glucksmann's system.

The behavior of embryonic joints and cartilage under the influence of motion in culture *in ovo* is paralleled by findings in the mature animal. For example, excessive repetitive motion at a fracture site (particularly lateral or torque shear), will result in the formation of a pseudarthrosis. In long standing pseudarthroses, most of the structural elements of a joint are present. Well-differentiated hyalin and fibrocartilage cap the bony ends, and the cleft ("joint cavity") is filled with a mucinous liquid similar to joint fluid. Re-establishment of bony continuity, both in a fibrous union and in true pseudarthrosis, centers on the elimination of motion by means of rigid fixation. This can be accomplished by application of compression screws and plates, a well-fitted intramedullary nail, transcutaneous pins or rods that fix the bone to a rigid, external frame or by onlay, cortical bone grafts. Once motion between the contiguous bony fragments has ceased, cartilage or fibrous tissue, or both, in the gap undergo gradual remodeling and are transformed into bone.

Regeneration of cartilage following resection of an articular surface also is dependent upon cyclic motion. New fibrocartilage is formed most effectively if movement is delayed until a sufficient population of mesenchymal cells is present in a structurally firm granulation tissue. When motion is prevented or started after an optimal time period, a firm fibrous scar develops. Similar findings are common in the studies of cup arthroplasties. Despite the prompt production of fibrocartilage in the adult, neither motion nor any other known factor is able uniformly to induce hyalin cartilage.

From the foregoing, it is evident that dynamic compression, tensile and shear forces are involved in the development of joints and their covering cartilage. The maintenance of normal chondrocyte behavior and of normal articular structure also requires the continuing operation of functional forces. When a joint is immobilized or its surface statically compressed or unopposed, rapid degeneration of the cartilage ensues. Opposing articular surfaces of rabbit knee joints that are in contact have been shown to degenerate within two weeks following compression and immobilization. Similar results have been obtained by immobilization alone, without significant compression. More recently, destruction of articular cartilage of tibial condyles has been observed following resection of the opposing femoral condyle. In a study, conducted recently in these laboratories by Thompson, of the simultaneous use of compression-immobilization and femoral condyle resection in a series of rabbit knees, differing mechanisms of cartilage destruction were found in the two systems. Histologic features in the compression-immobilization series were similar to those reported by previous investigators. They were characterized by progressive loss of metachromasia, disruption of collagen bundle architecture, including fibrillation, and by cloning of chondrocytes. In three week old specimens, almost all of the extracellular matrix was destroyed and replaced by a population of spindle-shaped and ameboid cells. These changes occurred progressively from the joint surface until ultimately the subchondral bone of opposing surfaces was in contact. In animals subjected to resection, breakdown of cartilage was effected primarily from the underlying bone. Marked osteoporosis of the unopposed tibial condyle appeared and was associated with an increase of the vascular bed, commonly observed in disuse osteoclasia (Geiser and Trueta, 1958). As the vascular elements broached the subchondral bone plate, cartilage erosion ensued and the articular surface was destroyed mainly from below. Attendant with these histologic changes, elevations of lysosomal enzymes were noted in the degenerating cartilage and synovial fluid. These observations of cartilage destruction are consistent with a scheme proposed by Chrisman (1969) for the development of arthritic changes in cartilage and are represented by a negative feedback system shown in Figure 16-1.

Apparently both cartilage and osseous cells respond promptly to changes in mechanical force patterns by altering their metabolic activities. Although evidence strongly suggests that mechanical stimuli also are involved directly in the specialization of cartilage cells, the underlying mechanisms have not been clarified. Some insight into these relationships will be provided in the section on mechanisms.

Epiphyseal Cartilage

Like the histogenesis and maintenance of articular cartilage the behavior of epiphyseal cartilage is dependent upon physical forces. Increased compressive forces, acting across the epiphyseal plate, result in decreased longitudinal bone growth (Blount and Zeir, 1952). When induced by staples or wires, these forces lead to characteristic histologic changes in the cartilage of the plate. Release of compression or introduction of tension, on the other hand, causes acceleration of growth (Arkin and Katz, 1965). When a growing epiphysis is subjected to stress, the rate or direction, or both, of the growth of that epiphy-

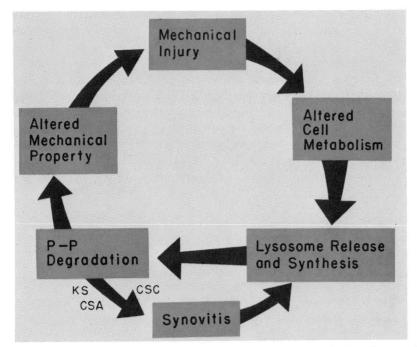

Figure 16—1 Scheme representing current concept of negative feedback cycle operating in development of osteoarthritis. P-P stands for protein-polysaccharide, KS for keratosulfate, CSA for chondroitin sulfate A and CSC for chondroitin sulfate C. (Drawn from Chrisman: Biochemical aspects of degenerative joint disease. Clin. Orthop., *64*:77, 1969.)

sis is modified so that it yields to the stress, particularly if the stress is static (as opposed to dynamic). Pressures applied in a direction parallel to the direction of epiphyseal growth inhibit the rate of growth. While considerable pressures are necessary to stop cartilaginous growth completely, slight or even intermittently increased pressures can slow or hinder it. Pressures applied in directions perpendicular to the direction of epiphyseal growth deflect the direction of such growth, resulting in lateral or spiral (torsional) displacement of the newly laid down bone. The ease with which angular or torsional deformities may be produced in a growing bone varies with its diameter; the narrower the bone, the greater its "plasticity."

MECHANICAL FORCES AND OTHER NON-CALCIFIED CONNECTIVE TISSUES

Although compression is the major mode of loading in bone and cartilage, tension is dominant in tendons, ligaments and arteries. The collagen bundles generally are arranged parallel to the axis of the tensile force. These tissues are very easily deformed by loading in modes other than tension and are particularly inefficient as structural units when compressed. Collagen comprises fully 86 per cent of the total solids in tendon and, together with elastin, 50 per cent of the dry weight of large arteries. In addition to collagen, mucopolysaccharides and water are essential components of these connective tissues and may account, in significant measure, for their physical properties. It has been suggested, for example, that the differences in tensile strength between tendons in the newborn and in adults may be caused by the greater amount of ground substance present in these two types of tendon. As with bone and cartilage, there is much evidence suggesting that the rate of synthesis, orientation and maintenance of collagen and other components in tendons, ligaments and arteries are, in part, stress dependent.

This fundamental concept is not new. In fact, over a hundred years ago Wilhelm His described the relationship between stress and the development of connective tissues.

At every place where connective tissue is exposed to a constant and often repeated pulling action, there is formed a fibrous band, e.g. a tendon, the direction of whose fibers is parallel to the direction of the pull; where a connective tissue layer experiences a supporting or oft repeated pressure in the same direction, there is formed a fibrous disc, of greater or lesser thickness, of laminated structure, with generally a cross fiber formation, the fibers of which run in planes perpendicular to the direction of the pressure.

Wilhelm Roux also believed at one time that function and action were primary factors in developing specific connective tissue structures. Later, however, he modified his views to include the concept that "directly inherited characters" determined the initial phases of organogenesis and that external stimuli (including stress) controlled the secondary modeling process.

Tendon and Ligament

The effects of physical forces on the histogenesis and maintenance of normal architecture in bone and cartilage are also reflected in tendons and ligaments. Both disuse and increased use lead to fundamental changes in these structures and function shapes their pattern of development, healing and maintenance. It has been noted that one month after nerve section the caliber of a healing tenotomy wound is much less than in control tenotomies of non-paralyzed muscle-tendon units, and that the girth of normal tendons is affected by immobilization. Furthermore, intermittent stress and motion are requisites for the maintenance of certain mucopolysaccharides at physiologic levels in periarticular connective tissue. A reduction of these complex sugars, together with the water they bind, quite possibly affects the physical properties of immobilized collagenous structures. Increased use of tendons in growing rabbits, on the other hand, leads to an enlarged cross-sectional area in primary tendon, without a parallel increase in tenocytes. There is also a significantly greater maximum load-failure capability and a longer linear portion of a stress-strain curve in tendons of rabbits subjected to training. At the same time, failure energy and the maximum load capacity of anterior cruciate ligaments of knees is increased significantly by training.

Although some of the improvement in the mechanical behavior of tendons from trained animals may be due to a larger collagen bulk, certain structural changes undoubtedly take place at the molecular level. For example, the normal 680 Å banding pattern of collagen observed with the electron microscope frequently is disrupted in heavily "trained" tendons. Some fibrils demonstrate increased period lengths; others demonstrate decreased lengths. An additional index of the molecular effects of physical forces is provided by high angle x-ray diffraction patterns of collagen from tendons subjected to prolonged cycles of tension. These indicate a more highly ordered structure.

During repair of a collagenous structure, such as tendon, the initial phase of fibroplasia is followed by a second phase of fiber reorientation, which begins approximately three weeks after wounding. The second phase, which is responsible for the major increase in tensile strength, is dependent upon the continuing operation of functional forces. This behavior shapes the clinical approach to tendon and ligament repair. A similar pattern also is evident in healing fascia and dermis. On the basis of these and other factors, Dunphy and Jackson (1962) postulated that functional use is the prime factor in bringing about fiber orientation and in changing the physical state of collagen, possibly by induction of increased numbers of cross links in fibrils.

Arteries

The laminar fabric of collagen fibers in osteons was thought by Gebhardt, in 1905, to result from radial transmission of tensile forces originating in the vessels of the haversian canals. Although it is doubtful that significant pulsatile waves exist in the small caliber vessels of longitudinally oriented cortical osteons, a similar structure is observed in the lamellae encircling large vessels that enter the cortex perpendicularly from endosteal and periosteal surfaces. This laminated pattern of collagen fiber alignment also is present in the walls of the arteries themselves. Recently, it has been reported that distensible tubes, introduced into the subcutaneous space of immature guinea pigs and rats, will induce formation of circumferential layers of cells and collagen fibers resembling those in arterial walls. This result was obtained only when the tubes were pulsed rhythmically by a pump. In the absence of pulsation, the tubes caused little cellular reaction and no preferred orientation of collagen fibers. These results can be interpreted as demonstrating an effect of physical factors (e.g., radially transmitted, pulsatile forces) on the metabolic activity of connective tissue cells and on their by-products.

Stress affects not only the behavior of collagen fibers in developing vascular structures, but also, apparently, their maintenance. If dense tubes of connective tissue, obtained from the submucosal layer of the small bowel, are transplanted to a non-functional site in the subcutaneous tissue, they promptly resorb. When inserted as grafts into the aorta, they are subjected to pulsatile hemodynamic forces. Under these circumstances, the full thickness of the graft wall is maintained and gradually replaced by an intense connective tissue infiltration.

Thus, it seems likely that synthesis of collagen and ground substance in bone, cartilage, tendon, ligament, artery and other connective tissues is controlled in some manner by mechanical forces. Since these structural, extracellular macromolecules are the by-products of cells, it is essential to determine how cells sense and respond to forces. It is hoped that the following section will provide some insight into possible mechanisms behind this behavior.

MECHANISMS

Many data have been presented in the preceding sections to demonstrate the variety of effects that mechanical forces exert on connective tissues. Repeated reference has been made to the role cells must play in translating these forces into appropriate action. Before embarking on a discussion of the possible mechanisms by which connective tissue cells "sense" and respond to mechanical factors, it is essential to describe briefly some of the characteristics of these cells. Furthermore, it would seem appropriate to summarize their role in synthesizing the macromolecules of which the different connective tissues are constructed.

Cells

An increasing body of information supports the view, expressed clearly for the first time by Maximov in 1927, that each of the connective tissues is produced and maintained by a specialized form of the mesenchymal cell. After embryogenesis, the perivascular connective tissue cell may be considered the prime source of these cells. Although Trueta (1968) favors the view that the endothelial cell is a major source of osteoblasts in postfetal osteogenesis, it seems likely that endothelium is too highly specialized to perform this function without a significant change in its habitus or organelles. In fact, endothelial cells in capillaries may leave their functional position as vascular lining elements and become perivascular, a less specialized form of existence. Together with other perivascular cells, and possibly with lymphocytes and monocytes, they constitute a pool of undifferentiated cells, which can develop a variety of specialized behaviors in response to changes in their microenvironment. Although evidence exists to suggest that the monocyte can develop the capacity to synthesize collagen and mucopolysaccharides under appropriate conditions, wound fibroblasts probably do not arise from hematogenous precursors but from adjacent connective tissue cells.

It still is not clear whether all cells of mesenchymal origin retain, after embryonic development, the capacity to produce all of the extracellular components of the various connective tissues. Recent experiments have been interpreted to show that despite a common genome, the competence of mesenchymal cells to specialize as osteoblasts becomes restricted in postfetal life to populations in specific areas of the body. Although this interpretation may be valid, it fails to consider the possible effects of differing microenvironments on cell behavior in those specific areas. Osteogenesis requires not only a cell with the proper competence (genetic endowment), but also a proper nutrition and an appropriate stimulus.

Until more specific data are available to the contrary, the pool of perivascular connective tissue cells can be considered as the major source of bone cells (osteoblasts, osteocytes and osteoclasts), cartilage cells (chondroblasts, chondrocytes and chondroclasts) and fibrous tissue cells (fibroblasts and fibrocytes). A possible scheme of the spectrum of cell behavior is demonstrated in Figure 16-2. This system provides a reversible pathway in each instance, thereby permitting cells in one type of tissue to re-enter the pool by a modulation of

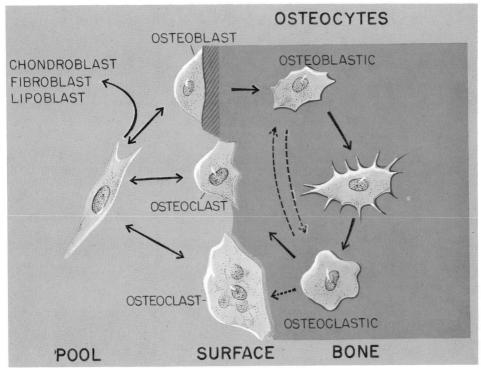

Figure 16–2 Diagram of current concepts of mesenchymal cell specialization. Mesenchymal "pool" cells, under the influence of specific microenvironmental stimuli, specialize as osteoblasts, osteoclasts (mono- or multinuclear), as chondroblasts, fibroblasts or lipoblasts. Once the surface-active osteoblast is incorporated in bone, it may continue to synthesize the organic fractions of bone (osteoblastic osteocyte), "rest" (osteocyte) or resorb (osteoclastic osteocyte). Since cells may reenter the "pool" from specialized function, a wide spectrum of activity is possible.

their behavior from specialized to "despecialized." The terms "modulate and specialize" are used to indicate a reversible or temporary change in function and are more appropriate in this application than the term "differentiate" which implies a fixed or permanent alteration. No attempt is made to prejudge the ultimate function of a cell by labeling it as a preosteoblast or an osteoprogenitor cell, a prechondroblast, or a prefibroblast. This emphasis seems justified by evidence that cells, while in the mesenchymal "pool," have a variety of potential specialization pathways available to them. Given a competence, which is genetically determined, the pathway each follows will depend largely on the microenvironment. For example, certain raw materials or nutrients are required by the cell in order for it to produce collagen or any of the several essential mucopolysaccharides. A host of factors will determine the availability of these nutrients. Some of the more important of these are as follows: (1) the nutritional status of the total organism, (2) the distance of the cell from its source of supply in the adjacent vessel, (3) the diffusion rate in the extracellular space (determined, in part, by fixed charge and filtrational characteristics), (4) the interposition of barriers to diffusion (e.g., other cells) between the cell and its source of nutrition, (5) the propulsion of extracellular fluids by cyclic deformation of tissues and (6) the electrophoretic "pumping" action arising from "stress potentials" (details are advanced in the following section). Cell nutrition is dependent not only on these extracellular factors, but also on properties of the cell itself. The rapidity of movement of the plasma membrane, the rate of pinocytosis, the fixed-charge characteristics and "pore size" of the plasma membrane, and the rate of intracellular streaming all may play a role in determining the type of raw materials available to the cell and all may be affected by factors in the microenvironment.

Although nutrition is of major importance in determining which macromolecules a given cell will synthesize, it is not the sole feature of the microenvironment. The direction and rate of cell migration are controlled by the properties and orientation of extracellular structures in its immediate vicinity. Furthermore, the microenvironment probably encompasses those mechanical or electrical stimuli, or both, responsible for alterations in the rate or pattern of cell division and function.

A significant body of information has been developed to support the view that specialization of mesenchymal cells can be determined by external factors, both in vitro and in vivo. A summary of the details of several studies will be used to demonstrate this point. Bassett (1962, 1964) reported that endosteal and reticular elements (mesenchymal cells) arising from explants of embryonal bone produced bone, cartilage or fibrous tissue or a combination of these, depending upon the conditions present in the tissue culture system. When cells were allowed to become compacted, through repeated excision of the zone of outgrowth and given adequate amounts of oxygen (35 per cent O_2 in the gas phase), bone formation resulted. The bone had histologic and ultrastructural characteristics of fiber bone and was well calcified. These cells, permitted to compact and subjected to low oxygen concentrations (5 per cent O_2 in the gas phase) produced only cartilage. Similar results have been reported recently by other investigators. If the zone of outgrowth was stretched repeatedly, so that compaction was not permitted, and adequate amounts of oxygen were present, highly oriented fibrous tissue, resembling young tendon or fascia, was obtained. From these studies it is clear that both nutritional (O_2) and physical factors (tension versus compaction-compression) determine, in part, the pathway of cell specialization and behavior. Also there seems to be little doubt that if the level of oxygen available to the cell is elevated significantly in culture, both osteoclasia and chondroclasia ensue. In all probability, this pattern of specialization is attendant, in part, upon the activation of lysosomal enzymes within the cells. A host of other factors including parathyroid hormone, thyrocalcitonin, Vitamin A, antibodies, and so forth, introduced into the culture environment also affect profoundly the functional capacity of mesenchymal cells (Fell, 1969).

In a recent paper entitled "Ultrastructural aspects of cartilage and membrane bone differentiation from common germinal cells," Hall and Shorey (1968) trace the patterns of organelle development in osseous and cartilage cells (Fig. 16-3). They conclude that the

"throwing of the morphogenetic switch from osteogenesis to chondrogenesis" involves a change in the rate of collagen synthesis by the germinal cells, a high level of synthesis leading to the differentiation of bone and a low level of synthesis leading to the differentiation of adventitious cartilage.

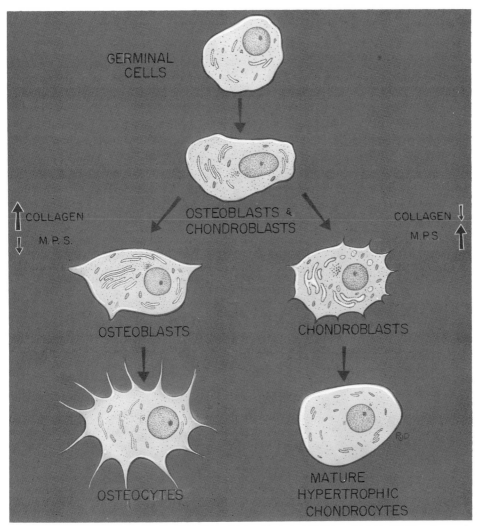

Figure 16–3 Scheme of specialization pathways for osteoblasts and chondroblasts arising from a common stem. Characteristic organelle changes take place along with metabolic changes reflected in increased collagen and decreased mucopolysaccharides (MPS) synthesis by osteoblasts and decreased collagen and increased MPS synthesis by chondroblasts. (After Hall and Shorey: Ultrastructural aspects of cartilage and membrane bone differentiation from common germinal cells. Aust. J. Zool., *16*:821, 1968.)

One of the factors responsible for "throwing the morphogenetic switch" may be the nutritional status of the cell. From tissue culture studies of chick cartilage it is evident that chondrocytes can be induced to form large quantities of collagen and, sometimes, to assume characteristics of osteocytes (Shaw and Bassett, 1967). Although Hall and Shorey (1968) did not find evidence of direct transformation of cartilage to bone or of "dedifferentiation" of cartilage and "redifferentiation" into bone, it must be remembered that they studied whole, normal chick embryos. There is evidence in other systems that fibrous tissue can be transformed into bone, chondrocytes can be transformed directly to osteocytes and the tissues in a pseudarthrosis (cartilage and fibrous tissue) can be transformed to bone without intercedent surgical excision or necrosis.

This pattern of cell behavior should not be surprising, if one considers that bone, cartilage and fibrous tissue have many biochemical similarities. Each contains collagen, mucopolysaccharides and minerals in different proportions, types and combinations. At the ultrastructural level, bone is characterized by an intimate relationship between collagen fibrils and calcium hydroxyapatite crystals. Although this specific association is not found normally in other mammalian mesenchymal tissues, both collagen and mineral may coexist in structures such as the calcified zone of the epiphyseal plate. It is conceivable, therefore, that major alterations in cell function probably are not necessary to produce a collagenous matrix that calcifies, as opposed to one that does not. For example, it is known that variations in the type and amount of mucopolysaccharide present during reconstitution of collagen fibrils may account for physical differences in the resultant fibrils. Furthermore, it now appears probable that a mucopolysaccharide matrix exists in native collagenous fibrils and that the protein-polysaccharides may bear a structural relationship to collagen in the interfibrillar space. At the present time, there seems to be little question that the switch from osteogenesis to chondrogenesis in a population of germinal cells is the result of alterations in the metabolic pathways open to these mesenchymal cells (Hall, 1968). These alterations are characterized by a suppresion of collagen synthesis and a stimulation of acid mucopolysaccharide, mucoprotein and glycogen production during chondrogenesis.

Stimuli

In most adult organisms osteogenesis, chondrogenesis and fibroplasia are in relatively "low gear." Yet with the proper stimulus, a myriad of osteoblasts can appear within a few hours, and the formation of primitive, multipotential granulation tissue is begun in full thickness wounds of cartilage or tenotomies within 24 hours. From these and the foregoing data it can be concluded that production and destruction of connective tissues probably is dependent upon at least three major factors. First, cells with the proper genetic endowment must be available; second, these cells must be properly nourished, and third, they must receive an effective stimulus. In the case of osteogenesis, the stimulus may be chemical, as in the case of egg-laying birds or in hypervitaminosis D, but it also may be mechanical or electrical.

ELECTROMECHANICAL FACTORS CONTROLLING CONNECTIVE TISSUE RESPONSES. The following proposal on the mechanisms underlying the response of connective tissue cells to mechanical factors is based mainly on data collected from studies of bone. It has been shown, however, that cartilage and other non-mineralized mesenchymal tissues have certain electromechanical properties similar to those of bone, and, as noted earlier in the second and third sections, these are affected by physical forces in much the same fashion as bone. Therefore, the mechanisms seem to be applicable to connective tissues in general. When behavior of the different tissues varies significantly, we will attempt to reconcile the variances in the following discussion.

It has been said that there is "little new under the sun." When the author began a study, in 1956, of stress generated electric potentials in bone, he did so at the suggestion of L. C. Johnson, made five years earlier, that bone had piezoelectric properties. Simultaneously and independently Japanese workers were investigating the same phenomenon. Despite extensive searches of published material, neither the author nor Fukada and Yasuda were aware until recently that in Italy Gayda had described the presence of stress induced electric potentials in bone, tendon and cartilage as early as 1912.

In simplest terms, piezoelectricity is electricity produced by pressure on crystals. When a crystal lattice is mechanically deformed, the electric centers of neutrality within the crystal are physically separated, and an electric charge can be detected on the surface. Generally the charge (potential difference) in non-viscoelastic or plastic materials is proportional to the amount of deformation. In a true piezoelectric crystal a converse effect can be demonstrated, i.e., application of an electric field to the crystal produces deformation (strain). For those interested in a more comprehensive discussion of piezoelectricity in biological and non-biological systems, the books by Bazenhov (1961) and Cady (1946) and articles by Bassett (1968, 1971) and by Cochran et al. (1968) are recommended.

On the basis of studies with whole, moist bone, Bassett and Becker (1962) proposed that the stress-generated electric potentials could influence the behavior of cells and affect the alignment and aggregation of their macromolecular by-products. This basic concept was expanded in 1964 to include a theory of bone regulation that is based on a cybernetic or negative feedback loop (Becker et al., 1964). The major points of this system are as follows:

1. Mechanical stress deformed apatite-collagen junctions in bone to produce electric potentials and current proportional to the stress.

2. These potentials and current altered cellular activity and caused alignment of collagen fibers.

3. As a result, structural changes were produced in an appropriate manner to reduce the mechanical stress, thereby closing the negative feedback loop.

Since this proposal was made, a number of modifications have been introduced (Bassett, 1968), and much evidence has been produced to support and clarify the nature of the proposed interactions (Fig. 16-4). For example, many investigators have demonstrated piezoelectric responses in dry bone, and an increase in electric conductivity has been observed when dry bone samples were suddenly deformed. Cochran et al. (1968) and others have made observations on stress potentials in moist bone. The main points of Cochran's work with cantilever-mounted, cortical bone strips can be summarized as follows:

1. Piezoelectricity is generated by extracellular osseous matrix and does not require the presence of living cells for its generation. The voltage waveforms (essentially non-symmetric, biphasic waves) are qualitatively similar for bone of several species and persist without significant alteration, despite a variety of mechanical, physical and chemical treatments, until the specimen approaches destruction.

2. The concave side of the specimen, which is under compression, is always negative, and the convex side, which is under tension, is always positive. It should be remembered that "negative" and "positive" can be relative terms and, therefore, analogous to heat and cold. Cold is the relative absence of heat;

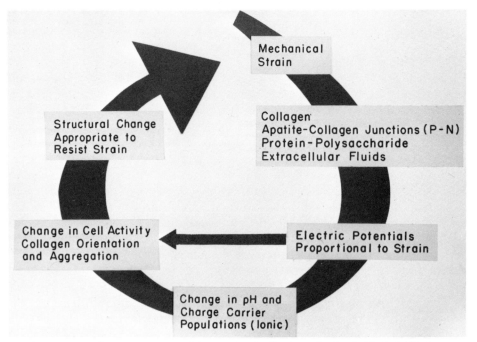

Figure 16–4 Current concepts of the negative feedback mechanism behind Wolff's Law.

positivity may be measured when there are fewer electrons at one electrode than at another.

3. The voltage caused by charge displacement is neutralized by "charge leakage," caused by neutralization of fixed charges by free, mobile charge carriers, during the period of deformation. As a result, another voltage of opposite polarity, but not necessarily of equal magnitude, is generated as load is removed and the specimen allowed to return freely to its resting position by virtue of elastic recoil. A bidirectional current flow, therefore, is generated in the system. The two phases of the current, however, are not necessarily equal. This highly stylized, biphasic system may have few or no counterparts in the living animal.

4. The amplitude of strain generated voltages varies markedly with the rate of deformation (due to "charge leakage") unless the rate is high.

5. Assuming a sufficiently rapid rate of deformation, the amplitude of voltage increases linearly with load (force required to produce the deformation) through the regions of viscoelastic and plastic behavior until fracture. The amplitude of voltage diminishes with load for a given deformation if fatigue is present. Voltage also varies as a function of the amount of deformation along a curve similar to that obtained from plotting the load (force) as a function of deformation.

6. Voltages are generated by feline tibiae, in vivo, in response to forces similar to those produced by normal walking.

Interestingly, electric potentials have been detected in $70\mu \times 100\mu$ sections of a single osteon, loaded rapidly in tension. Electric output from such small samples can approach 1 mv.

The data on the production of stress potentials in bone have been collected by means of a variety of techniques. They are consistent and demonstrate clearly that when the extracellular matrix of bone is deformed, electric potentials and currents result. At the present time there seem to be at least five possible sources of these potentials. Initially, let us consider four of these, which are based on mechanical deformation of crystalline materials with permanent or spontaneous dipole moments. Two of these four possible sources involve piezoelectric properties. First, dry collagen demonstrates classic piezoelectric behavior. Second, steady-state potentials have been reported in deformed bone, and behavior suggesting solid-state characteristics has been detected in hydrated osseous tissues. If semiconductor properties exist, it is conceivable that they, in themselves, may account for stress potentials, since it is known that solid-state devices can function both piezoelectrically and piezoresistively.

The third type of mechanically induced charge separation involves displacement potentials. These have been demonstrated in polyelectrolytes such as potassium hyaluronate. Since mucopolysaccharides are present in bone and other skeletal tissues, they too are likely sources of the total bioelectric response. A fourth type of charge separation involves ferroelectricity and ferroelasticity. Although none of the extracellular matrix components of the skeletal tissues has been demonstrated as yet to have these properties, their crystalline nature suggests the possibility. Many crystalline substances exhibit permanent, spontaneous polarization (dipole moments), which can be reversed by an electric field, and thereby demonstrate ferroelectric properties. One long chain crystalline biopolymer (RNA) has already been found to be ferroelectric. If, in addition to permanent spontaneous polarization, a material demonstrates a shift in polarization secondary to mechanical deformation and a tendency to return to its initial state on removal of the deforming force, it may be termed "ferroelastic."

These four mechanically induced charge separation phenomena may occur in the absence of water, but the fifth possible source of "stress potentials" in skeletal tissues is dependent upon extracellular fluids. It is known that a flow of liquids containing charge carriers (ions and dipoles) past sites of fixed charge (such as exist in extracellular matrix) can produce streaming potentials. The flow, which results in this "hydraulically" induced charge separation, may occur in several ways. First, fluids may be "massaged" through a deformable tissue by cyclically applied external forces and by inherent elastic recoil. Second, fluids may be propelled as they are in the circulatory system, where flow of blood past sites of fixed charge in the walls of vascular spaces will result in a "hydraulically" induced separation of charge. Third, within the cell itself, fluids are in a constant state of motion past sites of fixed charge in the plasma membrane and in the internal membranes bounding the organelles.

Streaming potentials have been demonstrated in tendon (Anderson and Eriksson, 1968), cartilage (Maroudas, 1968) and bone (Cerquiglini et al., 1967) on deformation. Although the total bioelectric response of tendon and cartilage has been interpreted as resulting from streaming potentials, work by these men and others indicates also the presence of mechanically induced charge separation phenomena of the piezoelectric type. Since both of these tissues are essentially avascular, "hydraulically" induced charge separation must result from "massage" of fluids through the extracellular matrix and from intracellular streaming. On the other hand, bone is quite vascular and demonstrates regions of significant potential differences even in the static state, probably on the basis of streaming potentials. The report of Cerquiglini et al. (1967) notwithstanding, it still has not been absolutely determined whether this type of potential also is generated in the relatively incompressible extracellular matrix or canaliculi of bone by deforming forces.

From the foregoing is should be evident that the *total* bioelectric *response to deformation* will reflect both mechanically and "hydraulically" induced charge separation. The relative amounts of each type will depend largely on the deformability or modulus of elasticity of the tissue. Thus, in cartilage or tendon streaming potentials may well account for a larger fraction of the total bioelectric response to deformation than will piezoelectric potentials. In bone, a tissue with a significantly high modulus of elasticity, the reverse probably will be true. Finally, in any cybernetic or feedback control system it is essential that the "correcting" signal be related or proportional to the "triggering" stimulus. It is probable, therefore, that only those potentials that are generated by repetitive deforming forces are involved directly in control of connective tissue orientation and mass. This proposal does not exclude, however, the probable interaction of these "deformation" or "stress" potentials with other bioelectric potentials arising in vessels, cells, nerves and muscles.

All of these factors indicate that the first portion of the proposed negative feedback system of bone regulation (production of electric potentials as a result of deformation) appears to have a firm foundation. The second portion, dealing with the response of cells and their by-products to stress induced electrical activity, has also gained additional support in recent years. One of the first demonstrations in the author's laboratory of a structural effect, centered on the alignment of collagen fibrils in vitro by weak electric currents in the range of 10^{-6} amps (Becker et al., 1964). Subsequently, these findings were expanded, and even weaker currents (10^{-8} amps) were found to be effective in producing orientation of collagen fibrils that were reconstituted from solution (Bassett, 1968). Fibrils with a normal 680Å banding pattern and unbanded fibrils formed at right angles to the field, near the cathode, along the front of a steep pH gradient. It appears, therefore, that one effect of electric potentials in bone might be to cause collagen to orient in a specific pattern on preexisting osseous surfaces where stress potentials are present.

Inherent in these observations is the possibility that long chain, piezoelectric biopolymers, such as collagen and cellulose, may possess an "auto-control" mechanism, which functions largely independently of the cell. As stress induced charge is generated, charged macromolecules and ions in the locality of the fibril or fiber would be attracted to or repelled from its surface. If polymerization of "coupling" then occurred, irreversibly, a "reverse" phase of a biphasic pulse might be inoperative. In this manner, extracellular structures conceivably could revise shape or orientation independently while providing the cell with stimuli that could alter its response (Bassett, 1968). Furthermore, as suggested by recent work in other laboratories, the growth rate of these extracellular crystalline materials can be controlled by the stress generated electric potentials. Teleologically, this pattern of "auto control" could serve Nature economically in limited ways. Cell action still would be required, however, to effect major changes and to provide the specific macromolecules necessary to fabricate extracellular matrix.

In the first three sections of this chapter the key issue was cited repeatedly: what is the mechanism by which mechanical forces are "sensed" by cells and translated into effective action? Two possible explanations exist. First, mechanical forces may affect cells directly. Second, since bone and other connective tissues function as transducers to convert a mechanical to an electric "signal," it is conceivable that this electric response is involved in the regulation of the cells in these tissues. The evidence to support the first of the two possibilities is meager. It is known, for example, that enzyme activity in bacteria can be affected by a marked increase in hydrostatic pressure. Furthermore, protein and nucleic acid synthesis is stimulated or inhibited in *E. coli* by changes in hydrostatic pressure over a range of 4000 to 10,000 p.s.i. Application of pressures up to 5000 p.s.i., however, has not affected DNA synthesis in sea urchin eggs.

In bone and other connective tissues there are no data to link increased or decreased pressures *directly* with cell responses. On the contrary, evidence supports the interpretation that statically increased pressures, over a range from 4000 to 12,000 p.s.i., are not accompanied by any discernible change in the activity of osseous cells. It would seem, therefore, that one could accept, almost by default, the second of the two possible explanations, namely, that mechanical forces affect cell behavior through their capacity to alter the electrical environment of the cell. Fortunately, however, this explanation no longer has to be accepted as an "act of faith" or as the result of teleologic reasoning, since there are abundant data to support it.

Before presenting data to demonstrate that change in the electric environment can affect the behavior of connective tissue cells, a few pertinent examples of conversion of mechanical to electric energy in other biological systems will be given.

"As the twig is bent, the tree's inclined," wrote Alexander Pope. Obviously, then, the cells of plants and trees must be sensitive to changes in physical forces and respond to them in an appropriate manner. Again the mechanism seems to involve the transduction of mechanical to electric energy by a two-phased, extracellular material (cellulose fibers and lignin). Waller (1901) first recognized that vegetable stalks demonstrated "stress potentials." Furthermore, wood and other cellulose based materials are known to have piezoelectric properties (Bazenhov, 1961), and this fact frequently is used in a practical way to determine when lumber is properly "seasoned." Even needle fascicles of pine seedlings and sensory hairs of the Venus flytrap produce electric potentials when they are sharply deflected. Plants generate relatively large differences in potential, and both the direction and amount of growth are affected by external electric fields (Lund, 1947). Marine invertebrates also are sensitive to small changes in hydrostatic pressure, and it has been suggested that this sensitivity has an electric basis. Finally, mechanoreceptors are thought to operate by conversion of mechanical deformation to an electric or chemical signal, which in turn triggers a neural response.

What is the evidence that electric stimuli can affect the behavior of connective tissue cells? Bassett et al. (1964) observed that following implantation of platinum electrodes into the medullary canals of adult canine femora, osteogenesis was markedly increased at the negative pole (cathode). This result was observed when the current exceeded 2×10^{-6} amps (2 microamps). The osteogenic response at the cathode was characterized by a significant increase in cellularity and in the number of mitotic figures during the interval from 14 to 21 days after the battery (1.35 v) resistor packs were implanted. Since then these results have been confirmed in a number of other laboratories. In a recent series of experiments in the author's laboratory a method has been developed to delay osteogenesis in circular cortical defects in canine femora by the insertion of teflon rings. These defects heal much more promptly and completely if stimulated by direct current from a cathode. The distribution of the newly forming bone in the medullary space strongly suggested orientation by the field. In another series of experiments, application of symmetrical, squarewave, alternating current (1 Hz at 3 microamps) failed to increase osteogenesis, whereas continuing direct current, interrupted (1 Hz) direct current and asymmetric alternating current increased the amount of new bone deposited about the cathode. Furthermore, galvanic stimulation will increase the regenerative capacity of limbs in non-regenerating reptiles and accelerate healing of soft tissue wounds.

Shortly after the in vivo studies of electric stimulation of osteogenesis were begun in the author's laboratory, an investigation of the effects of currents on bone formation and development was undertaken in tissue culture. However, polarization, with its attendant shifts in pH, mitigated against a clear-cut result and emphasis was shifted to electrostatic fields. Plastic Petri dish cultures containing 3-T-6 fibroblasts were exposed to both static and dynamic (1 Hz) electrostatic fields ranging from 100 to 2000 v per cm during the period of maximum collagen synthesis (7 to 14 days). In cultures treated statically with 1000 v per cm, DNA synthesis was increased 20 per cent above control values, and collagen (as judged both by total hydroxyproline in the cell sheet and medium and by incorporation of 3-H proline) was increased 40 per cent above the control. In dynamic fields, total collagen synthesis was increased more than 100 per cent. The results bore a discernible relationship to the polarity of the system, and demonstrated quantitative effects as a function of the strength of the applied field. Preliminary electronmicroscopic studies of the electrostatically stimulated cells revealed a strikingly greater number of ribosomes, increased numbers of mitochondria with thin cristae (state III as contrasted with state IV mitochondria in control fibroblasts) and many large secretory vesicles and vacuoles. The potential significance of these results has been buttressed by a study of the effects of electrostatic fields on osteogenesis in living animals. Both static and dynamic electrostatic fields (with a D.C. potential of 100 v and A.C. potentials of 200 v at 3 and 30 Hz) diminished the osteoporosis of disuse in rabbits.

The interaction between electrostatic fields and connective tissue cells is not unique, since apparently many stages of an organisms's life are affected by field effects. For example, electric field patterns have been detected on the surface of amphibia blastulas. It is believed that the surface field pattern of the early embryo has a significant influence on morphogenesis. Electrostatic fields also have been demonstrated to increase mitotic division in chick embryo fibroblasts in vitro. It has been proposed that this effect is based on the presence of electrostatic fields within the cell that result in polarization of mobile π electrons in DNA, which is known to have semiconductor properties.

The cumulative data indicate that connective tissue cells can be stimulated electrically and that the macromolecular by-products of their synthetic activity can be oriented by weak electric currents. Although the pattern of response clearly is consistent with the proposed negative feedback system to control the structure of connective tissue, it still is necessary to define the possible mechanism by which electric phenomena affect cells. This vast subject cannot be dealt with comprehensively in the space at hand, and, therefore, an attempt will be made to summarize the more salient features of these mechanisms. For a more comprehensive review, the reader is referred to articles by the author (Bassett, 1968. 1971).

POSSIBLE MECHANISMS OF ELECTRIC EFFECTS ON CONNECTIVE TISSUE CELLS. From the data cited above, and from many other studies, it appears that both electric currents and electric fields interact with cells to determine patterns of behavior. It is not clear, however, whether potential difference, capacitance or current density has the more important effect on the cell. Since extracellular fluids bathe the surfaces of all possible stress-sensitive, electric generators in the connective tissues (collagen, protein-polysaccharides, collagen-apatite junctions and, conceivably, apatite itself), there are ample numbers of mobile charge carriers to dissipate rapidly any potential difference created by deformation. This does not imply that currents generated during dissipation of potential may not have a profound effect on cells in the area; they probably do, as do the attendant shifts in pH. On first glance, however, this behavior would seem to be unconducive to charge storage and would result in transient electrostatic fields. At least two possible mechanisms exist, however, by which tissues could build up and store the electric charge created by stress for biologically significant periods of time. The first of these involves charge trapping in structural vacancies in the crystal lattice of apatite or other crystalline biopolymers (Bassett, 1968); the second involves electrets (electrically charged, dielectric materials). These materials retain a charge even if their surfaces are short-circuited. A charge will remain for indefinite periods if the insulator properties of the electret are sufficient. Interestingly, the charge is imparted by forming the proper material in an electric field.

The total electric environment of the osseous cell also, conceivably, may be affected by a variety of agents, particularly if bone proves to have solid-state properties. Becker et al. (1964) stated:

Substances such as Vitamin D and certain hormones which are active in minute amounts may function by being incorporated into lattice as impurities or by providing for charge transfer reactions. It also appears feasible to evaluate certain bone diseases from this point of view. Within a living system, the semiconduction mechanism may be altered by injection of large numbers of free charge carriers, by addition of new lattice impurities, or by administration of molecules having proper steric and electronic properties to react with the lattice.

In this regard it should be noted that cyclic AMP, which is a well-established extracellular messenger that mediates a variety of hormonal effects, increases the short-circuit current in isolated toad bladders. At the same time, transmembrane potentials are not increased as much, indicating a fall in electric resistance. On the other hand, parathyroid hormone apparently increases membrane resistance in toad bladders. These observations suggest that a thorough investigation of the effects of parathyroid hormone on the electric environment of osseous cells should be made.

The traditional view of cells assumes that ions are in solution in the cytoplasm of the cell and in the extracellular fluids. In this view, ions move in and out of the cell on the basis of diffusion gradients and by active "pumping" mechanisms. Recently this interpretation has been challenged by Cope (1967) and Ling and Cope (1969), who propose that ions—particularly sodium and potassium ions—are complexed to sites on macromolecules. These ions (and, presumably, others such as calcium) could "hop" from site to site through an icelike matrix, obeying laws analogous to those governing conduction of electrons in semiconducting solids. Ion equilibrium in such a system would depend on relative affinities that different ions have for complexing. Under such circumstances, both dissociation and ion migration would be greatly influenced both by currents and field effects, particularly if the complexing macromolecule itself were stress sensitive and capable of generating deformation potentials. Furthermore, dissociation of bound ions is pH and field dependent and, therefore, under the influence of electric phenomena. Certainly there seems to be clear evidence that the levels of both monovalent and divalent cations available within and without the cell have a profound effect on the cell's behavior. For example, ionic calcium may control many cell functions, from the contractility of the plasma membrane, to mitotic activity, to rates of respiration by mitochondria. Furthermore, ionic potassium is required for protein synthesis. The role of electronic and protonic conduction in biological systems, as a result of solid-state characteristics of the system, is under intensive investigation, and much has been learned about it. Undoubtedly integration of the data arising from this effort will greatly improve understanding of the mechanisms behind the control of cellular behavior. The reader will find comprehensive discussions in a recent conference report (Feigelson, 1969).

Before leaving this brief discussion of the possible mechanism behind the interaction between stress potentials and cell behavior, we should mention a few words about nutrition. Earlier in this presentation the capacity of a cell to synthesize specific macromolecules was related to its nutritional status, to its genetic endowment and to specific stimuli. Furthermore, it was proposed that nutrition was influenced by factors both outside the cell and resident within the cell itself. In fact, the nutrition of osteocytes by simple diffusion through the canalicular system was questioned, and a mechanism of "electrophoretic pumping" has been proposed (Bassett, 1965). Stress generated charge on the bony surfaces surrounding the osteocyte would alternately attract and repel dipoles and ions in such a system. This concept need not be limited to bone, but may well apply in any tissue. All tissues are deformable by a variety of mechanisms (muscular activity, breathing, changes in the center of gravity, impact of a body with its environment and through hemodynamic forces) and all contain biopolymers that can generate charge on deformation (collagen, protein-polysaccharides and, probably, other structural macromolecules). It is likely, therefore, that cell nutrition is both affected and effected directly by movement of substances in the extracellular fluids by electrostatic fields and electrophoresis. The reader is referred to an article by Heinmets and Herschman (1961) in which both the practical and theoretical aspects of the behavior of ions and dipoles in superimposed electrostatic and electromagnetic fields are reviewed. If such a mechanism exists outside the cell, it probably operates inside the cell as well.

Electric phenomena influence not only nutrients reaching the plasma membrane, but probably affect qualitatively and quantitatively the entrance of nutrients into the cell. Theoretically, a large amount of energy is required to transport ions across the plasma membrane. As the size and net charge of a particle increase, the energy expenditure for transport also increases. It has been proposed that "pores" and "carriers" can lower the energy barrier significantly. Specifically, the cell membrane may deform under the influence of electrostrictive forces at the point of ion crossing (in association with a small protein molecule). It is now clear that electrostatic forces are strong on the scale of molecular interactions that stabilize a membrane. Electrostrictive forces, however, may deform the membrane to effect transient changes in membrane permeability during flow of ions across it. In such a system the influence of externally generated "stress potentials" would be great. Furthermore, the plasma membrane itself may have piezoelectric properties (Bassett, 1968). Since cells are in a constant state of motion and can be deformed by external physical forces (both electrical and mechanical), such an intrinsic property would have profound effects on "permeability." Finally, it should be noted that cell membranes and other complex biological systems exhibit electronic conduction, which is indicative of the presence of materials with solid-state characteristics. These characteristics conceivably may be responsible for a piezoelectric response and thereby may be involved in regulation of cell nutrition and in "energy conservation."

Osteogenic Induction

At first glance the reader may wonder why this topic has been placed in its present position and not included with the earlier sections pertaining to bone formation. Although attention in the past has been directed for the most part toward chemical agents that might influence mesenchymal cells to become osteoblasts, there is increasing evidence to suggest that electrical factors also may be involved in osteogenic induction. It seemed advisable, therefore, to provide some details on electric effects and cell behavior prior to a discussion of this topic.

Earlier in the chapter emphasis was placed on three primary factors required for bone formation, namely, cells having the proper genetic equipment, an adequate nutrition, and a proper stimulus. Should any one of these three factors be missing, it is unlikely that osteogenesis will ensue. In this light, the three factors can be considered to exert a permissive action on bone formation. When osteogenic induction is being investigated, therefore, a negative result is not necessarily indicative of the absence of a proper induction principle.

The definition of osteogenic induction is based on concepts of cell interactions that occur during embryogenesis. These can be summarized as a mechanism of cellular differentiation in which there is interaction between one tissue — the inductor — and another — the responding tissue; as a result of this interaction the responding tissue takes a course of development it would not have followed if the interaction had not occurred. An extensive study of bone induction led Urist to postulate, in 1968, two mechanisms by which the differentiation of bone could occur. One embraced the concept of transmission and reflux of a complex group of non-covalently bound macromolecular agents through circumscribed channels in ground substance surrounding mesenchymal cells. The second, which was based on the electric theories (Bassett and Becker, 1962; Becker et al., 1964; Bassett, 1966; and Becker and Murray, 1967), assumed the characteristic structure of bone matrix to be covalently locked in place and that nothing more specific than an electric signal was involved in the bone induction principle. Under these circumstances, Urist theorized, only solid-state properties for diffusion of electrons from the inductive substrate to the plasma membranes of competent mesenchymal cells were required for bone induction. At the present it is impossible to identify precisely, however, which of these two postulates is correct, or whether both or neither are. There is a large body of information suggesting that diffusible chemical factors play a role in bone induction and in the stimulation of connective tissue cells. For example, bone can be induced in ectopic sites following transplantation of bladder mucosa and outside millipore chambers containing bladder mucosa, bone and osteosarcomas. Furthermore, ectopic bone has been induced in gelfoam sponges soaked in aqueous extracts of bovine metaphyseal bone. Collectively, these and other studies point to the first of Urist's postulates — i.e., a chemical induction principle — as a logical assumption. On the other hand, data from a variety of sources suggest just as strongly that electric phenomena are involved directly in osteogenic induction. Although some of these have been cited in previous sections, a recapitulation here may help to buttress the preceding statement.

The observation that the rate of collagen synthesis by fibroblasts can be increased sharply by exposure of the cells to electrostatic fields may have great significance in osteogenesis if Hall and Shorey's (1968) concepts of bone and cartilage differentiation from germinal cells are correct. These authors, it may be remembered, stated that

the "throwing of the morphogenetic switch from osteogenesis to chondrogenesis" involves a change in the rate of collagen synthesis by the germinal cells, a high level of synthesis leading to the differentiation of bone and a low level of synthesis leading to differentiation of adventitious cartilage."

Additional support for this link is provided by the work of Becker and Murray (1967). These investigators observed changes in electric potentials in the bullfrog (*Rana pipiens*) tibia following fracture. Within 24 hours, nucleated red cells within the fracture hematoma underwent a series of morphologic changes, suggesting "dedifferentiation." Similar alterations in the nucleated red cells of the peripheral blood of frogs without fractures could be induced in vitro by the passage of small amounts of current (2×10^{-10} amps). Cells transformed by this technique were capable of synthesizing collagen in tissue culture, whereas normal peripheral red cells were not. Recently, histochemical changes have been reported to occur in these cells, some of which suggest alterations similar to those reported above for fibroblasts exposed to an electrostatic field.

Finally, several diverse observations should be cited to support further the theory that electric phenomena may be involved in bone induction. First, cells from a variety of tissues have low-resistance, intercellular junctions and are electrically coupled. Substances having molecular weights up to 70,000 can pass across these junctions of the plasma membranes. It is possible, therefore, for a colony of interconnected cells to share intracytoplasmic information and electrical experiences. In such a system the behavior of one cell may well determine the behavior of the other cells of the colony. Certainly such a possibility exists in the syncytial arrangement of the cell membranes of osteocytes. Theoretically, if some chemical or electrical "transfer" is required for osteogenic induction, undifferentiated mesenchymal cells could be "induced" when they make contact with cell processes of osteocytes, extending to the surface through canaliculae in bone. Second, inductive information, in the form of electric stimuli, could be passed to cells on osseous surfaces that do not contain living cells, if the bone were being cyclically deformed. It is known that electrons can be conducted through a crystal, subjected to microbending, by means of lattice distortions and edge dislocations. This factor is considered elsewhere in some detail (Bassett, 1968). Furthermore, it is possible that through charge trapping apatite might behave as a "condenser" to store charge and, thereby, produce an electrostatic field (Bassett, 1968). Third, direct transmission of information from the substrate to adjacent mesenchymal cells may also conceivably take place as the result of steric imprinting. If bone (or other connective tissues) is demonstrated to have electret properties, as seems possible, a mechanism for copying the surface would be available. The electret state will occur in superficial layers of a crystal when sufficiently strong electric fields are present. Electron microscopy studies have confirmed the presence of a variety of charge point defects on the surface of semiconductor crystals, the electric field intensity of which may reach thousands of Kv per cm over atomic dimensions. These charge point defects at specific loci on the surface of the crystal impart an "electrical memory" that can transmit structural information by "copying." If bone, other connective tissues and biopolymers (such as DNA) can behave as electrets, the recent identification of ferroelectric properties in RNA may take an added significance in bone induction and a variety of other biological transcription processes. Ferroelectrics, which display dielectric hysteresis, are characterized by the presence of spontaneous dipole moments which can be oriented by the application of electric fields to the material. In such a material, the state of polarization represents a memory of its electrical history.

The degree to which a cell is differentiated undoubtedly determines its latitude of function. Germinal cells might be expected to have more avenues open for specialization than perivascular connective tissue cells in the adult, unless specific behavioral "information" were imparted to the more mature cells. Both chemical induction agents and electrically based "copying" mechanisms may function by directly "programming" a cell for a specific response, or they might "reactivate" certain genetic information repressed by differentiation. In this manner, a cell may gain the potential for bone formation. It still will require adequate nutrition and, possibly, an added stimulus to set its synthetic machinery in motion.

It would be remiss to leave the reader with the impression that electromechanical and other environmental factors are the sole determinants of the shape of a bone. Tissue culture experiments have demonstrated repeatedly that rudiments removed from embryos, long before shape is apparent, have the capacity of developing contours characteristic of the adult bone. Development occurs in an environment completely devoid of neural or major mechanical influences. Clearly, genetic factors must direct this shaping process.

PRACTICAL CONSIDERATIONS IN PHYSICAL AND REHABILITATION MEDICINE

Several guiding principles for the care of patients emerge from the basic information provided in the previous sections. The first of these concerns bone mass. Since stress is dependent upon the cross sectional area of a material and the load it bears, both factors must be considered when forming a clinical opinion on when function is to be permitted and how much is to be allowed. If advanced osteopenia is present and the patient is urged to become excessively active, an acute, gross fracture, a microfracture or a stress fracture will result. Each will bring pain, which will, in turn, limit function. It is essential, therefore, to tailor any rehabilitation program to the capacity of bone to respond to increased demands. This requires time and close supervision of the pattern of loading. Since electrical "signals" seem to be intimately involved in the function of osteoblasts, osteocytes and osteoclasts, the mechanical factors governing the generation of these signals probably are important in shaping rehabilitation programs. In this regard, it is known that the rate of loading must be sufficiently rapid to produce potentials of significant magnitude. Impact loading, therefore, is more effective in promoting osteogenesis than is gradual loading and should be incorporated into programs if the total amount of loading is within the structural (stress concentration) capabilities of the remaining skeleton at any given time. Furthermore, from the limited experience gained in the NASA program and in bed rest studies, cyclic axial compression loading may have an important place in rehabilitating patients with osteoporotic bone or in preventing the sequellae of immobilization or prolonged bed rest. On the basis of this information, a rehabilitation program has been developed, the results of which can be seen in a complex case demonstrated in Figure 16-5.

This program involves the use of an apparatus demonstrated in Figures 16-6 and 16-7. Initially, gradual loading to 10 pounds is applied by the therapist or patient in line with the axis of the extended extremity; this is repeated 4 times a minute for 15 minutes, 4 times a day. After the first week, gradual loading is replaced by rapid or "snatch" loading to 10 pounds, on the same schedule, for an additional week. At weekly intervals thereafter, the levels are raised to a total of 50 to 100 pounds, depending on the patient and his problem.

This general plan of rehabilitation has been used successfully in a variety

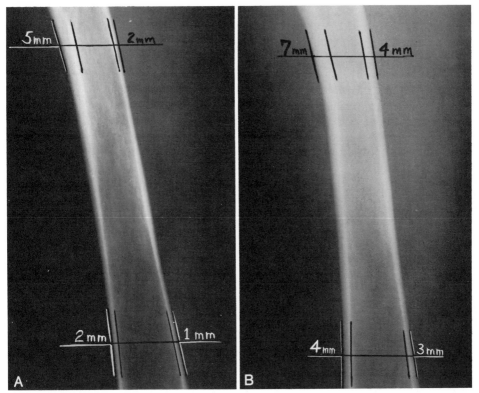

Figure 16–5 *A*, Right femur of 14 year old boy with severe osteoporosis secondary to biliary atresia, cirrhosis and disuse. Note marked thinning of femoral cortices. *B*. Same patient six months after beginning axial compression exercises and graduated weight bearing, partially buoyant in pool. Note that cortices at isthmus of femur now account for one half total diameter (as opposed to less than one third six months previously) and that distal cortices have doubled in thickness.

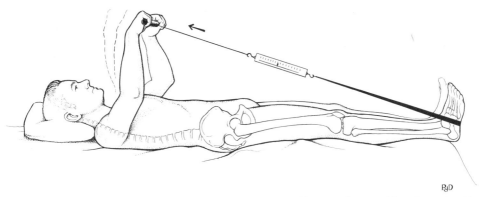

Figure 16–6 Scheme of axial compression exercise used in recumbent position. Arms should be held as close to central axis of body as possible and both feet are included in stirrups. Scale can be graded from 25 to 100 lbs. and may be loaded slowly or rapidly for different effects.

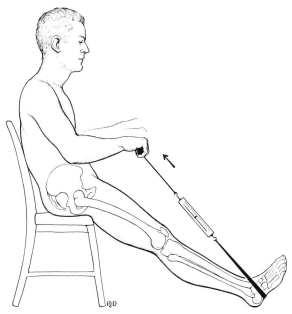

Figure 16–7 Scheme of axial compression exercise for lower extremity. Handle should be kept as close to front of thighs as possible.

of clinical problems. For example, following leg lengthening by the Anderson technique, the newly formed bone in the cortical gap has been subjected to functional stresses within the limits of its mechanical tolerance with beneficial results. Individuals with extensive postimmobilization osteoporosis, as a consequence of fracture and plaster casts, frequently find partial weight bearing too painful to permit rapid return to function. In these patients axial compression exercises have been most helpful prior to weight bearing. Principles involved in the use of this simple device for applying compression probably can be incorporated to better advantage in therapeutic beds. The oscillating bed employed by Whedon and his collaborators was a step in the right direction for individuals confined to bed for long periods. Loading in such an apparatus is gradual, however, and results might well be improved if the loading rate could be increased or perhaps if proper vibration can be substituted.

It seems reasonable to hope that increased understanding of mechanisms behind the electric control of cell behavior eventually may permit adaptation of electric stimulation to rehabilitation of patients with osteoporosis, fractures and growth problems. Before that time, much remains to be done to define the various types of energy which can be used to this end. Electric currents, electrostatic fields, microwaves and radio frequencies should all be investigated. Furthermore, it is essential to determine whether potentials generated by muscle activity interact with bone cells in the maintenance of osseous mass. In the end, we must understand basic functions in biological systems in order to be able to offer patients the best therapeutic programs.

REFERENCES

1. Anderson, J. C. and Eriksson, C.: Electrical properties of wet collagen. Nature, *218*:166-168, 1968.
2. Arkin, A. M. and Katz, J. F.: The effects of pressure on epiphyseal growth. The mechanism of plasticity of growing bone. J. Bone Joint Surg., *38-A*:1056-1076, 1956.
3. Bassett, C. A. L.: Current concepts of bone formation. J. Bone Joint Surg., *44-A*:1217-1244, 1962.
4. Bassett, C. A. L.: Environmental and cellular factors regulating osteogenesis. *In*: Frost, H. M. (ed.): *Bone Biodynamics.* Boston, Little, Brown and Company, 1964, pp. 233-244.
5. Bassett, C. A. L.: Electrical effects in bone. Sci. Amer., *213* (4):18-25, 1965.
6. Bassett, C. A. L.: Biologic significance of piezoelectricity. Calcified Tissue Res., *1*:252-272, 1968.
6a. Bassett, C. A. L.: Biophysical principles affecting bone structure. In: *The Biochemistry and Physiology of Bone.* New York, Academic Press, Inc., 1971.
7. Bassett, C. A. L. and Becker, R. O.: Generation of electric potentials by bone in response to mechanical stress. Science, *137*:1063-1064, 1962.
8. Bazenhov, V. A.: Piezoelectric properties of wood. New York, Consultants Bureau, 1961.
9. Becker, R. O., Bassett, C. A. and Bachman, C. H.: Bioelectrical factors controlling bone structure. *In*: H. M. Frost (ed.): *Bone Biodynamics.* Boston, Little, Brown and Company, 1964, pp. 209-232.
10. Becker, R. O. and Murray, D. G.: A method for producing cellular dedifferentiation by means of very small electrical currents. Trans. N.Y. Acad. Sci., *29*:606-615, 1967.
11. Birge, S. J., Jr. and Whedon, G. D.: Bone. *In*: McCally, M. (ed.): *Hypodynamics and Hypogravics: The Physiology of Inactivity and Weightlessness.* New York, Academic Press, 1968, pp. 213-235.
12. Blount, W. P. and Zeier, F.: Control of bone length. J. Am. Med. Assoc., *148*:451-457, 1952.
13. Cady, W. G.: *Piezoelectricity: An Introduction to the Theory and Applications of Electromechanical Phenomena in Crystals.* New York, McGraw-Hill Book Company, 1946.
14. Chrisman, O. D.: Biochemical aspects of degenerative joint disease. Clin. Orthop., *64*:77-86, 1969.
15. Chvapil, M.: *Physiology of Connective Tissue.* London, Butterworths, 1967.
16. Cochran, G. V. B., Pawluk, R. J. and Bassett, C. A. L.: Electromechanical characteristics of bone under physiologic moisture conditions. Clin. Orthop., *58*:249-270, 1968.
17. Cope, F. W.: A theory of cell hydration governed by adsorption of water on cell proteins rather than by osmotic pressure. Bull. Math. Biophys., *29*:583-596, 1967.
18. Drachman, D. B. and Sokoloff, L.: The role of movement in embryonic joint development. Develop, Biol., *14*:401-420, 1966.
19. Dunphy, J. E. and Jackson, D. S.: Practical applications of experimental studies in the care of the primarily closed wound. Am. J. Surg., *104*:273-282, 1962.
20. Enlow, D. H.: Wolff's law and the factor of architectonic circumstance. Am. J. Orthodon., *54*:803-822, 1968.
21. Feigelson, P.: Electronic aspects of biochemistry. Ann. N.Y. Acad. Sci., *158*:1-438, 1969.
22. Fell, H. B.: The effect of environment on skeletal tissue in culture. Embryologia (Nagoya), *10*:181-205, 1969.
23. Frost, H. M.: *The Laws of Bone Structure.* Springfield, Ill., Charles C Thomas, 1964.
24. Fukada, E. and Yasuda, I.: On the piezoelectric effect of bone. J. Phys. Soc. Japan, *12*:1158-1162, 1957.
25. Geiser, M. and Trueta, J.: Muscle action, bone rarefaction and bone formation. J. Bone Joint Surg., *40-B*:282-311, 1958.
26. Hall, B. K.: *In vitro* studies on the mechanical evocation of adventitious cartilage in the chick. J. Exp. Zool., *168*:283-305, 1968.
27. Hall, B. K. and Shorey, C. D.: Ultrastructural aspects of cartilage and membrane bone differentiation from common germinal cells. Aust. J. Zool., *16*:821-840, 1968.
28. Hattner, R. S. and McMillan, D. E.: Influence of weightlessness upon the skeleton: a review. Aerospace Med., *39*:849-855, 1968.
29. Heinmets, F. and Herschman, A.: Considerations on the effects produced by superimposed electric and magnetic fields in biological systems and electrolytes. Phys. Med. Biol., *5*:271-288, 1961.
30. Issekutz, B., Jr., Blizzard, J. J., Birkhead, N. C. and Rodahl, K.: Effect of prolonged bed rest on urinary calcium output. J. Appl. Physiol., *21*:1013-1020, 1966.
31. Jansen, M.: *On Bone Formation: Its Relation to Tension and Pressure.* London, Longmans, Ltd., 1920.
32. Johnson, L. C.: The kinetics of skeletal remodeling. A further consideration of the theoretical

biology of bone. *In*: Symposium on Structural Organization of the Skeleton. Birth Defects Original Article, Series 2 (*1*):66-142, 1966.

33. Ling, G. N. and Cope, F. W.: Potassium ion: is the bulk of intracellular K$^+$ absorbed? Science, *163*:1335-1336, 1969.

34. Lund, E. J.: *Bioelectric Fields and Growth*. Austin, University of Texas Press, 1947.

35. Maroudas, A.: Physiochemical properties of cartilage in the light of ion exchange theory. Biophys. J., *8*:575-595, 1968.

36. Morris, J. M. and Blickenstaff, L. D.: *Fatigue Fractures: A Clinical Study*. Springfield, Ill., Charles C Thomas, 1967.

37. Murray, P. D. F.: *Bones: A Study of the Development and Structure of the Vertebrate Skeleton*. Cambridge (Eng.), University Press, 1936.

38. Shamos, M. H. and Lavine, L. S.: Piezoelectricity as a fundamental property of biological tissues. Nature, *213*:267-269, 1967.

39. Shaw, J. L. and Bassett, C. A. L.: The effects of varying oxygen concentrations on osteogenesis and embryonic cartilage *in vitro*. J. Bone Joint Surg., *49-A*:73-80, 1967.

40. Thompson, D'A. W.: *On Growth and Form*, 2nd ed. Cambridge (Eng.), University Press, 1942.

41. Trueta, R. J.: *Studies of the Development and Decay of the Human Frame*. Philadelphia, W. B. Saunders Company, 1968.

42. Urist, M. R., Dowell, T. A., Hay, P. H. and Strates, B. S.: Inductive substrates for bone formation. Clin. Orthop., *59*:59-96, 1968.

43. Weiss, P. A.: From cell dynamics to tissue architecture. *In*: Advanced Study Institute on Structure and Function of Connective and Skeletal Tissue, St. Andrews, Scotland, 1964. London, Butterworths, 1965, pp. 256-263.

44. Wolff, J.: *Das Gesetz der Transformation der Knochen*. Berlin, Hirschwald, 1892.

Chapter 17

PHYSIOLOGY OF THE SKIN

by Bard Cosman, M.D.

INTRODUCTION

The skin is a complex organ whose basic function is holocrine secretion of itself. It lives to die, and in its carefully regulated decease produces the cornified layer that covers us. It is bipartite, being composed of epidermis and dermis, each of different embryological origin. The skin organ is a vital one of giant size. Its 20,000 sq cm of surface in an adult and its average thickness of approximately 2.5 mm make it the human body's largest organ.[47, 67] With the best of modern supportive treatment, a 60 to 70 per cent loss of the integument, as in a burn, is associated with a 50 per cent mortality rate. In this chapter we will discuss some of the functions of the skin which make it so vital, and the consequences of its loss, which are so heavy.

ORIGIN OF SKIN

The epidermis is derived from the embryological ectoderm. It first consists of a single cell layer, but by the second intrauterine month the single layer has become two—a superficial flattened but nucleated layer (the periderm or epitrichium) and a basal layer of cuboidal cells (the stratum germinativum).[66] Underlying these is the corium, which is derived from the mesoderm. Initially present as a single layer of flattened cells, by the third month it has become two multicelled layers, the more superficial of which is the dermis, and the deeper layer of which is the subcutaneous tissue. By the third month the basal epidermal layer proliferates a stratum intermedium which, at four to five months,

317

becomes stratified, forming the stratum spinosum. Those areas which in later life will be most heavily used—the palms and soles—are first to show this differentiation. Curiously enough, the perialar areas also participate in this early maturation. Simultaneously, the dermis differentiates its ridges or papillae which fit, like lock and key, into undulations on the inner surface of the epidermis. These undulations are the skin markings, most highly developed on the hands and feet, that constitute the finger, palm, hand, toe and foot prints. The vernix caseosa forms from the epitrichium in the fourth to fifth month, helps to lubricate the emergence of the child at birth and is subsequently lost. The periderm is replaced by the stratum corneum.

Hair is the first of the accessory epithelial structures to differentiate. In the second month or early in the third month hair follicles first appear as downward growths from the epithelium into the dermis in the regions of the eyebrows, upper lip and chin. General hair development begins at the fourth month.[57] At about the same time nails develop as thickenings of the epidermis beneath the epitrichium on the dorsal surface of the terminal phalanges. This thickening is called the primary nail field. As this area enlarges it sinks down into the dorsal surface of the digit and is bounded laterally and proximally by an elevated fold of epidermis—the nail fold. The material of the true nail develops at a later stage from the underturned epithelium of the nail fold rather than from the initial nail field.[54] Sweat glands develop as downward growths from the epithelium in the fourth to fifth months. Sebaceous glands develop as protuberances on the posterior aspects of the hair pegs at about the same time. The rudiment of an apocrine gland also appears on the hair peg as an epithelial swelling. The apocrine buds are present over almost the entire body, but within a few weeks they disappear from everywhere except the axilla, navel, anogenital area, nipples and ears.[47] The phylogenetic recency of appearance of the eccrine sweat gland system in primates is suggested by the fact that the sweat gland ducts do not open on the skin surface until the seventh month.

DERMATOGLYPHICS

Both the study of the ridges of fingers, palms and feet and the structures themselves are termed dermatoglyphics.[8, 55] It is of interest that no two individuals possess identical print patterns. General configuration may be similar, but even in identical twins details differ. Aside from the teleologic reasoning that the ridged skin gives an advantage in grasping, the origin of the ridging is obscure. Dermatoglyphics are found on the volar skins of man, apes and monkeys. Lower primates have incomplete ridge formations. Three groups of New World monkeys have dermatoglyphics on the ventral skin of their prehensile tails. Outside the primate order, dermatoglyphics are, like the eccrine sweat glands, found principally among marsupials. Observations that certain dermatoglyphic patterns in man are frequently associated with chromosomal defects, such as Down's syndrome (mongolism), Turner's syndrome and trisomies, especially of chromosomes 13, 14 and 15, have given major impetus to the study of these skin features.

CONGENITAL DEFECTS

Syndromes in which abnormalities of the skin play a part are legion. One of these is congenital absence of skin, which occurs in limited areas. The lesion is most often in the scalp (60 per cent). The area is covered with a fine membrane like that of the two month embryonic skin. Breakdown of the area occurs, with epithelization from the sides, in about three months. If bone is absent and venous sinuses are present beneath the scalp defect, early operation for skin flap closure of the defect is necessary.[52] Similar early skin flap coverage may be needed for the skin defects overlying myelomeningoceles, since perforation of their membranes exposes the cord structures.

GENERAL ANATOMY

Figure 17-1 is an idealized diagram of the skin organ. The epidermis consists of five layers. Most superficial is the stratum corneum, the horny layer. This consists of flakes of compressed keratin, the transversely flattened remnants of the epithelial cells of the basal layer at the end of their upward migration. Most microscopic preparations show the stratum corneum as a loose meshwork of lamellae with large spaces between them; recent work has demonstrated the layer to be a compact one, consisting of lipid and keratin in nearly equal amounts. Its component cell remains are cemented together in a manner that is not completely understood, but they form a true barrier, not a network. The cementing mechanism weakens at the surface, and flaking away of the surface lamellae occurs invisibly or visibly, as in dandruff.

Just beneath the stratum corneum is the stratum lucidum. Only in the especially thick epithelium of the palms and soles is this layer clearly demonstrated. Special preparations, however, suggest its existence generally throughout the body. It is the transition zone in which the epithelial cells complete their keratinization and lose water, their nuclei and their lives, and from which they move into the stratum corneum.

Next in from the surface is the stratum granulosum, where the epithelial cells begin to take the flattened form and the transverse orientation of the horny layer's lamellae. Keratohyalin droplets accumulate on the tonofibril network within and at the periphery of the cells, giving the layer its name.

The bulk of the epidermis as seen in transverse section lies in the next layer, the stratum spinosum. Nucleated and clearly alive, these cells are characterized by the presence of the "prickles" seeming to join each to each. In the past, these have been viewed as bridges through which cell contents were in continuity, but this no longer appears to be true. The prickles seem to be complexes consisting of laminated intercellular attachment plaques at which the cell membranes touch and into which tonofibrils condense and insert. These areas are called desmosomes.[70] They play an important role in keratinization and may persist as the attachment devices of the cornified layer.

The basal layer or stratum germinativum lies at the bottom. More columnar in appearance, these cells are the parents of all the others, although mitoses also take place in the stratum spinosum as well. Scattered among the basal cells

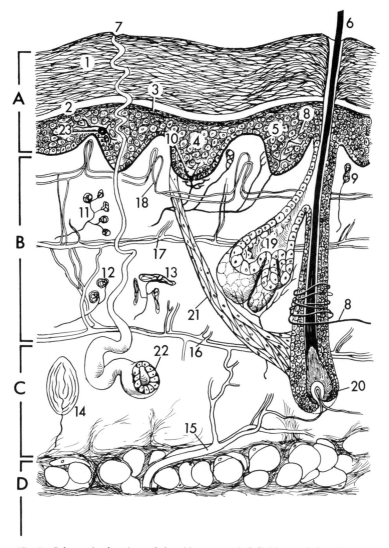

Figure 17 – 1 Schematic drawing of the skin organ. Subdivisions of the skin organ: (A) epidermis; (B) dermis; (C) subdermis; (D) subcutaneous tissue.

Parts of the epidermis: (1) stratum corneum or horny layer; (2) stratum lucidum; (3) stratum granulosum or granular cell layer; (4) stratum spinosum or prickle cell layer; (5) stratum germinativum or basal cell layer.

Features of the epidermis: (6) terminal hair shaft; (7) sweat duct pore opening on an epidermal ridge.

Innervation of the skin organ: (8) free nerve endings in epidermis and around hair root. Free endings also present around sebaceous gland (19) and sweat gland (22). (9) Meissner corpuscle; (10) Merkel tactile discs; note free endings, Meissner, and Merkel endings arising from common trunk. (11) Krause bulbs; (12) Golgi-Mazzoni corpuscles; (13) Ruffini corpuscle; (14) Pacinian corpuscle.

Blood supply of skin organ: (15) subcutaneous artery and vein plexus; (16) hypodermal plexus; (17) dermal plexus; (18) subdermal plexus; note prolongation as blind loops (papillary loops) up into the dermal papillae between the rete pegs of the epidermis.

Accessory epithelial structures: pilosebaceous unit: (19) sebaceous gland; (20) hair root with bulb and vascular papilla; (21) arrector pili muscle. Sweat gland: (22) coiled gland and straight duct with spiral through epidermis.

Pigment system: (23) melanocyte with dendrites in basal layer of epidermis.

are the melanocytes, cells originating from the neuroectoderm, which are equipped with long dendritic processes that appear to contact adjacent basal cells. The basal cell layer is the only one in close contact with the capillary tufts of the dermal papillae. Metabolic exchange in the rest of the Malpighian layer (spinosum and granulosum) is maintained by a system of intercellular spaces filled with tissue fluid. This space is sealed off at the surface by the stratum lucidum and corneum.

The dermo-epidermal junction and the basement membrane thereof are anatomical features whose interpretation is still to be resolved. Some observers have described the basal cells as sending protoplasmic processes into the dermis, and others have described elastic fibers of the dermis continuing around and into the basal cells. The compact reticulum or basal lamella beneath the basal cells has been ascribed to the secretion of the basal cells themselves or to the dermal cells acting under the influence of the basal cells.[24]

The dermis is equally complex, although it is not so clearly layered. It has a superficial papillary layer, molded into valleys and ridges corresponding to the underside of the epidermis, and a deep reticular layer. The papillary layer has more delicate collagen, elastin and reticulin fibers. The reticular layer is coarser, with irregular layers of fibers lying mostly parallel to the surface but at angular directions to each other. A few fibers extend down to participate in the formation of the retinacula cutis, which separates the subcutaneous fat into lobules.[46] The fibroblasts of the dermis lay down this system of fibers in a matrix or ground substance containing sulfated mucopolysaccharide, for which they are also responsible. The organization of the fibers of the dermis bears a relationship to the stress to which the skin is subjected and will be discussed later. Elastic fibers run between the collagen bundles, and in the middle dermis they are convoluted and spiral around the collagen fibers.[18] Reticulin fibers, a precollagen material, make up a branching network and probably are a stage in the development of mature collagen fibers. Fibroblasts, histiocytes, chromaffin cells and mast cells are the major cellular types of the dermis.

Plunging into the dermis are those derivatives of the epithelium called the accessory epithelial structures. The coiled sweat glands are found throughout the skin, with their bodies situated in the dermis and their ducts spiraling upward to end in the summits of the skin ridges. The sebaceous glands exist wherever there are hairs, and their ducts open into the superficial part of the hair follicle. They exist independently of the hair only in a few locations, such as the glans penis and the mammary areola. They are absent on the palms and soles and between the toes. Their secretion consists of the broken down bodies of their inner cell lining. They are thus holocrine glands, as opposed to the eccrine sweat glands that secrete sweat without loss to their own cell bodies. Forming a part of the pilosebaceous apparatus are the arrectores pilorum (smooth muscle fibers). Attached to the hair follicle deeply, they pass upward close to the sebaceous glands and end in the dermal papillae or basement membrane of the dermo-epidermal junction. Contraction of the arrectores pilorum elevates the hair, compresses the sebaceous glands, expressing their contents, and produces "goose pimples."

Nourishing the epidermis is the subepidermal capillary plexus continued as papillary loops into the dermal papillae.[45, 62] Lymphatics at this level collect fluid from the epithelium and form their own plexus. Blockage of this plexus, as in the cutaneous spread of breast carcinoma, produces the "peau d'orange" appearance. Much remains to be learned about the flow of lymph in the skin as well as elsewhere, and new concepts are being developed.[5] At a deeper level in the dermis is the dermal capillary-venule-arteriole plexus—usually called the dermal plexus. At the dermal and subdermal junction a third plexus, the hypodermal plexus, transmits and collects blood for the dermal capillaries. It is the venules of these last two plexuses that dilate and proliferate, showing the major response to the graded anoxia of a "delay" procedure in the formation of a skin flap for tissue transfer. Still deeper, the major artery-vein supply runs at the dermis-subcutaneous tissue level, and valved lymphatics exist.

Free nerve endings are found scattered in the stratum germinativum and extend in places into the stratum spinosum. They appear to constitute the peripheral pain end organs.[62] A subepithelial as well as an intraepithelial plexus can be distinguished. Free nerve endings also occur around sweat glands and in the papillae and root sheaths of the hair follicles. A variety of special nerve end organs also exist, whose classical functional attributions are much more exact than modern evidence can sustain. They are present in the glabrous skin but mostly are absent in the hairy skin of the scalp, which, however, has no deficiency of feeling. Bulbous corpuscles (Krause) occur in the skin and have been found in groups beneath "cold spots." Similar appearing endings (Golgi-Mazzoni bodies) are said to subserve pressure sense. Deeper in the dermis and subdermis the lamellated corpuscles of Pacini are found; these are also said to be pressure transducers. Oval shaped corpuscles (Meissner) and disclike endings (Merkel) occur in both epithelium and dermis and are said to be tactile sensors. Long oval or fusiform endings (Ruffini) are present in similar locations; some are said to be associated with the sensing of warmth and some with pressure.

REGIONAL MODIFICATIONS

Within the general anatomy of the skin are many regional differences and specializations. As was already mentioned, areas of the skin subject to consider-able motion or periodic volume changes have a well-developed dermal fiber feltwork organization designed to return the skin to its predistortion state.[18] Accordingly, the skin is under a certain degree of intrinsic tension. The direc-tion of this force tends to be perpendicular to the line of pull of the underlying muscles. When the dermal continuity is disturbed by a penetrating wound, this intrinsic tension manifests itself by distortion of the wound along the axis of tension. Thus, a round wound is elongated into an oval. This phenomenon was noted by Langer, who traced these lines of tension on the cadaver, making multiple perforations and plotting their distortion.[7, 35] In the living body the skin wrinkle lines are manifestations of this fiber organization, and wounds made parallel to these lines tend to spread less than wounds cutting across them. The surgeon making elective incisions keeps this in mind.[33]

The skin both is modified and modifies itself for manipulation in several ways. The epidermal ridges of hands and feet have been mentioned. The cornified layer is, in general, thicker where it is exposed to repeated contact, as in the hands and feet. The dermis is thicker where the contact is of a more diffuse, environmental type, as on the extensor and dorsal surfaces generally. When contact is more local and more intense, the cornified layer maintains itself and does not flake as easily. The result is callus formation. The stimulus may cause increased production of cornified layer or hyperkeratosis. A special manipulation-associated specialization is found in the palmar and plantar fasciae, with their extensions upwards into the dermis binding the skin in those locations to the underlying structures and preventing the slippage that ordinarily occurs between skin and subcutaneous tissue. The significance of this specialization becomes apparent in the manipulative difficulty suffered by a patient whose palmar or digital skin has been replaced by an abdominal pedicle flap and whose tissue lacks this modification.

Different areas of the skin are specially modified for emotional expression. The sweating of the hands and feet and the sweating and blushing of the face are instances of this. Thermal stimuli may actually reduce rather than increase sweating on the palms and soles. Emotion-related odor signals are given by skin structures in many animals. Although human beings do not have musk glands, they have apocrine glands, the large sweat gland-like structures attached to the hair follicles of the axilla and groin especially. Their secretion is stimulated in sexual arousal. These glands are anatomically extensive, ramifying systems, and chronic infection within one may often spread to the others, producing a condition (hidradenitis suppurativa) which may require total area excision and replacement.[32]

SKIN MEMBRANE FUNCTION

The skin, as the interface between our body and the world, performs some of the general functions of other such biological membranes, in addition to some functions that are specific to it. The skin acts as a gate. Some things it keeps in, some it lets out, some it keeps out completely, some it lets in at least in part. The skin must maintain itself, and to this end it has the ability to replicate itself, but it has only limited ability to replace itself when its substance has been lost. We shall discuss these various functions in turn.

Keeping in Water

The most important substance "kept in" by the skin is water. When a fish first wriggled up onto the shore, it faced the problem of desiccation which its aqueous environment had previously obviated. The development of a stratum corneum was one answer and is the one upon which we now rely. The water barrier of the human skin lies within the stratum corneum as a whole, is not localized to a single level within the horny layer and depends upon both the keratin and the lipid content of the layer.[31]

Keratinization and the Water Barrier

Keratinization is the process by which the horny layer forms. It has remained a subject of active study as better techniques succeed in revealing new complexities.[51, 63] The process appears to start in the basal cells with the laying down of tonofilaments, predominantly near the periphery of the cells but throughout the cell substance. As the cells move into the stratum spinosum the filaments condense into bundles called the tonofibrils. In the upper stratum spinosum, small spherical granules appear and enlarge, producing distinct droplets by the time the cell arrives in the stratum granulosum. The keratohyalin granules accumulate at the interstices of the tonofibril meshwork. These fibrils are concentrated at the desmosomes, as was previously noted, and these appear to act as centers from which the keratinization spreads.[70] Relatively suddenly, within the stratum lucidum, the entire cell becomes keratinized and passes into the stratum corneum.

The keratins are fibrous polypeptides distinguished by great resistance to peptic and tryptic digestion as well as to acid and alkali hydrolysis. Hair formed more than 30,000 years ago preserves its basic structure.[19] In amino acid content keratins do not differ markedly from the cell proteins from which they derive, except in their high cystine content. The cystine-sulfur in the keratin molecule appears in the form of disulfide cross links and the formation of these bonds, probably catalyzed by a copper-containing group of enzymes, is a vital part of keratinization, since it is these bonds which appear to give keratin its unique properties. Breakage of these links permits the solution of keratin and the demonstration that the molecule can be separated into two parts, one rich in sulfur and the other one poor. The latter is a fibrous molecule, the former a globulin molecule.[17] From this has arisen the concept of the complete keratin fiber as comprising two parts, one truly fibrous, the other a cross-linking cement or matrix. The fibrous molecule has the alpha helical configuration shared by many other biological fibers.

Accompanying these changes in protein state, the cell itself undergoes dehydration. The cell's lipids and lipoproteins may well become bound in some way to the keratinizing fibrils. It is certain that lipid forms a large part of the total mass of the cornified layer. In addition, nuclear decomposition ordinarily occurs at this point, but in certain abnormal states, the nucleus persists—a condition known as parakeratosis. These are the events which occur in the cell's passage from basal layer to stratum corneum. Despite these changes in state, the keratin flakes of the horny layer still truly adhere to each other, and the layer can be removed intact and still preserve its continuity.

The stratum corneum is the water-retaining barrier of the skin. Sandpapering off the horny layer and using such skin as a cover to a chamber containing water shows that the water is lost by diffusion essentially as fast as if the entire epidermis were removed. With intact skin, very little water is lost, and the same proves true if the horny layer alone is separated and used to cap such a chamber.[31] Water loss through intact skin is the same for living as well as dead skin—further evidence that metabolic activity per se does not play a significant role in preventing water transpiration. Regional differences do exist, however; palm and sole skins allow greater water loss than skin elsewhere.

Clinical Importance of the Water Barrier

The skin water barrier becomes clinically important in burn patients and in those with large exposed wounds, such as multiple decubitus ulcers. Water loss has been related to the hypermetabolic state of burn patients via the thermal load placed on the body by the accelerated insensible water loss suffered through the burned or absent skin. The normal rate of insensible transpiration (excluding that of palms and soles) is only 1.3 per cent of that which occurs through denuded dermis. A man 175 cm in height and 75 Kg in weight normally loses 6.5 to 10 gm of water per hour or 240 gm of water per day. However, an individual of this size with 55 per cent burns has been observed to lose 7500 ml per 24 hours, with a loss of approximately 4400 Kcal, traceable to the evaporation of this huge water loss.[15] Others have reported fluid losses of 100 to 300 ml per square meter of burn surface per hour, and at 560 Kcal/liter at 30°C, caloric loss ranges between 1200 and 4000 Kcal/24 hr.[44]

Lipid and the Water Barrier

Recent studies have suggested that the water retaining element in the cornified layer resides in the lipid component thereof. This lipid has been purified and when reapplied to an eschar or to a collagen film will reduce water vapor transmission almost to intact skin levels.[27] These findings suggest a new importance for the lipids of the cells undergoing keratinization, and the elucidation of the lipid-keratin relationship in the stratum corneum may shed new light on this fundamental skin function of keeping water in.

Keeping in Heat

Although the more important function of the skin relative to thermoregulation is in letting heat out, the skin nevertheless plays a part in conserving heat. To what extent it is itself an insulator has not been explored. However, the human skin shows neither of the two major insulation modifications common to other animals. The hair and feathers that are such efficient insulating layers are absent. Indeed, our hair has regressed to the point of functional insignificance. The blubber layer, a subcutaneous fat derivative, has never developed in man. However, by its vascular responses, the skin does conserve heat effectively. Also, the skin can produce heat via the activity of the arrector pili muscles. As a heat sensor, the skin initiates some of the complex mechanisms that are discussed more fully in Chapter 7.

Keeping the Inside In

The skin is less important as a limiting membrane than as either a water barrier or a heat insulator. It is relatively impotent in the limiting of volume, unless it is aided and abetted by underlying scar tissue, as in burn contractures. Normal skin stretches slowly and offers no impediment to the development of huge hernias or tumors, so long as their size increases slowly. The skin's intrinsic tension is greater in childhood than in old age. The elastic behavior of the skin — its resiliency — shows a similar relationship to age in that skin rebound in response to indentation is closer to 100 per cent in the young than in the old. The tensile strength of skin — that is, the measure of the force needed to tear the skin — is a different aspect and also varies with age. Cadaver skin tensile strength averages 1.8 Kg/sq mm. In infants it is only 0.25 to 0.30 Kg/sq mm, and in young adults it is 1.61 Kg/sq mm.[62] Skin stretched acutely, but not so strongly as to rupture, undergoes "fracture" of the dermal feltwork and does not fully recover. Striae are the external manifestations of this event. High corticoid levels, achieved in medical treatment or autogenously as in pregnancy, predispose the skin to such partial breaks. That these mechanical features are not vital for skin function is amply demonstrated, however, by the absence of significant functional defects in patients who have abnormal distensibility of the skin, as in Ehlers-Danlos syndrome, pseudoxanthoma elasticum or cutis verticis gyrata.

Keeping Out Particulate Foreign Bodies

The mechanical properties of the skin are of some minor importance in keeping gross foreign bodies out. Clearly, however, human skin is not comparable to an armadillo's body armor. In fact, finely divided, inert particulate foreign bodies are often well tolerated by the dermis. Such is the case with tatoos. Slightly larger foreign bodies tend to be extruded through the skin when they have been placed just beneath or within it. This is the course taken by most of the fragments of glass implanted in the facial skin in an automobile accident, for example.

Keeping Out Pathogenic Organisms

Mechanical Factors

Of infinitely greater importance is the protection the skin affords against bacteria and fungi. Whether or not the skin presents any barrier at all to viruses is a moot point. The skin's protection takes several forms. Generally agreed upon is the mechanical aspect: The stratum corneum is impermeable to bacteria from the outside, and fungi can live only in its outermost layers. The relative dryness of most of the skin is also a relevant feature; bacteria are most numerous on moist areas of the skin.[41] In addition, the constant flaking off of the surface squames or keratin lamellae serves to carry away a portion of the potential bacterial colonists.

The Aqueous Barrier

A second feature of the barrier against bacteria is the aqueous "acid mantle" afforded by the eccrine sweat, although much more importance was given to this factor in past years than is given at present. Lactic acid is the main acid in sweat, and it is synthesized by the glands, not merely filtered from the blood. On most parts of the body, the pH range is 4.2 to 5.6.[62] Heat-induced sweat becomes more acid as it evaporates; nonthermal sweating is less acid from onset. This slight acidity of the skin surface has been credited with discouraging the growth of many bacterial species. Most mammals have alkaline sweat (pH 7.8 to 8.9) similar to the secretion produced by the human apocrine glands.

The Sebaceous Barrier

Other factors have also been credited with inhibiting bacterial and fungal growth. The sebum produced by the sebaceous glands, partially emulsified by the eccrine sweat, contains many lipids, some of which by themselves, and others by way of their fatty acid breakdown products, inhibit fungi and bacteria.[62] The presence of the ubiquitous "athlete's foot" fungus infection in the intertriginous toe areas and the regression of scalp ringworm at puberty have been adduced in proof of this. It is argued that lack of sebaceous glands between the toes and the adolescent increase in sebum production, respectively, explain these clinical findings.

Sebaceous gland function is said to be controlled by a form of feedback mechanism in that the glands tend to continue secreting until a certain amount of sebum is present on the skin surface, at which point gland activity stops. The saturation level is said to be constant for a given temperature. Wiping the surface or removing the sebum will stimulate the glands until they have produced enough to reach saturation level again. Increased temperature leads to sweating and dilution of sebum, it is said, and consequently to greater glandular activity to rebuild the sebum level. Males produce more sebum than females and blacks produce more than whites. The increases in size of sebaceous glands as well as in secretion rates that occur in puberty are well known. Testosterone is known to have these effects, and the fact that they occur in females as well suggests that progesterone acts similarly. Some believe that there is a dietary effect and that a high carbohydrate diet increases sebum production. The question of what effect the innervation of the sebaceous glands exerts remains unsolved. The meaning of the local sebaceous gland hyperplasia in post-encephalitic Parkinson's disease, for instance, is obscure. It is only fair to point out that some investigators believe that all these theories relative to the importance of the sebaceous glands are false, and that the glands should be viewed as useless remnants of the days when we had hair for them to lubricate.[30]

SEBUM AND NORMAL SKIN ECOLOGY.   The sebaceous gland secretion is a main source of nutrients for the normal skin inhabitants.[42] In most cases these surface dwellers appear to be "freeloaders," but in some instances they appear to help the skin function in protecting against invasive pathogens. Only one animal form is truly indigenous on human skin—the follicle mite *Demodex folliculorum*, which lives, mates, and breeds in and around the eyelashes and the hair follicles of the outer nasal folds and the chin. A few fungi, such as that responsible for "athlete's foot," and a few yeasts are fairly normal inhabitants.

The dominant members of the ecologic community on the human skin are Gram-positive bacteria.[41] Two groups are present: the cocci, chief among them being *Staphylococcus aureus,* and the diphtheroids, among them *Corynebacterium acne,* the "acne bacillus." Gram-negative bacteria are also found normally. The densest bacterial populations are found on the face, neck, axilla and groin, while the trunk and back have smaller populations. The mean population of the axilla in an adult male has been calculated as 2.41 million bacteria per square centimeter of epidermis, compared to only 314 bacteria per square centimeter on the back. The metabolic activity of the Gram-positive cocci may be significant in breaking down sebum into unsaturated fatty acids, which in turn help to inhibit pathogenic bacteria. Depression of Gram-positive organisms is associated with a rise in the Gram-negative population, so that the original bacterial density is reattained.

Keeping Out Chemicals

The skin is also of service in preventing the penetration of chemicals and various other liquids and gases with which it comes into contact. The degree of its impermeability is greater than that of most other biological membranes. The stratum corneum is, again, the basic barrier, as can be demonstrated by the immediate loss of impermeability function following stripping of this layer. This fact was recognized long before the technique of hypodermic injection was developed; the application of medicine to a blistered area of skin was a well-known means of achieving percutaneous passage of a drug that otherwise was impossible to administer via the intact skin. It is the lack of the keratinized layer that accounts for the permeability of the mucous membranes. Even in cornified skin, however, regional variations exist; scrotal skin, for example, has been shown to be more permeable than abdominal skin.[62]

Percutaneous Absorption

There are two groups of factors that can enhance percutaneous absorption: those that act by physical means to increase absorption through an intact stratum corneum, and those that increase the permeability of the barrier cells or disrupt the layer itself. The first category includes temperature, hyperemia, high skin surface concentration of the involved agent and electrophoresis. With the exception of the last, the effects of these are small. Of all the gases the skin is most permeable to CO_2, and appreciable amounts may be absorbed from saturated solutions. The vehicle in which a substance is dissolved may be included here. Its effect appears to be the enhancing of lipid penetration through the pilosebaceous apparatus (transappendageal transport) rather than through the stratum corneum itself (transepidermal transport).

The second group of factors enhancing percutaneous absorption includes physical stripping, abrasion, injurious vesicant chemicals, inflammatory processes and moisture.[40] All appear to remove some of the stratum corneum. The mechanism whereby moisture accomplishes this is not clear, but the demonstration that a significant fraction of the horny layer is made up of water-soluble substances may suggest that the leaching of these components may interfere with the adherence of the keratin flakes and so compromise the integrity of the cornified layer. This may be the means whereby "maceration" leads to skin injury.

Keeping Out Radiation

Another entity the skin keeps out is the sun's radiation. The most biologically injurious of the sun's rays to reach the earth's surface is ultraviolet light. The short wavelength end of the sun's radiation spectrum—from x-rays to ultraviolet rays—is hazardous. Attenuation of these by passage through the atmosphere permits survival. Ozone in the outer atmosphere filters ultraviolet rays of wavelengths up to 2900 Å, but a substantial amount at wavelengths of 2000 to 3200 Å does penetrate to the earth's surface. The skin achieves its protective function by virtue of its pigment barrier.

The Pigment Barrier

There are five primary skin pigments: melanin, oxyhemoglobin, reduced hemoglobin, melanoid and carotene. A sixth pigment, trichosiderin, is limited to red-haired people and contains iron, as its name suggests. These pigments, their physical distribution and the thickness and optical qualities of the overlying tissues affect the final observed skin color. Of all these pigments, it is melanin which acts as the ultraviolet screen.

Melanin is an oxidation product of tyrosine. It is produced in the melanocytes with the aid of the enzyme tyrosinase. Oxidation of tyrosine produces dihydroxyphenylalanine (dopa). Dopa reduces the copper ions in tyrosinase and makes the enzyme fully active. In succeeding reactions, dopa yields three active quinone compounds: dopa quinone, dopachrome and indole-5,6-quinone. These substances combine with protein molecules and oxidize to form melanin pigments. In its final polymerized form, the pigment is bound to protein molecules aggregated in granules. The melanin granules found in the basal and spiny layer cells are the result of cytocrine injection by the melanocytes via their dendrites.[16] The melanin granules themselves are actually discrete particles approximately 0.1 to 2 microns in diameter and are composed of melanin in combination with a pseudoglobulin. These are suspected of being actual mitochondria, and the phenomenon of pigment spread from transplanted black mouse skin into surrounding white mouse skin has been used to suggest that the granules may be self-replicating.

Sun Tanning

Pigment spread is involved in the phenomenon of sun tanning, the reaction of the pigment barrier to incident ultraviolet light. There is an immediate darkening—the Meirowsky phenomenon—which appears to be a direct photo-oxidation of preformed reduced melanin. A subsequent upward migration of melanin occurs as the result of dispersion of granules into the dendrites. New melanin formation, as well as activation of previously inactive melanocytes, occurs about 2 days after the initial exposure and reaches a maximum effect after 19 days.[38] The controlling factors of this portion of the reaction are not known. Hormonal influences on pigment are complex and are in the process of being worked out in laboratory animals. The pituitary and pineal glands play some part, but the problem is still obscure in humans.[11] At the local skin level, a decrease in tyrosinase-inhibiting epidermal sulfhydryl groups has been postulated to occur as a result of sun exposure with resultant increase of tyrosinase-catalyzed melanin production and melanocyte injection of pigment into the epidermal cells. The melanin in a well tanned or naturally dark skin is so effective a shield that the amount of ultraviolet penetrating to the underlying dermis is reduced by 90 per cent or more.[9]

Additional Reactions to Light

In addition to melanin pigment, the skin has certain other means of keeping out ultraviolet radiation. The horny layer, which scatters and absorbs ultraviolet radiation, responds to exposure by becoming thicker. Another protective agent is said to be urocanic acid, a substance found in the epidermis which changes from a *trans* to a *cis* form on ultraviolet exposure and, on reverting, dissipates the acquired energy harmlessly.[9] The precise anatomical localization of this reaction is not yet clear.

Certain compounds applied to the skin, injected, or produced endogenously can sensitize skin cells to radiation of wavelengths other than ultraviolet. Antibiotics like demethylchlorotetracycline HCl have been linked with such photosensitization. Furocoumarins sensitize skin to light of 3200 to 3800 Å wavelength, which is within the range of visible radiation. The porphyrins in the skin of the patient with porphyria bring about sensitization and urticarial reactions to light of 4000 Å wavelength. Light-induced damage to the abnormal skin of persons with xeroderma pigmentosa leads to the formation of multiple skin cancers.

Sunburn

These abnormal sensitivity reactions are, however, merely exaggerations of the events attending acute sun exposure in the untanned skin or severe sun exposure even in the already tanned skin. Within 12 hours, the victim may be "beet red," have fever and chills, feel nauseated and, in the ensuing days, blister and peel. The mechanism of this syndrome may be found in the damage that ultraviolet radiation does to intracellular lysosomes, causing them to break down and release hydrolytic enzymes, leading in turn to cell death and release of still other tissue enzymes, which produce the dilatation of blood vessels and the fever.[9] Long-term ultraviolet damage may be related to subtle changes in the DNA of surviving cells. These changes may, in the course of decades, lead to accelerated age-related changes in the skin, including thinning, patchy pigmentation, chronic redness, senile elastosis, keratosis and the development of skin cancers.

Letting in Sunlight

The ultraviolet screen of the skin is not absolute. Ultraviolet radiation is vital for the production of the skin's major hormone, calciferol, somewhat misleadingly called Vitamin D.[37] Calciferol plays a vital part in controlling the entrance of calcium into the body and is therefore one of the controlling hormones in the metabolism of bone. Ultraviolet radiation brings about the synthesis of a form of calciferol, Vitamin D_3, through the conversion of the 7-dehydrocholesterol produced in the skin. A particular daily dose of radiation at 2970 Å — a dose that is only 5 per cent of the amount needed to produce a visible sunburn — applied to only 200 sq cm of skin has been found to be sufficient to cure rickets.[9] Fish can synthesize calciferol without ultraviolet light, but man cannot. Inhabitants of smoke-shadowed cities and dwellers of temperate and Northern climes where the sun remains lower than 35 degrees above the horizon receive insufficient ultraviolet light in winter and must obtain calciferol in their diets or suffer rickets.[37] It has been suggested that the development of dark- and light-skinned races came about through the necessity of peoples in temperate climates to decrease their pigment screen so as to maximize their ultraviolet absorption in winter and through the opposite need of tropical man to decrease his absorption to avoid Vitamin D intoxication. That the latter occurs from sun exposure, however, does not seem true; white dwellers in the tropics do not show signs of Vitamin D overdosage.

Letting in Sensation

The skin may be said to "let in" sensations of heat, cold, pain, pressure and touch. The specialized and unspecialized nerve endings that subserve these functions, as well as the paradox of the paucity of specialized endings in the hairy skin without apparent absence of the functions that are ascribed to them, have been mentioned. In addition, differing forms of stimulation of the same area can produce different central sensations. Threshold activation of pain spots causes merely contact sensation and, sometimes, an itching sensation. Cold spots, however, no matter how stimulated, lead to a perception of cold. For all modalities, the skin surface is a mosaic of sensitive points.[62] Variations in the density and size of touch spots determine the limits of two-point discrimination. On the forearm, for instance, the touch spots are irregularly shaped areas up to 5 mm in diameter. Cold spots occur in groups, each 3 to 8 sq mm in area, with the groups spaced 10 mm apart. Warmth spots are more difficult to map. Pain spots are more densely distributed than the spots of other modalities. The relationship between the nerve-ending systems and the sensation of itching remains difficult to define despite much study. In general, itching seems related to the pain fibers with undifferentiated endings but is produced only by certain levels and types of stimuli applied to them. Pain and itch spots are relatively, but not absolutely, congruent.

Abnormalities of Sensation

Abnormalities of skin sensation are of many degrees and types. Three of great severity are hyperpathia, meralgia paresthetica and causalgia.[62] Hyperpathia is a most intense pain occurring during recovery from peripheral nerve lesions and with some cutaneous scars. In this state, needle prick pain is not felt as a quick flash but as a slow, expanding, burning sting associated with an extremity withdrawal reflex, sweating and peripheral blood vessel dilatation. Skin in hyperpathic areas is actually found to be hypoalgesic, however. Meralgia paresthetica is marked by paresthesias in the outer surface of the thigh, in the distribution of the injured femoral cutaneous nerve, and consists of burning, tingling, stabbing pain or unpleasant numbness. The area is hyperexcitable to itch stimuli. Causalgia is a special case of hyperpathia in which extreme vasodilation accompanies the reaction. It appears after trauma to peripheral nerves. The severe burning pain is exacerbated by any stimulus. Skin and nail changes occur with vasodilation and sweating. Disuse atrophy complicates the rehabilitation even after relief of the syndrome, which can sometimes be accomplished by sympathectomy.

Letting Out Heat

Heat is the most significant of the entities "let out" by the skin. The skin plays its part in thermoregulation through its eccrine sweat glands, through vascular reactions and through sensing of heat.

The sweat glands of the palms and soles produce sweat constantly, and their secretion is not increased by a thermal stimulation.[34] Otherwise, except for the emotion-stimulated glands of the face, the sweat glands of the trunk and extremities are quiescent unless stimulated by a heat load. The so-called "insensible perspiration," as measured by the weight loss of the body at rest, is the sum of (1) water loss via the lungs, (2) actual sweating of palms and soles, and (3) transpiration of water vapor through the epidermis in other areas. Its magnitude is of the order of 1000 gm/day, of which nearly half is from the lungs. There is a critical level of skin temperature—between 32° and 34°C—at which a sudden outbreak of visible sweating (thermal sweating) occurs over the whole body surface. This also takes place, although at a higher threshold, if only a part of the body is heated; the condition is then called "reflex sweating." The number of glands functioning, as well as the intensity of their function, is affected. Well over 2 million sweat glands are present in an adult. This distribution ranges between less than 500 per sq in on the back to over 2500 per sq in on the palm. While there appear to be few racial differences in sweating ability, people adapted to the cold have fewer functioning sweat glands compared to members of heat-adapted groups, who show a quicker, more intense response. Sweat glands are usually under nervous control—anatomically sympathetic but physiologically and pharmacologically cholinergic. The tendency to excessive perspiration in hyperthyroidism and in some other diseases appears to reflect change in the central settings of this nervous control rather than any local alteration in the sweat glands themselves. The situation in cases of local hyperhidrosis is unexplained.

Sweating and Heat Diseases

The eccrine sweat is an aqueous solution composed of 99 to 99.5 per cent water and 0.5 to 1 per cent solids. Half of the solids are inorganic salts, mostly NaCl, and half are organic substances, with urea forming more than 50 per cent of this remainder. Sweat is hypotonic, but at high secretion rates it may be nearly isotonic. Abnormally large amounts of sodium and chloride may be lost by patients with mucoviscidosis and with Addison's disease. Such patients are especially prone, therefore, to heat exhaustion, one of the four major clinical syndromes related to high environmental temperature and sweating. *Heat stroke* is the most severe of these syndromes. Sudden cessation of sweating peripherally is associated with failure of central hypothalamic regulatory centers. High body temperatures cause thermal and anoxic damage to various organs of the body. The process seems to be initiated by sweat gland "fatigue" after continuous exposure to high temperatures.[62] *Heat exhaustion* is the syndrome which follows loss of large amounts of salt and water via prolonged sweating. It is characterized by pallor, vomiting, muscle cramps and syncope. Body temperature is usually normal. Water and salt replacement reverses the process. *Heat cramps* are a mild form of heat disease marked by painful skeletal muscle contractions, which can be prevented by dietary salt supplementation. The *sweat retention syndrome* is the mildest of the four and the most local. In hot, moist environments, unacclimated men may develop mild malaise and low grade fever and may show large nonsweating areas over the body. Miliaria rubra develops in these areas. It has been shown that under these climatic conditions a keratin plug forms in the sweat duct orifice, leading to backup of sweat, cessation of production and breakdown of the duct in the dermis, causing local inflammatory reaction and possible permanent loss of the involved gland.[64]

Other Means of Letting Out Heat

The evaporation of sweat accounts for only about 40 per cent of the heat lost by the body under ordinary climatic conditions, although this percentage can be increased markedly. Under usual atmospheric conditions, about 60 per cent of the total heat loss is by radiation.[62] As a radiating surface, the skin of both black and white persons radiates in the infrared region as an essentially perfect black body. The amount of heat available for radiation by the skin is profoundly affected by the blood supply of the skin. Its vascular system is integrated into the central control mechanisms for thermoregulation, which were described in Chapter 7. Convection as a means of heat loss is markedly dependent on the microclimate produced by clothing and ambient conditions. Neither convection nor conduction is important in the heat loss of the skin under usual conditions. Evaporation of sweat and vascular reaction are the major effectors of thermoregulation.

SELF-REPLICATION

All the components of the skin are in the process of constant self-maintenance and replication. The epidermal cells are constantly being added to from the basal layer while being lost from the horny layer's surface. The period required for a single basal cell to migrate through the epidermis and be cast off at the surface is called the epidermal renewal time. It is an indirect measurement of mitotic activity. In ordinary circumstances, this period appears to be about 26 to 28 days, although in certain skin diseases, it may be as little as 3 to 4 days.[31] There has been much speculation regarding the apparently low rate of mitotic activity in the skin, a rate which on first consideration seems inadequate to the skin's need for replacement. However, the fully keratinized epidermal cell is a flake with a diameter of 25 to 30 microns, while the basal cells are cuboidal and only 5 to 6 microns in diameter. Thus, a single basal cell accounts for a larger surface area in the stratum corneum than it did in the basal layer. In addition, the stratum germinativum undulates, as opposed to the plane surface of the horny layer, so there is a greater area source of basal cells than initially appears. These two factors seem sufficient to explain the apparent discrepancy.[56] The lifetime of skin cells is reduced with age, although mitotic rate is not much altered. Accordingly, there is an absolute thinning of skin with age. There are also diurnal variations in mitotic activity with a peak at 10 P.M. and a low at 5 to 10 A.M., as measured in the excised foreskins of circumcised infants.[56]

Little is known of the replication rates of sweat and sebaceous glands. Hair has been better studied in this regard. Human hair shows the growth phases of anagen, catagen and telogen that were first noted in lower animals. Scalp hair replacement in man occurs in scattered mosaic fashion. The average period of a scalp hair's growth is 1000 days, and the resting phase lasts 100 days. One may expect to shed 100 scalp hairs per day.[53] Human nail growth has also been studied; it shows age variation as well as some long-term cyclic variations suggestive of the seven-year skin renewal concept of popular legend. A value of linear nail growth of 0.83 mm per week in the first three decades of life, compared to 0.52 mm per week in the ninth decade, has been recorded.[53]

RESPONSE TO INJURY

Nonpenetrating Trauma

Nonpenetrating injuries to the skin in the form of tension or pressure cause direct and indirect vascular reactions without other overt changes.[62] Direct vascular reactions are limited to the area stimulated. The indirect responses either spread slowly from the area of stimulation and are caused by a locally liberated substance that diffuses out, or spread more rapidly and are the result of locally initiated nerve impulses. In the category of direct response is the constriction of local blood vessels in a stretched area producing local skin blanching and known as the "white line" effect. If the stimulus is more intense, a "red line" develops after a short latent period and reaches a maximum in 0.5 to 1 min. This reaction is caused by the active dilation of the smallest blood vessels having muscular elements. Both "white" and "red" reactions occur in denervated areas. A white border accompanying a red line response is often seen, since the stimulating force grades down peripherally.

Development of an erythematous wheal is a step beyond the red line response, and is an example of indirect reaction. Local alterations in capillary permeability occur and fluid is lost into the skin, producing an elevation 1 to 3 min after the stimulus is applied, with a maximum response height achieved in 3 to 5 min and a duration of 2 to 4 hrs. Susceptible individuals exhibit this reaction so easily that "writing" on their skin, a phenomenon called dermatographia, is possible. The release of histamine or a substance like it from damaged epidermal cells appears to be the basis for this response, with the changes in capillary permeability occurring in response to the released substance. The same mechanism, associated with an axon reflex, is said to account for the more elaborate "triple response" in which, following injury, a local vasodilation causes local reddening, then wheal formation, after which a vasodilation axon-reflex with arteriolar dilation and development of a red flare surrounding the wheal occur.

Nonpenetrating Injury with Cell Loss

When the injury is nonpenetrating but does result in the loss of epidermal cells—as in stripping of the epidermal surface, or, more commonly, abrasion—the response of the skin, after a lag period of about 24 hours, is a burst of mitotic activity in the basal and spinous layers, with the rapid reconstitution of the stratum corneum.[14] Two hypotheses exist to explain this. It has been suggested that damaged cells release a "wound hormone" which, as it diffuses out from the site of injury, stimulates mitosis.[1] On the other hand, it has also been hypothesized that the skin cells are always ready to divide but normally produce a mitosis-inhibiting factor, probably a protein, termed chalone.[4] Damage or loss of tissue leads to decreased production of chalone, with subsequent increase in mitotic rate. As tissue regenerates, chalone production rises, and the situation again reaches an equilibrium. Chalone appears to operate as an unstable chalone-epinephrine complex. A decision between these views has not yet been reached and, indeed, both may be applicable.[2]

Abrasion commonly involves small areas of loss deeper than the epidermal layer. As long as accessory epithelial structures remain, a new basal layer and, subsequently, the full epidermal structure will be reconstituted by dedifferentiation of the cells of the sweat glands and pilosebaceous units and their migration over the dermal surface. The same phenomenon brings about the healing of the donor site of a split-thickness skin graft. In these situations, we can speak of skin healing by replication. When epithelial structures are lost and the injury penetrates into the dermis, the healing process differs and involves the substitution of scar tissue.

PENETRATING INJURIES

Incised Wounds—Histologic Events

The healing of the incised skin wound constitutes the paradigm of wound healing studies. The histologic events are well known. The blood from severed vessels clots in the wound, and fibrin strands are formed from the fibrinogen molecules of the blood. These strands make a network that weakly unites the wound edges. At the wound surface, in the gap between the wound edges that have retracted from each other as a consequence of the intrinsic tension of the skin, the clot dehydrates, and the fibrin, blood serum proteins and dehydrated superficial dead dermis form the scab. The injury to the cells in the wound leads to their release of substances—histamine among them—which cause adjacent uninjured blood vessels to leak serum into the area. This is the inflammatory response of injury.

Some 6 hr later neutrophils begin to move through the capillary walls and into the wound area.[61] Substances released by the damaged cells may serve as the chemical messengers, which inform the white blood cells of the need for their services. Leukotaxine is one such postulated substance.[43] In the wound, the neutrophils ingest bacteria if they are present and subsequently the white cells disintegrate, releasing a series of enzyme granules which contain the group of enzymes called cathepsins. These aid in the dissolution of the extracellular necrotic debris present in the wound. Within the next 6 hr monocytes arrive via the bloodstream and migrate into the wound. Some of the dermal macrophages may also participate in this second cellular movement into the wound. The blood-derived monocytes become macrophages and ingest the cellular and extracellular debris.

At about two days following injury, substantial numbers of capillary buds begin to invade the wound—mostly from its depths. They become a prominent feature in the healing wound and are called "granulation tissue."[65] Accompanying them, possibly arising in some instances from these actively dividing cells, and also in small part from surrounding similar cells, are the fibroblasts which enter the wound.[23] Simultaneously, at this period the epidermal cells of the basal and spinous layers adjacent to the wound undergo changes. They begin to slide into and along the surface of the wound on the front of the upward-rising granulation tissue. Cellular movement predominates, although cell division occurs as both old and new epidermal cells join in this flow.[28, 71] They undermine the scab at appropriate skin level, seemingly producing a collagenase in the process as they cut through the surface debris. They will not grow downward into a wound to any considerable extent, nor will they grow far "uphill." Rather, the cells await the filling in of the gap with granulations and pass across that tissue to reconstitute the skin surface. With granulations to grow upon, epithelium migrates from each side of the wound at a rate of 0.1 to 0.5 mm per day. The cells grow faster on a moist surface than on a dry one. Epithelial coverage occurs at a rate of about 1 to 3 cell diameters per hour.[71]

By one week, in such a simple wound, the fibroblasts have laid down considerable numbers of reticulin fibers. Concomitant with laying down of these protocollagen fibers, and starting long before the mature organization of the fibers, the rather mysterious process of wound contraction has begun. Depending on location, mobility of local tissue and wound shape (rectangular wounds contract faster than round wounds), contraction accounts for at least 50 per cent of the actual spontaneous closure of a wound, the rest being brought about by the epithelial migration. In man contraction occurs at its fastest rate over the first six days after wounding but continues thereafter at a slower rate.[59] The rate of contraction appears to be a species constant given similar wound circumstances.[3] Its mechanism is unknown. The driving force appears to lie in a "picture frame" area around the edge of the wound, since central granulation tissue excision does not alter the rate of contraction, while peripheral excision stops the process.[69] Evidence points to the fibroblasts themselves rather than collagen fibers or other mechanisms as being responsible for the movement.[29] This wound contraction, which is a normal and necessary part of wound healing, is not to be confused with "contracture," the abnormal scar band that may lead to functional impairment long after the wound has healed. This latter problem arises consequent upon excessive scar being produced along the line of persistent motion, as, for example, across a joint. Subject to constant but varying pulls, the scar tissue undergoes microinjuries and responds with more scar formation.

At the end of the initial healing period, possibly signaled by the cell contact or by other means as yet unknown, the epidermal cells cease their motion and devote themselves to thickening and restratifying their layer. The epidermal contact is apparently also a part of the means for signaling the fibroblasts, so that they gradually cease to lay down new collagen and ground substance and devote themselves to the reorganization of the dermal structure. The collagen fibers, which tended to lie perpendicularly in the wound, are reoriented to lie roughly in transverse direction.[20] The amount of collagen is returned to more normal quantities by means not yet well understood, but which may involve a collagenase. The number of blood vessels in the wound decreases. Over the course of weeks only a slight increase in local fibrous tissue—the scar—remains to mark the site of the wound on the surface. Histologically a slight thinness of epithelium lacking skin appendages over the scar tissue may be noted, and the area may be picked out in the dermis by the slight break in the organization of the dermal fibers.

Biochemical Events in Wound Healing

Biochemically, the wound is the site of an initial mucopolysaccharide accumulation. The serum appears to be the source of this material. This mucopolysaccharide pool serves as a bank upon which the fibroblasts draw in the production of collagen fibers and in their production of new ground substance. Hexosamine is the chief component in this mucopolysaccharide production phase. Rapid incorporation of radioactive sulfur into the wound area testifies to the formation of the sulfated mucopolysaccharides characteristic of ground substance.[20] The height of the hexosamine response is reached between the third to sixth day, while the production of collagen is beginning. Thereafter, the level begins to fall back toward normal.[68] Collagen production becomes apparent by the second day and the concentration of hydroxyproline, the amino acid unique to collagen and thus followed as a marker of its production, begins to rise. By the sixth to seventh day, hydroxyproline concentration is climbing very rapidly. Histologically, masses of reticulin fibers have been produced. With the organization of these into a mature collagen network, the concentration of hydroxyproline begins to return toward normal.[2]

Tensile Strength as Related to Biochemical and Histological Events

The initial tensile strength of a wound is that which the fibrin clot or the sutures, or both, give (Fig. 17-2). Loss of tensile strength occurs as the sutures pull through and the fibrin clot is lysed during the formation of the granulation tissue. With the production of reticulin and the beginning maturation of the collagen fibers, the wound tensile strength rises abruptly. The part played by the epidermis in this early acquisition of tensile strength is still uncertain, but it may be more important than has previously been suspected. By the seventh day the wound can support itself in most cases, and suture removal can be carried out. Tensile strength has by no means been regained fully, however, and the process continues. By about the fourteenth day the tensile strength rate of gain has, strictly speaking, leveled off, although it is still slowly increasing. Even beyond the period of scar maturation, the wound does not quite achieve a completely normal tensile strength. In addition, the hydroxyproline content remains slightly higher than normal. This suggests that the wound area is the site of continued "repair" and remains different from unwounded tissues. That this is true is demonstrated by the fact that old wounds in patients

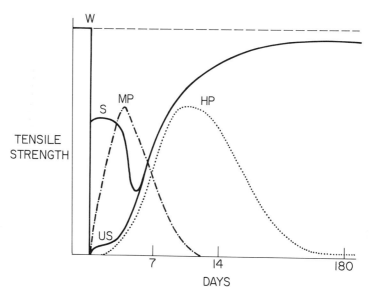

Figure 17−2 Skin wound tensile strength and histochemical events. Curves of the accumulation of mucopolysaccharide−MP (dot-dash line)−and hydroxyproline−HP (dotted line)−are superimposed on the curve of tensile strength (solid line) following a wound−W. Arbitrary units are employed for the sake of schematization. After wounding, tensile strength falls to nothing; if the wound is unsutured (US), tensile strength rises slightly immediately because of the fibrin clot. If sutured (S), the wound possesses considerable, though not normal, tensile strength. Mucopolysaccharides accumulate rapidly (MP), but begin to return toward normal even as hydroxyproline production (HP) rises. Tensile strength gain accelerates at approximately the same rate as the increase in HP, and by seven days about one-half normal strength has been achieved. The sutured wound (S) falls from its initial level of strength as sutures begin to pull through, but then rejoins the climb of tensile strength. The height of HP levels has been reached by 12 to 13 days after wounding, but wound tensile strength continues to climb, albeit at a slower rate, as collagen fibers mature. Neither tensile strength nor hydroxyproline levels are quite normal even at six months after wounding.

who develop scurvy tend to reopen. Needing continued "repair" and deprived of it, the seemingly healed wound breaks down before the normal tissues do. Some of the failure to achieve normal tensile strength also seems to lie in the very imperfect regeneration of elastic fibers in the wound, with a general failure to re-establish the elastic fiber–collagen fiber network that characterizes the normal dermis.[18]

The Deceptiveness of Wound Healing

The apparent perfection of the healing of an incised wound is really misleading.[50] As has been noted, a normal collagen and elastin fiber feltwork is not re-established. The collagen fibers do not show a normal alignment, and the elastin fibers are deficient in number and organization. The dermis lacks a normal papillary layer beneath the surface scar. The capillary and lymphatic networks likewise are not normal. The epithelium over the scarred dermis is

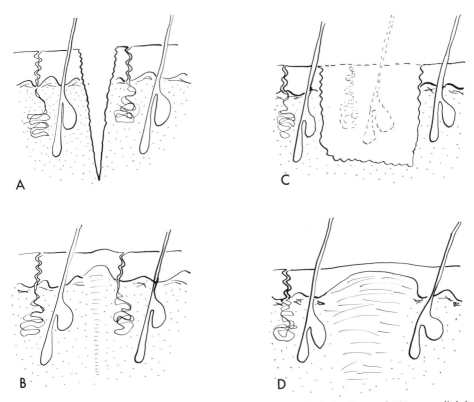

Figure 17–3 Wound healing—appearance and reality. An incised wound (A) gapes slightly, consequent upon the intrinsic skin tension. In healing, the wound surfaces are reapposed (B) so well that no loss seems to have occurred. In reality the scar tissue can be seen interrupting the organization of the dermis, the epidermis is thinner and elastic fibers are deficient along the line of cicatrix.

The situation in a wound with loss of substance (C) illustrates this more clearly. The accessory skin structures lost are not regenerated. The papillary layer is not re-formed, the rete pegs are missing and the nerve, blood and lymphatic supply of the scar is not as it was. Scar tissue has substituted for the missing tissue which has not been re-formed.

aberrant in that it lacks hair follicles, sebaceous glands and sweat glands. It is usually thinner than normal and has no rete pegs. The scarred skin is not normally innervated. The specialized endings that may have been present do not regenerate. What has really occurred is the drawing together of adjacent normal tissue cemented together by an area of new tissue (scar tissue). Healing has actually been by substitution, not replication (Fig. 17-3). The greater the loss of substance in the initial wound, the more conspicuous is this substitutive healing.

Factors Interfering with Wound Healing

Local and systemic factors may interfere with wound healing. Locally, excessive bleeding into the wound (hemorrhage) delays healing by enlarging the "dead space" of the wound, that area requiring filling with granulation tissue. Such a collection of blood in the wound — called a hematoma — also predisposes to the development of infection. Bacterial enzymes can break down early collagen structures, thrombose the healing capillaries, prolong the phase of neutrophil invasion and delay the onset of macrophage cleanup and fibroplasia. Motion of the wound edges shears the new capillary connections, causing microhemorrhages. Edema, if marked, may expand tissue spaces and delay healing early in the process, but not terminally.[49] Seroma has the same effect as hematoma. Lack of blood supply (ischemia) can retard or even prevent healing.

Neurogenic influence is sometimes cited as a local factor but its importance or existence seems in doubt. Healing occurs in a denervated area as well as in a fully innervated one. This appears to be true whether the denervation is a local peripheral one or a central defect, as in a cord transection. Donor sites of skin grafts have been placed above, below and straddling the sensory level in the same paraplegic patient. Healing in all areas was identical. However, when neurologic damage is associated with vascular damage, healing may be greatly delayed, owing more likely to the ischemia than to the sensory deficit.

Vitamin C deficiency or scurvy is the most profound of the systemic factors that interfere with healing. The interruption occurs in the laying down of normal collagen. Fibroplasia, mucopolysaccharide production and the formation of reticulin procollagen material are not inhibited, but mature collagen synthesis is halted. The defect is corrected within 24 hr after the intramuscular administration of ascorbic acid.[12] Protein deficiency must be very severe to retard wound healing significantly. The wounds of a starving but nonscorbutic man heal. However, of all the amino acids, only methionine, when added to a protein-free diet in specially depleted experimental animals, restores the accumulation of mucopolysaccharides and the formation of new collagen fibers to normal levels.[68] The effect of anemia on wound healing is not clear. Chronic anemia seems mildly deleterious to wound healing during the phase when ground substance is elaborated, but it does not adversely affect rate of gain in tensile strength during the phase of collagen production. Except in severe anemias the magnitude of these effects is small.[25] It appears that most wounds are well able to heal in an environment that is poor in oxygen and that they actually do so.[26] Metabolic diseases such as diabetes or cirrhosis appear to

exert their effects through local mechanisms. Diabetics may show delayed healing on an ischemic basis if small vessel disease is present locally. Wounds in
cirrhotics may heal slowly as a consequence of wound hemorrhage or edema,
both of which are secondary to deficient liver production of clotting factors,
proteins and albumin. High levels of corticosteroid administration can interfere
with granulation and fibroplasia, although the interference is not manifested if
an acute local inflammatory response is produced.[36] Epidermal migration seems
more resistant to cortisone retardation. The relationship of other hormonal
influences on wound healing is much less well defined and seems of little
practical importance. The ill-defined clinical impression that healing can be
influenced by the patient's "mental set" has been the subject of some fascinat-
ing observations.[60]

Factors Accelerating Wound Healing

A host of factors have been claimed as stimulating wound healing. Such
claims have to be examined critically. The evolutionary importance of wound
healing suggests that it probably proceeds optimally under most normal circumstances. Surprisingly, a small degree of bacterial contamination in a wound
or other injurious stimulus is needed for normal healing rates. Germ-free
animals wounded aseptically develop wound tensile strength more slowly than
normal animals. Wounds teated with pepsin-digested powdered heterologous
cartilage have been shown to produce greater tensile strength by the fifth to
seventh day than normal wounds, but at nine to 14 days, the differences are
not noticeable.[58] The effect seems to be independent of the inflammatory
effect of the powder per se. The effects of secondary, local and distant wounds
on healing remains controversial. Disrupted and resutured wounds regain
tensile strength at an accelerated rate compared to undisturbed primary
wounds. This appears to result from the previous mild inflammation associated
with the initial wound, leading to a greater "readiness" of the tissues to heal. It
has been reported that a healing wound in one part of the body accelerates the
healing rate of another wound subsequently inflicted in a different part of the
body, but this observation has not been confirmed.[13] Embyronic tissue extracts,
amniotic fluid, zinc salts, and many other agents administered locally or systemi-
cally have had claims made for them which time and repetition have not
borne out. It seems more desirable to set the conditions for normal healing
than to seek for supernormal responses.

Aberrations of Wound Healing

Despite the finely honed evolutionary significance of wound healing already noted, aberrations in the ideal process are not infrequent. The commonest is the failure of the fibroblasts to cease the production of collagen fibers.
Whether this is a consequence of failure to send the message of healing completion, an error in the message sent, faulty transmission or reception or inability
to act upon the message is unknown. Many wounds show excessive scar forma-

tion, termed scar hypertrophy. Such scars are marked by continued abundant blood supply as well as the symptom of pruritus, the mechanism of which is unknown. However, over the course of 6 months to 1 year or more, a slow process of maturation occurs, the excessive collagen tends to be partially resorbed and the symptoms disappear.

Another aberration, differing in degree or possibly in kind, exists, which is called keloid formation. A keloid not only remains active but also grows in size and extends beyond the initial wound, coming to involve previously untraumatized normal tissue.[6] Huge quantities of collagen are laid down. Regression does not ordinarily occur. Periodic intermittent growth continues for many years, accompanied by symptoms of tenderness and of pruritus. The cause of this condition is unknown. The collagen formed is aggregated histologically in the form of giant fibers recognizably different from normal scar tissue. However, the fibers have a normal histochemistry and under the electron microscope show a normal collagen periodicity of 640 Å. The tendency to form keloids is not necessarily systemic; one wound and not another may heal in this way. The tendency is only occasionally familial; however, it is often genetically determined in that the abnormality is much more frequent among those with pigmented skin, be they black, yellow or white of Mediterranean basin origin.

Healing of Wounds with Loss of Substance

Wounds with loss of substance are of several types. Traumatic avulsions and amputations are one group. Thermal, electrical and chemical burns with large, full-thickness skin losses are another. A third group may be termed ischemic. The decubitus ulcer is a major type within this last group. It is of special interest and so will be discussed in some detail both for its own sake and as a representative of this category of wounds.

Decubitus Ulcers

A decubitus ulcer usually follows excessively long compression of skin and subcutaneous tissue between an underlying bony prominence and the surface upon which the patient is lying or sitting. The pressure not only expresses blood from the tissues but also prevents it from reaching the tissues. The resulting anoxia leads to death of the tissue (necrosis). The dead skin and other tissue—called the eschar—sloughs and a break in the surface of the body, termed an ulcer, is produced. The length of time and the pressure involved in bringing this injury about have not been quantitated. Since ischemic tissue announces its plight by pain, the development of these lesions depends upon an interference in the perception of pain or the ability to act upon the perception. The spinal-injury patient is deficient in both regards, as is the unconscious patient. On the other hand, the weak, elderly patient felled by a hip fracture, for example, suffers only the latter disability.

Predisposing to the development of decubiti are advanced age, probably associated with small vessel arteriosclerosis and decreased local circulation, malnutrition with edema, and possibly, specific drug effects, as have been implicated in both narcotic and carbon monoxide intoxications.[39] A tendency to develop hemorrhage into tissues, with subsequent hematoma formation and separation of tissues from their vascular supply which leads to necrosis, occurs in some patients receiving anticoagulants. Local chronic skin breakdown following friction or maceration, while it is not caused by pressure, is often included under the heading of decubitus ulcer. Such lesions usually do not show the deep, conelike extension into the subcutaneous tissue typical of true pressure-induced ulcers. Their chronicity is usually consequent upon lack of recognition and persistence of the initiating conditions.

Natural History of a Decubitus Ulcer. The events following the necrosis of the compressed tissue are essentially the same as after wounding. The separation of necrotic material begins with an intense neutrophilic response. The margin between the living tissue and the necrotic tissue becomes well defined by this response, a process called demarcation. The necrotic tissue becomes dehydrated and blackened, further differentiating it from the inflamed surrounding skin. Tissue enzymes serve to sever the connections between the dead and the living tissue. With the sloughing of the eschar, granulation, epithelization and contraction can begin. Given enough time and the cessation of the initiating pressure, the ulcer will heal spontaneously. In some instances it does not heal but undergoes a peculiar reaction whereby the ulcer cavity becomes lined with a layer of flattened fibroblasts, and the space becomes the site of tissue fluid accumulation. This is termed a pseudobursa, and the cause of its development is unknown. Its formation is noted clinically as the wound heals to a small ostium but refuses to close completely thereafter, except for brief periods during which fluid collects (Fig. 17-4).

Location of Decubitus Ulcers. Decubiti are most frequent over the ischial tuberosity (30 per cent), the greater trochanter (20 per cent), the sacrum (15 per cent) and the heel (10 per cent). These locations represent the major pressure points for the recumbent and for the seated spinal patient.[10] Almost any other area can be involved, however, depending upon the specific circumstances of injury.

Treatment of Decubitus Ulcers. The treatment of decubitus ulcer depends on the physiological facts of wound healing already discussed. On the basis of the profound tendency of wounds to heal, one can choose to allow spontaneous closure. However, a large wound may require many months to heal. A large, exposed area is a site of low grade inflammation, with the possibility of bacterial invasion. The wound surface is a site of blood and protein losses as well as water loss, and multiple decubiti can be the sources of significant metabolic losses.[48] Damage to underlying structures—bone, tendon, nerve, muscle—may occur via the open wound. Since the ultimate repair will be substitutive, a large defect will yield a large, scarred area with the decreased tensile strength, the thin epithelium and the other disabilities of scar tissue already noted. Depending on the area involved, this may lead to functional disability. Accordingly, spontaneous closure is usually allowed only when the defect is small, the area is not likely to suffer functionally, or other factors in the patient's problems preclude intervention.

The forms of intervention are several: direct surgical closure, skin grafting and skin flap coverage (Fig. 17-5). Direct closure does for the defect what

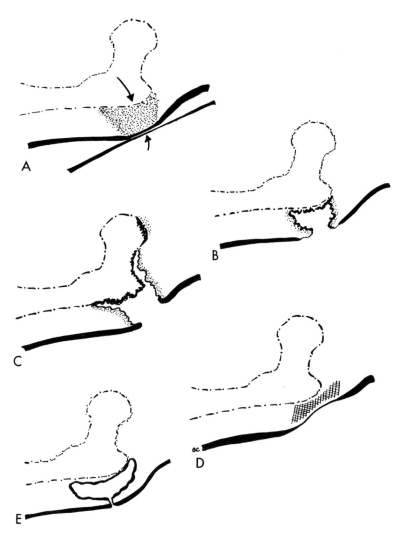

Figure 17–4 Natural history of decubitus ulcers. (A) Soft tissue between the greater trochanter of a hip and the surface upon which the hip is lying is compressed. The blunt cone of injury (stippled area) is shown to be greater in the subcutaneous tissue than in the skin itself. (B) Slough of the necrotic tissue has left a decubitus ulcer with characteristic undermined edges. (C) If exposure and infection persist, the bone and joint may become involved. The roughened, eroded edge of the trochanter indicates the osteomyelitis, and the similar roughening of the articular surface of the femoral head indicates the pyoarthrosis that has occurred. (D) More usually, the decubitus, if recognized and treated, will heal, leaving scar in the area with its physiological limitations as a substitute tissue. (E) Occasionally the ulcer cavity becomes lined with flattened fibroblasts and the area fills with tissue fluid. Surface healing always seems just about to occur, but persistent reaccumulation of fluid and breakdown occur instead; a pseudobursa has been formed.

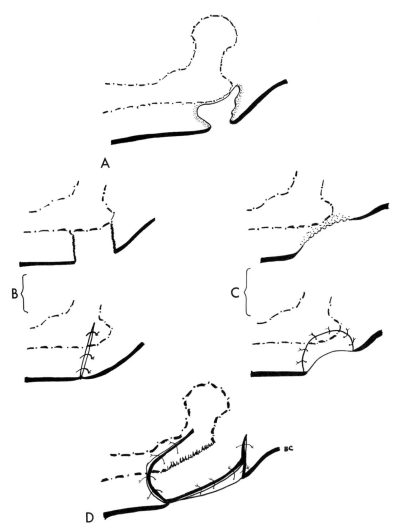

Figure 17-5 Treatment of decubitus ulcers. (A) A characteristic ulcer over the greater trochanter with granulation tissue lining the cavity. (B) Direct closure. The ulcer and the chronically inflamed tissue have been excised and the wound directly closed and sutured. (C) Skin graft. The ulcer has been allowed to heal partially; granulation tissue has filled in most of the defect. A skin graft is then applied and is shown sutured in place. (D) Skin flap. The ulcer has been excised, the trochanter has been osteectomized and a skin flap from the side of the thigh rotated to fill the defect. The donor area of the flap is covered with a skin graft.

the forces of wound healing will ultimately do—draw the normal adjacent tissues together. However, the amount of force needed to bring this about at once rather than over a long period of time is far greater than the tensile strength of the tissue itself. A wound so sutured will most likely pull apart as the sutures cut through the wound edges.

The use of a skin graft is the next consideration. The donor site of a split-thickness graft has already been discussed; it will heal by replication, so that no loss is suffered by the donor area. The "take" of an autogenous graft is a special case of wound healing. The graft initially has no blood supply and survives because its low metabolic needs are satisfied temporarily by diffusion from the clot plasma lying between it and the recipient site. Subsequently blood vessels from the granulation tissue find their way to their counterparts in the graft's dermis, supply the graft via its own vasculature, and then ultimately replace the graft's vessels partially or totally. However, no significant quantity of subcutaneous tissue can be transplanted in this way. Since subcutaneous tissue has been lost extensively at the site of the decubitus, and it is usually necessary to supply cushioning at that point, it may be mandatory to resupply subcutaneous tissue. In addition, the skin graft is only a partial functional replacement for the skin that is lost. The sweat glands and sebaceous glands of a skin graft usually either do not survive transplantation or do not function. It may be added that the skin graft never achieves the sensation normal for the area into which it is transplanted. It remains deficient despite the ingrowth of some of the local nerve endings. Further, if bone or tendon has been exposed by the death of the overlying tissue, its exposed surfaces may have insufficient blood supply to allow for the "take" of the skin graft.

For these reasons, the use of a skin flap which brings with it a full subcutaneous tissue layer and which possesses its own blood supply in its base is the most usual method for closing a decubitus ulcer. To make the repair as permanent as possible, the conditions that led to the ulcer are altered as much as possible. The bony prominence underlying the defect is removed if at all possible.[22] If a pseudobursa has formed, its removal must be complete. The maceration or friction which may have initiated skin breakdown must be recognized and avoided. The use of various devices, seats, pillows, etc., must be considered. Of greatest importance is behavioral modification aimed at avoiding recurrent, prolonged pressure. The 20 to 30 per cent recurrence rate suffered, however, is testimony to the limitations of therapy. And, since the flap is both bounded and underlain by scar tissue, not least among the causes for recurrence are the physiologic limitations of the imperfect tissue of healing—the scar.

CONCLUSION

The skin is the largest organ of the body. Its composite nature has been demonstrated by a review of its embryology and anatomy. The skin functions as a biological membrane. In this regard it acts as a gate—keeping water in; keeping pathogenic organisms and most radiation out; letting sensation in; letting heat out. The solid keratin barrier, the aqueous sweat production, the lipid sebaceous film, the pigment shield, the vessel and nerve networks by which skin accomplishes these functions and so acts to assure the body's homeostasis have all been detailed. As a living membrane the skin also has the characteristics of self-replication and of self-repair in response to injury. The differences between these two responses and the substitutive nature of the repair of major skin losses have been emphasized. Some of the physiological limitations of the scar—which is the tissue substituted—have been discussed. The implications of these limitations have been illustrated in the choice of treatments for decubitus ulcers, one of the forms of major skin injury.

REFERENCES

1. Abercrombie, M.: Localized formation of new tissue in an adult mammal. Soc. Exper. Biol. Symp., *11*:235-254, 1957.
2. Abercrombie, M.: Behavior of cells towards one another. In: Montagna, W. and R. E. Billingham (eds.): *Wound Healing. Advances in Biology of Skin*, Vol. V, pp. 95-112. New York, Macmillan Co., 1964.
3. Billingham, R. E., and Russell, P. S.: Studies on wound healing, with special reference to phenomenon of contracture in experimental wounds in rabbits' skin. Ann. Surg., *144*:961-981, 1956.
4. Bullough, W. S.: Growth control in mammalian skin. Nature, *193*:520–523, 1962.
5. Calnan, J. S., Pflug, J. J., Reis, N. D., and Taylor, L. M.: Lymphatic pressures and the flow of lymph. Brit. J. Plast. Surg., *23*:305–317, 1970.
6. Cosman, B., Crikelair, G. F., Ju, D. M. C., Gaulin, J. C., and Lattes, R.: The surgical treatment of keloids. Plast. Reconstr. Surg., *27*:335–358, 1961.
7. Cox, H. T.: The cleavage lines of skin. Brit. J. Surg., *29*:234–240, 1941.
8. Cummins, H.: Dermatoglyphics: a brief review. In: Montagna, W., and W. C. Lobitz, Jr. (eds.): *The Epidermis*, pp. 375-385. New York, Academic Press, 1964.
9. Daniels, F., Jr., van der Leun, J. C., and Johnson, B. E.: Sunburn. Scient. Amer. *219*:37-46, 1968.
10. Dansereau, J. G., and Conway, H.: Closure of decubiti in paraplegics: report on 2000 cases. Plast. Reconstr. Surg., *33*:474-480, 1964.
11. Deutsch, S., and Mescon, H.: Melanin pigmentation and its endocrine control. N. Eng. J. Med., *257*:222-226, 1957.
12. Dunphy, J. E., Udupa, K. N., and Edwards, L. C.: Wound healing: a new perspective with particular reference to ascorbic acid deficiency. Ann. Surg., *144*:304-317, 1956.
13. Edwards, L. C., and Dunphy, J. E.: Wound healing. I. Injury and normal repair; II. Injury and abnormal repair. N. Eng. J. Med., *259*:224-233, 275-285, 1958.
14. Epstein, W. L., and Sullivan, D. J.: Epidermal mitotic activity in wounded human skin. In: Montagna, W., and R. E. Billingham (eds.): *Wound Healing, Advances in Biology of Skin*, Vol. V, pp. 68-75. New York. Macmillan Co., 1964.
15. Fallon, R. H., and Moyer, C. A.: Rates of insensible perspiration through normal, burned, tape stripped and epidermally denuded living human skin. Ann. Surg., *158*:915-923, 1963.
16. Fitzpatrick, T. B., Seiji, M., and McGugan, A. D.: Melanin pigmentation. N. Eng. J. Med., *265*:328-332, 374-378, 430-434, 1961.
17. Fraser, R. D. B.: Keratins. Scient. Amer., *221*:86-96, 1969.
18. Gibson, T., and Kenedi, R. M.: Biomechanical properties of skin. Surg. Clin. N. Am., *47*:279-294, 1967.
19. Gillespie, J. M.: Mammoth hair: stability of α-keratin structure and constituent proteins. Science, *170*:1100-1102, 1970.
20. Glücksmann, A.: Cell turnover in the dermis. In: Montagna, W., and R. E. Billingham (eds.): *Wound Healing. Advances in Biology of Skin*. Vol. V, pp. 76-94, New York, Macmillan Co., 1964.
21. Gottschalk, P. G., and Thomas, J. E.: Heat stroke. Mayo Clin. Proc., *41*:470-482, 1966.
22. Griffith, B. H.: Advances in the treatment of decubitus ulcers. Surg. Clin. N. Am., *43*:245-260, 1963.
23. Grillo, H. C.: Origin of fibroblasts in wound healing: an autoradiographic study of inhibition of cellular proliferation by local X-radiation. Ann. Surg., *157*:453-467, 1963.
24. Hay, E. D.: Secretion of a connective tissue protein by developing epidermis. In: Montagna, W. and W. C. Lobitz, Jr. (eds.): *The Epidermis*, pp. 97–116. New York, Academic Press, 1964.
25. Hugo, N. E., Thompson, L. W., Zook, E. G., and Bennett, J. E.: Effect of chronic anemia on the tensile strength of healing wounds. Surgery, *66*:741-745, 1969.
26. Hunt, T. K., Zederfeldt, B., and Goldstick, T. K.: Oxygen and healing. Am. J. Surg., *118*:521-525, 1969.
27. Jelenko, C.: Purification of the water-holding lipid of intact skin and burn eschar. Am. Surgeon, *35*:864-870, 1969.
28. Johnson, F. R., and McMinus, R. M. H.: The cytology of wound healing of body surfaces in mammals. Biol. Rev., *35*:364-412, 1960.
29. Jones, D. W.: Wound contraction—a synthesis. In: Montagna, W., and R. E. Billingham (eds.): *Wound Healing. Advances in Biology of Skin*, Vol. V, pp. 216-230. New York, Macmillan Co., 1964.
30. Kligman, A. M.: Uses of sebum? In: Montagna, W., R. S. Ellis, and A. F. Silver (eds.): *The Sebaceous Glands. Advances in Biology of Skin*, Vol. IV, pp. 110-124. New York, Macmillan Co., 1963.

31. Kligman, A. M.: The biology of the stratum corneum. In: Montagna, W., and W. C. Lobitz, Jr. (eds.): *The Epidermis*, pp. 387-433. New York, Academic Press, 1964.
32. Knaysi, G. A., Jr., Cosman, B., and Crikelair, G. F.: Hidradenitis suppurativa. J.A.M.A., *203*:19-22, 1968.
33. Kraissl, C. J., and Conway, H.: Excision of small tumors of the skin of the face with special reference to the wrinkle lines. Surg., *25*:592-600, 1949.
34. Kuno, Y.: *Human Perspiration.* Springfield, Ill., Charles C Thomas, 1956.
35. Langer, A. K.: Über die Spaltbarkeit der Cutis. Sitzungs b.d.k. Akad. der Wissensch. Math.-Naturw., *43*:233, 1861.
36. Lattes, R., Martin, J. R., and Ragan, C.: Suppression of cortisone effect on repair in presence of local bacterial infection. Am. J. Path., *30*:901-911, 1954.
37. Loomis, W. F.: Sun-pigment regulation of vitamin-D biosynthesis in man. Science, *157*:501-506, 1967.
38. Lorincz, A. L.: Pigmentation. In: Rothman, S. (ed.): *Physiology and Biochemistry of the Skin,* pp. 515-563. Chicago, University of Chicago Press, 1954.
39. Mandy, S., and Ackerman, A. B.: Characteristic traumatic skin lesions in drug-induced coma. J.A.M.A., *213*:253-256, 1970.
40. Malkinson, F. D.: Permeability of the stratum corneum. In: Montagna, W., and W. C. Lobitz, Jr. (eds.): *The Epidermis,* pp. 435-452. New York, Academic Press, 1964.
41. Marples, M. J.: *The Ecology of the Human Skin.* Springfield, Ill., Charles C Thomas, 1965.
42. Marples, M. J.: Life on the human skin. Scient. Amer., *220*:108-115, 1969.
43. Menkin, V.: Biology of inflammation; chemical mediators and cellular injury. Science, *123*:527-534, 1956.
44. Moncrief, J. A., and Mason, A. D., Jr.: Evaporative water loss in the burned patient. J. Trauma, *4*:180-185, 1964.
45. Montagna, W., and Ellis, R. A.: *Blood Vessels and Circulation. Advances in Biology of Skin,* Vol. II. Oxford, Pergamon Press, 1961.
46. Montagna, W.: *The Structure and Function of Skin,* 2nd edition. New York, Academic Press, Inc., 1962.
47. Montagna, W.: The skin. Scient. Amer., *212*:56-66, 1965.
48. Mulholland, J. H., CoTui, F., Wright, A. M., Vinci, V., and Shafiroff, B.: Protein metabolism and bedsores. Ann. Surg., *118*:1015-1023, 1943.
49. Myers, M. B., Cherry, G., Heimburger, S., Hay, M., Haydel, H., and Cooley, L.: The effect of edema and external pressure on wound healing. Arch. Surg., *94*:218-222, 1967.
50. Needham, V. A. E.: Biological considerations of wound healing. In: Montagna, W., and R. E. Billingham (eds.): *Wound Healing. Advances in Biology of Skin,* Vol. V, pp. 1–29. New York, Macmillan Co., 1964.
51. Odland, G. F.: Tonofilaments and keratohyalin. In: Montagna, W., and W. C. Lobitz, Jr. (eds.): *The Epidermis,* pp. 236-249. New York, Academic Press, 1964.
52. Ollivier, D., and Janvier, H.: Congenital cutaneous agenesis: six new cases. Ann. chir. plast., *14*:39-44, 1969.
53. Orentreich, N., and Selmanowitz, V. J.: Levels of biological functions with aging. Trans. N.Y. Acad. Sci., *31*:992-1012, 1969.
54. Patten, B. M.: *Human Embryology,* 2nd edition, pp. 235-237. New York, McGraw-Hill Book Co., Inc., 1953.
55. Penrose, L. S.: Dermatoglyphics. Scient. Amer., *221*:72-84, 1969.
56. Pinkus, H.: Biology of epidermal cells. In: Rothman, S. (ed.): *Physiology and Biochemistry of the Skin,* pp. 584–600. Chicago, University of Chicago Press, 1954.
57. Pinkus, H.: Embryology of hair. In: *Conference on the Biology of Hair Growth, London, 1957:* Montagna, W., and R. A. Ellis (eds.): *The Biology of Hair Growth.* pp. 1–32, New York, Academic Press, 1958.
58. Prudden, J. F., Nishihara, G., and Baker, L.: Acceleration of wound healing with cartilage – I, Surg., Gynec. Obstet., *105*:283–286, 1957.
59. Ramirez, A. T., Saroff, H. S., Schwartz, M. S., Mooty, J., Pearson, E., and Raden, M. S.: Experimental wound healing in man. Surg. Gynec. Obstet., *128*:283–293, 1969.
60. Reeves, R. B., Jr.: Healing and salvation: some research and its implications. Union Seminary Quarterly Review, *24*:187-197, 1969.
61. Ross, R.: Wound healing. Scient. Amer., *220*:40-49, 1969.
62. Rothman, S.: *Physiology and Biochemistry of the Skin.* Chicago, University of Chicago Press, 1954.
63. Rothman, S.: Keratinization in historical perspective. In: Montagna, W., and W. C. Lobitz, Jr. (eds.): *The Epidermis,* pp. 1-14. New York, Academic Press, 1964.
64. Sargent, E. S., and Slutsky, H. L.: The natural history of the eccrine miliarias: a study in human ecology. N. Eng. J. Med., *256*:401-408, 451-459, 1957.

65. Schoefl, G. I., and Majno, G.: Regeneration of blood vessels in wound healing. In: Montagna, W., and R. E. Billingham (eds.): *Wound Healing. Advances in Biology of Skin*, Vol. V, pp. 173–193. New York, Macmillan Co., 1964.
66. Serri, F., and Huber, W. M.: The development of sebaceous glands in man. In: Montagna, W., R. A. Ellis, and A. F. Silver (eds.): *The Sebaceous Glands. Advances in Biology of Skin*, Vol. IV, pp. 1–18. New York, Macmillan Co., 1963.
67. Southwood, W. F. W.: The thickness of the skin. Plast. Reconstr. Surg., *15*:423–429, 1955.
68. Udupa, K. N., Woessner, J. F., and Dunphy, J. E.: The effect of methionine on the production of mucopolysaccharide and collagen in healing wounds of protein-depleted animals. Surg., Gynec. Obstet., *102*:639–645, 1956.
69. Watts, F. T., Grillo, H. C., and Gross, J.: Studies in wound healing. II. The role of granulation tissue in contraction. Ann. Surg., *148*:153–160, 1958.
70. Wilgram, G., Caulfield, J. B., and Madgic, E. B.: A possible role of the desmosome in the process of keratinization. In: Montagna, W., and W. C. Lobitz, Jr. (eds.): *The Epidermis*, pp. 275–301. New York, Academic Press, 1964.
71. Winter, G. D.: Movement of epidermal cells over the wound surface. In: Montagna, W., and R. E. Billingham (eds.): *Wound Healing. Advances in Biology of Skin*, Vol. V, pp. 113–127, New York, Macmillan Co., 1964.

Psychosomatic Considerations

Chapter 18

MOTIVATIONAL FACTORS AND ADAPTIVE BEHAVIOR

by William N. Thetford, Ph.D., and
Helen Schucman, Ph.D.

In this chapter human motivation and adaptive capacities are considered primarily in the light of human ecology—the study of man in interaction with his environment. Early in the 20th century, the botanist J. W. Bews suggested that the ecological approach in biology, the branch which deals with the interaction of organisms and environments, might profitably be extended to the study of human behavior. Man lives in an environment with which he is in constant communication and to which he is constantly adapting. Biological, social and cultural factors combine to make up his world, and a disturbance in any one of these highly interdependent aspects cannot fail to exert an influence upon the others. A physical injury such as the loss of a leg or a severed spinal cord not only handicaps the person, but affects his group standing, his human relationships and his whole interpersonal and personal environment.[19]

In recent years, the ecological approach has been used to study human health and illness in the broadest sense. Areas of investigation have included disturbances of mood, thought, behavior and a variety of disorders of adaptation and adjustment. The study of health and illness in man's natural context demands consideration not only of individual behavior, but also of the whole communicative interchange between the person and the environment. Cross cultural studies have shown that virtually every aspect of human behavior varies between different cultures, and that man's functioning is intimately interwoven with the society and the culture into which he is born. The human ecological approach considers all behavior in terms of person-environment interaction.[26]

353

HUMAN DEVELOPMENT IN A CULTURAL SETTING

The term "development" encompasses all of the sequential stages — physical, social and emotional — through which every intact member of a species progresses. Each stage is characterized by changes in biological organization that alter behavior. While some individual differences are possible at each developmental level, the general sequence is universal. The new-born human infant has no innate guide to human behavior. His personality will be shaped by the multidimensional, multilevel interaction of his biological equipment, his family, his society and his culture.

A family is the basic social unit, existing in all societies although in different forms and with different key figures. A society is a self-sustaining, continuing community whose members cooperate for their mutual benefit. A culture includes all the customs, values, beliefs, institutions and practices which the members of a society share. Genetic endowment and constitutional organization are not culture-determined as such, yet the society and the culture often exert an indirect influence. For example, marriages are prearranged in some societies, and social considerations may influence marriage in many other ways so that the genetic endowment of the child is often affected by a culture-based selection process.

Although biological factors may impose limitations on what the individual *might* become, what he *does* become depends largely on his interaction with his social milieu. Environmental factors will largely determine whether the person develops or neglects his potentialities and whether he emphasizes or minimizes his limitations. Physically or mentally limited individuals in general can work productively in suitable job situations, but society must provide them with both opportunities to develop their skills and situations in which to utilize them. While society does not create potential, it does provide the setting in which potential is realized.

The term "maturation" refers to sequential stages in biological development which are independent of learning. In the human maturation pattern, most children crawl backward before they go forward, creep before they walk, and walk before they talk. Maturation limits the kinds of learning that can be acquired at a given period in life, since readiness for learning depends on it. Yet culture and maturation combine in determining the particular behavior patterns which are actually learned. A child cannot be taught to wave goodbye until he has gained the necessary control of arm and hand. The symbolic meaning of the gesture, however, is entirely culturally determined. Similarly, the ability to sustain attention, a prerequisite for learning, depends to a large extent on maturational organization. Society, however, becomes a major force in directing attention towards certain goals and away from others. Endowment and maturation are thus the raw materials on which socialization depends.

"Socialization" is the process by which the individual learns to behave as a member of a family, a society and a culture. The process, directed from birth by representatives of the culture, enables the infant to proceed from a passive dependent state to active social interaction and to learn what society expects of the child, the adolescent, the adult and the aged. Each individual is exposed to a special set of people, circumstances and events that contribute to the uniqueness of his socialization. However, social learning is also transmitted from one generation to the next. The individual learns the attitudes, values and beliefs of his society and the larger common heritage of his culture. Directly or indirectly, the culture influences both the forms of behavior which he adopts and which he inherits. At each stage of his life, the socialization process stamps a cultural impress upon what he does, what he thinks and how he adapts.

Communication and Socialization

Communication, both at verbal and non-verbal levels, is the medium by which socialization is accomplished. The highest and most complex form of communication involves the use of words. As with other forms of social learning, the basic equipment for human communication is biologically given, and the level at which the individual can perform depends on maturation. Maturational readiness is attained in a predictable sequence in verbal development. For example, the use of vowels precedes the use of consonants, and short words are used before longer words. However, the child must learn to associate particular sounds with specific events. The child must also learn which gestures and sounds lack communicative value and which constitute the specific tools of communication in his society. Being the means on which socialization rests, communication is also the crucial factor in human adaptation. Communication and adaptation are so intimately related that if either is impaired the other will inevitably suffer.

Man's highest integrative functions are utilized in symbolic language. Symbolic communication enables him to share his experiences with others and to participate in theirs. A common language establishes a basis for genuine solidarity, enabling individuals to enter into truly social living and to maintain sustained social interaction. The ability to deal with reality symbolically makes it possible for man to reduce his environment to meaningful units and deal with them conceptually. Concepts such as time, distance and direction are symbolic means of imposing order and continuity on the total perceptual field. Symbols permit man to detect similarities in divergent events, to recognize recurrent aspects of human experience, to deal with people and events beyond his immediate perceptual field and to remember the past and anticipate the future. Society as well as the individual preserves its past and plans for its future through the use of oral and written symbols.

When an individual's symbolic communication is impaired, his major communication channels are blocked and his entire life is disturbed. An injury that results in loss or serious impairment of speech may well pose a special hazard to effective adaptation. The person whose communication with his society is impaired is in much the same position as nations in a state of communications failure; disturbed relationships and even open warfare are likely to result. In fact, all forms of maladjustment may be said to involve some kind of disturbance in social communication, with resulting disequilibrium in the individual-environment relationship. The human ecological view of malfunctioning emphasizes that not only will the individual himself suffer from a lack of communicative harmony with his society, but because he is alienated from the environment at the most basic level, the entire person-environmental matrix will be disturbed.

ADAPTIVE BEHAVIOR

Adaptive behavior, broadly defined, refers to any constructive change the organism undertakes to help him meet the demands of his environment and improve the quality of his interaction with it. To adapt effectively, the individual must make continual adjustments to bring him into increasing harmony with his environment. Some degree of adaptation is necessary for the survival of all organisms. Man, however, is unique in this respect. Except at the level of very simple reflexes, instinctive behavior patterns provide him with little if any basis for the highly complex adjustments he must make. He must learn to solve problems at many levels, often simultaneously, and develop a large repertory of skills to cope with the many demands that continually confront him. He must learn to anticipate and predict. He must gain control and even mastery over some aspects of the environment through his ability to plan, to consider alternative approaches to problems and to evaluate their probable outcomes without random trial and error. He must adapt to a wide range of climates, to different kinds of foods and to a variety of environmental changes. His ingenuity enables him to survive many situations which other organisms could not. Because of his symbolic communication skills, he can build on the experience of preceding generations and transmit his learning to those who come after him.

The very assets that have provided man with such advantages in adaptive potential have, however, also enabled him to develop a vastly increased potential for destruction. He has established societies to help him attain greater satisfaction and safety, but these societies often cannot live at peace with one another. He has built increasingly efficient tools with which to cope with his environment and decrease its potential threat, but he has also turned his ingenuity toward increasingly destructive instruments of warfare. He has done much to control disease and minimize pain, but he has brought about conditions that can cripple and even kill him.

Many hazards which man has made for himself, and which Erich Fromm calls "historical dichotomies,"[8] can at least theoretically be averted by more adaptive use of human abilities. Man, however, is also faced with "existential dichotomies," which remain immutable. He knows he will die. He can lengthen his life span by his inventiveness, but he cannot change the inevitable end. He must accept this fact about himself and adapt to the loss of loved ones and the decline of his own abilities as he ages or suffers injuries. He is uniquely equipped to attain protection and pleasure, to express himself imaginatively, aesthetically and creatively, and to enjoy such expressions on the part of others. Yet he must also accept tragedies he cannot escape and prepare for the future as best he can. Change is continual and adaptation is the constant requirement of living.

It is apparent that not all behavior is equally successful in aiding the individual to meet internal and external demands constructively. Maladaptive behavior, while retaining the purposive, goal-directed intent of adjustment, leads to a deteriorating person-environment interaction. Claude Bernard, the 19th century French biologist, was among the first to regard even physical disease as the result of such unsuccessful adaptive attempts. While Bernard's interpretation of disease was largely limited to biological reactions, the human ecological approach extends this point of view to the entire range of man's adaptive responses. Episodes of irrational and sometimes destructive behavior, which even the most well-adjusted manifest at times, as well as the "blind spots" and other relatively minor distortions of the neurotic, and even the delusions and hallucinations of the psychotic, can be regarded as inappropriate adaptive attempts. The importance of genetic determinants and predisposing constitutional factors in behavior are clearly recognized. Nevertheless, the adaptational aspects of behavior remain the central focus of the human ecological approach.

MOTIVATION

Man is essentially a striving organism. He has needs, desires, urges and drives which, since they all serve to initiate behavior, can be classified as motives. A motive can be defined as any internal condition that induces striving, purposive behavior toward a goal. The behavior is purposive in that its aim is to reduce the tension aroused by the motive. Certain fundamental needs appear to be universal, although their expression may take the form of complex and highly divergent behavior patterns. To satisfy hunger, for example, men may climb trees to obtain coconuts, catch fish or go to a restaurant. All such behavior patterns involve a motivational sequence in which a common need arises, a goal is perceived, the possible means for achieving the goal are considered, a plan of approach is decided upon and release from tension and the achievement of satisfaction are sought accordingly.

Human behavior is more than a series of passive reactions to external and internal pressures. The very fact that man makes a large number of decisions about what to respond to and what to disregard indicates that he assumes an active role in his own behavior. Motives as such are essentially inferences, objectively evaluated by the behavior that results and the goals which are sought. It has been pointed out[1] that motives are both inferred from and taken to account for behavior, so that there is danger of circular reasoning in using the motive to explain the result. Those authors make a distinction between the kinds of motives which can be used to describe behavior and those which can be used to explain it. Motives are regarded as explanatory when the conditions which aroused them are known or independently measurable. For example, thirst can be inferred as a motive for drinking and can also explain the behavior, since what gives rise to the motive is known and its physical indicators can be measured in reasonably accurate biological terms.

The Classification of Motives

Motivation is not clearly understood, and there is wide difference of opinion even over its classification. Of the many classification systems that have been devised only a few will be mentioned here. No system advanced as yet is sufficient to account for the whole range of human behavior. One method is to divide motives into the two major categories—"primary" and "secondary." A primary motive includes those physiological and innate needs which members of a given species share. Such motives arise regardless of environmental factors, and are largely genetically determined. However, the kinds of behavior that the motive generates and the specific goals that the individual seeks will vary from one species to another and with man from one society to another. For example, to survive the cold, man can find a cave, build an igloo or move into a temperature-controlled apartment. In this type of classification, motives other than primary biological needs are considered secondary and are induced through the process of conditioning.

Motivation can also be classified in terms of various painful or unpleasant states which propel an individual toward tension reducing behavior; motives thus become primarily agents for restoring a disturbed equilibrium. A number of theories related to this tension reducing mechanism have been advanced. These may be subsumed under the general heading of the pleasure-pain classification, in which goal-directed behavior is stimulated by either the seeking of pleasure or the avoidance of pain. This general view has taken the form of a reward and punishment model, as well as the related dichotomous classification of motives into deficiency and abundancy categories.[15] Deficiency categories induce various kinds of avoidance behavior, such as responses aimed at the alleviation of hunger, thirst, excessive temperatures, fatigue, pain and other unpleasant states. Some investigators have expanded this concept to include the avoidance of danger, fear producing situations and feelings of inferiority, failure, shame, guilt and depression. Motives of this kind are generally related to safety or survival. Abundancy motives are mainly concerned with stimulation and satisfaction and give rise to behavior geared toward attaining bodily comfort, pleasant sensory experiences, material possessions, companionship, personal independence, self-enhancing experiences and a sense of personal achievement.

Other motivational theorists regard man as an energy system that responds to stimulation so as to maintain homeostasis. This approach, originally set forth by Cannon[3], has been extended by some theorists to include virtually all areas of disturbance or imbalance. The purpose of motivated behavior is regarded as an attempt to restore psychological as well as physiological equilibrium.

In all the classifications of motives there is general agreement about biological factors, such as hunger, thirst, sex and other bodily functions arising from physiological sources, which initiate behavior directed toward individual and species survival. At this level, human needs are similar to those of animals. However, such needs are rarely sufficient to promote human happiness. Man experiences many needs not experienced by other species, such as achievement, aesthetic satisfaction and creativity. Goals of this kind can supersede the aim of physical well-being and even of survival. The explanation of behavior initiated by motives of this kind is still controversial. Some theorists maintain that such motives are merely extensions of biological needs. Others regard them as being socially conditioned and learned or acquired. Still others attribute all human behavior to one basic motivating force which expresses itself at various levels. For example, it has been maintained that the primary human motivation is the basic drive to maintain and develop the potential of the individual and to enhance his self-esteem.

From the human ecological viewpoint, stimuli requiring an adaptive response may occur anywhere in the person-environment system, so that any classification which fails to involve motivational areas is inadequate. The individual may react adaptively or maladaptively to any kind of perceived threat, or to any event which symbolizes danger to him. Whether his response is appropriate or inappropriate, constructive or destructive, he is always motivated by the need to adapt so as to improve the person-environment relationship as he perceives it.

CONFLICT AND FRUSTRATION

Conflict results whenever incompatible motives arise and the individual must decide which goals to pursue. Until the conflict is resolved, the person is in a state of biological and psychological tension. At the biological level, conflict is manifested in the bodily changes associated with the "emergency" state. The psychological concomitants include various unpleasant feelings, such as a sense of strain, discomfort and frequently anxiety and depression. Conflicting motives make some amount of frustration or interference in goal-directed behavior inevitable. The interference may arise from opposing pressures from the environment, from contradictory desires in the individual himself or from incompatible interests in the environment and in the person.

The human ecological viewpoint considers an individual's response to conflict and frustration in the context of his total functioning as an organism.[23] This raises the question of the particular stimuli in the total perceptual field to which the person responds. It is essentially his perceptions of this field which become the reference points for decisions he will make in dealing with conflict and frustration. His perceptions will inevitably reflect his particular values, attitudes and needs, as well as his underlying sensory-neural processes.[24] Thus, the view of an individual toward a given situation depends on his perceptions and motivational system, rather than on objective properties of the situation itself.

No one responds with equal intensity to different stimuli. Some aspects of the total perceptual field must be emphasized at the expense of others in order for the individual to function. To a large extent, all unified behavior depends on this process of selectivity. For example, reading requires the ability to select certain stimuli from a page and to disregard others.

Rapid perceptual shifts continually occur at many levels and often without conscious choice. Habits, for example, which are relatively automatic response patterns, play an important part in facilitating effective behavior and saving time, but habit patterns cannot resolve conflict situations. If previously learned responses had been sufficient to settle the problem, a state of conflict would not have arisen.

Conflict Resolution

Conflicts can be compensated for or resolved through rebellion, compromise, or withdrawal,[2] but they cannot be resolved until the individual arrives at a decision. This enables the person to pursue the goals which his decision dictates, so that an adaptive response becomes possible and tension dissipates or at least diminishes. Making a decision does not necessarily mean that it is the best one available, or even the one which the individual would make after reconsideration. It does mean, however, that once he has decided on a course of action, his anxiety begins to lessen.

The crucial factor in decision making is the person's ability to accept frustration and to give up less desirable goals in order to achieve those which are more important to him. The ability to relinquish some satisfactions in order to achieve others is a necessary condition for maintaining effective adaptation. If the benefits perceived by one course of action clearly outweigh the gains of the others, there will be little difficulty in resolving the conflict and initiating a suitable response. It is only as the motives which propel the individual toward different courses of action approach each other in his value system that the conflict becomes increasingly intense. If the two incompatible goals are perceived as equally desirable, conflict resolution becomes impossible. Fortunately, this state is seldom reached under normal conditions. In pathological conflict, however, a person cannot allocate priorities to alternatives, so that no satisfying course of action can be undertaken.

Conflict is inherent in living. Hundreds of decisions must be made daily. If efficient functioning is to be maintained, the alternative goals which an individual perceives must be realistically obtainable and lend themselves to meaningful hierarchical ordering, thus facilitating suitable action. If his major solutions are not reality-oriented, conflict resolution becomes unlikely, ability to adapt is weakened and the individual remains in chronic tension and distress.

STRESS

The concept of stress in psychology was borrowed from physics and extended to the biological and behavioral sciences by the endocrinologist Hans Selye.[18] Stress has been defined as "a dynamic state within an organism in response to a demand for adaptation"[30] and is described as a condition that is present whenever the adaptive mechanisms of the organism are taxed. Conflict, frustration and stress are closely allied concepts. It is the implied frustration of a need that gives rise to the tension in a conflict situation, and frustration is inherently stressful. Since living requires continuous adaptation, the organism is constantly faced with stress. However, the stresses which different individuals face, and even those which confront the same individual at different times, fall into unique patterns. This is inevitable because people perceive similar situations in different ways, and because no two individuals are ever in exactly the same situation.

There are many adaptive behavior patterns that society expects of its members. Among the factors contributing to these expectations are age, sex, educational and occupational levels and shifts in social roles.[6] No society can reasonably require a child to respond as an adult. Lapses in toilet training, for example, are usually condoned in a child, but are unacceptable in an adult except under special circumstances. A child may be permitted to burst into tears in situations which the adult is expected to meet without a display of emotion. Boys and girls, and later men and women, often encounter different adjustment problems and are expected to cope with them in different ways. In many societies, the woman is encouraged to adopt dependent problem solving methods, while increased initiative is expected of the man. The unskilled laborer must cope with some situations unlike those which confront the theoretical physicist. The demands on a single adult alter considerably when he marries and begins to raise a family.

In addition to the general changes in adaptive patterns that are required of the individual, he must also adjust to the particular events in his life. However stable his life situation may be, he will have to make many special adjustments to unexpected events, such as physical injury, the loss of a job or the death of a loved one. He may lose his previously learned skills and be forced to acquire new ones. He may be called on to relocate and to adjust to a whole new set of adaptive demands. Each individual must thus learn to cope with the many stress patterns that are reasonably common in his society and with the more personal difficulties that arise in the course of his own life as well.

Areas of Stress

Stress may occur at different levels, from different sources and in different degrees. It may be biological, psychological or social, each calling for appropriate defense or coping mechanisms. The stress induced by physical illness, for example, evokes biological defenses, although there may be psychological concomitants as well. Adverse emotional reactions such as depression and anxiety, although associated with bodily changes, are experienced primarily as unpleasant psychological states and call forth so-called "ego defenses." Defenses of this kind, although sometimes initially constructive, can become extremely costly, since they introduce distortion into the person's perception of the situation. If a person is faced with an extreme personal tragedy, he may need an initial period in which he uses defenses such as denial and repression before he is able to deal with the situation realistically. Brief appeal to mechanisms of this kind may be compared to the reaction of fainting when a person experiences severe physical pain. During the shock period which follows personal tragedy the temporary appeal to certain ego defenses, such as denial, may actually contribute to a constructive long-range adaptation.[16] It is largely when such coping methods become a person's characteristic way of reacting to stress that more adaptive problem solving is seriously hampered. The individual's energies may then become increasingly invested in neurotic goals and maladaptive defenses, which are extremely difficult to undo.[20]

Physical injuries, impaired abilities, social and economic disadvantages and many other areas of limitation, although not always stressful in themselves, may easily become the focus of a more generalized sense of frustration and a continuous source of stress. Adverse environmental conditions and events may induce stress reactions not only in individuals, but also in groups, societies and even nations. Stress is associated with such inclusive environmental disasters as earthquakes, floods and famines. War confronts nations with dangers and deprivations at many levels. Particularly in times of rapid and extensive change, the individual needs a wide range of adjustive responses and considerable facility in achieving new ones in order to maintain a well functioning adaptation. There is, however, a point beyond which stress becomes overwhelming. Under conditions of prolonged tension and internal turmoil adjustive capacities become over-taxed, producing disturbances in the whole person-environment system, and leading ultimately to the breakdown of realistic problem solving abilities and to general behavioral disorganization.

Areas of Stress-Induced Impairment

Working with normal subjects and various clinical groups, including patients with brain damage, schizophrenia, neurosis, as well as with "psychosomatic" disturbances, Wolff and his associates studied the effects of stress on the highest integrative functions.[4] They identified and described a number of areas of potential impairment of highest integrative function and their behavioral concomitants in patients with known amounts of cerebral hemispheric tissue loss. These areas, which are outlined below, were investigated by laboratory procedures and extensive evaluations of patient functioning in the life situation. Although individual responses varied, these same areas were also found to be vulnerable to stress in other patient and non-patient groups as well.

LOWERED THRESHOLDS FOR DEPRIVATION AND FRUSTRATION. Patients became easily upset, showed more severe disorganization following frustration and deprivation, required longer periods for recovery and depended more heavily on external support and direction.

REDUCED OR INAPPROPRIATE EMOTIONAL RESPONSES. Diminished expressions of affection and sympathy were noted, as well as decreased spontaneity, communication and general expressiveness, with frequent outbursts of hostility and aggression.

IMPAIRED ALERTNESS AND VIGILANCE. Defects in attention and concentration were observed, with increased distractibility and difficulties in more complex perceptual organization.

WEAKENED ASSOCIATIVE, ABSTRACT, AND INITIATIVE ABILITIES. Creativity and imagination were reduced, as were curiosity, explorative behavior and self-initiated activities. Suggestibility was increased, and challenging situations were avoided. Abilities to plan, predict, extrapolate and identify relationships were impaired.

REDUCED CAPACITY TO FULFILL RESPONSIBILITIES. Failure to fulfill social, vocational and interpersonal responsibilities was apparent, along with waning concern about self-care and more fragmented attitudes toward ethical, religious, political and aesthetic values.

DIMINISHED STRIVING BEHAVIOR AND ALTERED ACTION PATTERNS. Pursuit of food, warmth, shelter and sexual satisfaction declined, with decreased interest in communication and recreation. Frequent rest periods were needed and fatigue occurred readily.

INEFFECTIVE DEFENSIVE AND COMPENSATORY REACTIONS. Poorly-organized, inappropriate or exaggerated defenses were found, with intrusions of irrational, personalized, socially unacceptable and sometimes even bizarre defensive and compensatory behavior.

DISTURBED ORIENTATION AND MEMORY FUNCTIONS.   Spatial and temporal orientation were adversely affected, and defects in long- and short-range memory were apparent. Even current experiences were inadequately recorded.

REDUCED EFFICIENCY IN LEARNING, SENSORY-MOTOR, AND OTHER SKILLS. Learning behavior became slower, impoverished and more unstable. Perseverative reactions increased, with impulsiveness and deviation from conventional social mores becoming more frequent. Conscious control was necessary for complex sensory-motor patterns, which were previously automatic, and level of skills in general declined.

FAULTY PERCEPTION OF SELF, ENVIRONMENT AND THE PERSON-ENVIRONMENT RELATIONSHIP.   Self evaluations became unrealistic, and awareness of self in relation to others was disturbed. Perception of the environment grew vague, poorly organized and distorted.

From these observations and related studies, Wolff and his associates[5] concluded that man's highest integrative functions can be jeopardized when the person-environment interaction is undermined by excessive or prolonged stress. While the extent to which such impairment is reversible is not known, there is evidence that restitution may occur with improvement in the person-environment relationship.

Following Wolff's work, there has been increased interest in the human ecological orientation, which sees man in the full context of his environment — social, cultural, physical and psychological. In the past decade, there has been a growing emphasis on ecological patterns of adjustment in response to perceived stress. Examples of such investigations are the present authors' studies of patients exhibiting somatic reactions such as migraine headaches, ulcerative colitis and conversion reactions.[21] [22] [28] [29] The results suggest that environmental conditions in interaction with certain basic traits in the individual may predispose him to fairly predictable types of somatic stress reactions. Consistent with these findings are the observations of Friedman,[7] Kolb,[14] and others,[27] who state that functional headaches tend to fall into two general types. One type is that found in patients whose headaches are psychophysiological reactions to underlying anxiety and conflict, the migraine being perhaps the most dramatic example. The second type, sometimes differentiated from the migraine as the "psychogenic headache," is presumably more closely related to conversion reactions. There is a growing tendency to regard such somatic reactions as ineffective modes of adaptation.

The Individual Nature of Stress

A stress situation is one in which the individual regards his well-being as endangered. Stress is not inherent in a given situation, but is a reaction of the individual to the situation. Although some conditions are more likely to induce stress than others, no one circumstance is maximally stressful to everyone. Even life threatening conditions are not the ultimate in stress, since many people commit suicide. Hunger is a powerful motive for avoidant behavior, yet people have gone on hunger strikes even to the point of death. The intensity of the stress situation a person experiences is proportional to the threat he sees in the situation. A perceived threat severe enough to engender marked or prolonged stress disturbs the whole individual-environment relationship.

The level of stress an individual can sustain without serious disruption of his adaptive capacities is his stress tolerance. This threshold varies with the individual and the situation; differences in physical and psychological make-up are involved, including the person's state of health, his general level of anxiety, his vulnerability to its disruptive effects and his characteristic methods of dealing with them. The entire life history of the individual may well be relevant. Traumatic experiences in childhood may leave his adaptive capacity vulnerable to particular stresses. As an example, intense fear aroused in a young child by a fire in the home may later be reflected in excessive stress reactions to situations even remotely related to fire and quite apart from any actual danger. Similarly, disruptive family experiences in childhood may lower a person's stress tolerance to the point at which a presumably mild stress becomes catastrophic to him.

Anxiety becomes greater when stress is prolonged or when the individual faces a variety of stresses simultaneously. However, the intensity of the stress is decreased if the person feels he can cope with it. For example, the reactions of an amputee who can no longer function in his previous occupation may become more adaptive in a new occupational situation which he knows he can handle well. For a given person, a maximal stress situation is one in which he perceives intense threat combined with complete inability to deal with it. In fact, Goldstein[9] regards the "catastrophic reaction" of the brain-damaged patient as a total reaction of an individual who sees himself in a situation he cannot handle. He is in a "state of failure," and his behavior becomes disorganized and chaotic. A minimal stress situation is one in which little threat is perceived, and the person quickly recognizes that he can cope with it. Situations of this kind are more likely to enhance self-confidence, and the outcome in terms of overall adaptive capacity may well be beneficial.

Although human and animal studies generally emphasize the disruptive effects of stress on adaptation, there may also be constructive results, especially if only mild to moderate tension is generated. The attainment of specific goals is often facilitated by some increase in tension, the individual becoming more goal-directed and less diffuse in his activities. As attention and vigilance become more focused, activity levels may rise as well, permitting more effective and energetic striving behavior. There may also be increased alertness to alternate ways of achieving need satisfaction. The channeling of behavior which is permitted by mild to moderate tension will sometimes enable a person to overcome barriers he himself would ordinarily regard as insurmountable. Beyond a certain point, however, the intensity of the stress exceeds the individual's tolerance and becomes increasingly disruptive.

Stress and Physical Illness

There is evidence that much physical illness is a reaction to stress. Working within the human ecological framework, Hinkle and his associates[11] studied the relationships between stress and disease in groups of similar ethnic, socioeconomic, occupational and general environmental backgrounds and experience. They found that illness episodes are not randomly distributed. Within each of these apparently homogeneous groups the same general pattern emerged: 25

per cent of the group members experienced 50 per cent of the illness in the entire group throughout a 20 year "prime of life" period, while another 25 per cent experienced less than 10 per cent. The first group also had a greater variety of disease syndromes, involving more organ systems and etiologies. In brief, they appeared to have a greater "general susceptibility to illness." This general susceptibility began early in life and was regarded as constitutional in part. However, the incidence of disease was also found to be significantly related to individual personality characteristics.

Some of the individual characteristics found to be associated with illness episodes were studied in a special group of displaced Chinese[10, 25] who were unexpectedly prevented from returning to their homeland. The study of this group, which had to make extensive and unexpected adjustments at many levels simultaneously, highlights the relationships between the individual's perception of his situation and his general physical and emotional health. The more frequently ill regarded their lives as hard, demanding and unsatisfactory, while the seldom ill considered theirs as interesting, varied and reasonably satisfactory. The frequently ill also saw their past life in an essentially negative light, while the seldom ill spoke of theirs in largely positive terms. Finally, the frequently ill were more introverted, self-absorbed and aware of emotional and interpersonal problems, while the seldom ill were predominantly outgoing, experienced little conflict or anxiety in their interpersonal relationships and were relatively unaware of experiencing emotional difficulties.

It is of particular interest that approximately the same distribution of illness episodes and general susceptibility to illness had previously been found among skilled and unskilled urban American workers, college students and recent graduates and refugees from the Hungarian revolution. The characteristics of the frequently and seldom ill within these groups were also consistent with those found in the study of the displaced Chinese. The investigators concluded that the differences in illness susceptibility were both genetically and environmentally determined, and that the person's life situation was less relevant to his bodily and emotional responses than his perception of it.

It is apparent that some people manifest disturbances in mood, thought, behavior and bodily function under circumstances which others would regard as innocuous. Others exhibit few if any symptomatic reactions to what might be considered far more serious disruptions. Stress reactions, like other behavioral reaction patterns, are strongly influenced by the individual's perception and the characteristic modes of adaptation which his attempts at adjustment may take.

CHANGE AND ADAPTATION

Adaptation to change is a lifelong requirement. The individual is persistently faced with the necessity of adjusting to a changing person-environment relationship. Periods of rapid change bring special stresses and strains which are largely absent when expectations are readily transmitted, understood and accepted. Well-established guidelines and clear-cut social roles foster smooth transitions from one stage of life to another. As a child's sense of security may suffer from over-permissiveness as much as from over-restriction, so a pervasive overthrow of guidelines from the past forces the individual to adapt to virtual chaos. In contemporary society, well-defined differences in parent-child, teacher-pupil and male-female roles are becoming increasingly obscure. Moral and religious precepts are being overthrown and have not yet been replaced by workable alternatives. Long accepted values and attitudes have been questioned, and no new system of shared beliefs has been substituted. Common language groups are split by age, subcultures and special interests, with increasing difficulty in communication.

While the individual has been freed from many of the conflict producing restrictions from which earlier generations suffered, he has no consistent guide for handling his freedom. The closely knit family, the prescriptions of religion and the many other shaping factors of human development of the past have lost their control over large segments of our society. The lack of security that such rapid and extensive changes tend to induce plays an important part in the current increase in the incidence of so-called "stress disorders."

Change and the Life Cycle

Change is potentially stressful because it represents a continual demand for adaptation. Change may occur in both the individual and the environment and often takes place in spurts, interspersed with intervals of relative stability and continuity. Some of these changes are predictable. For example, a growing child must adjust to new adults and contemporaries, new expectations and often to new physical surroundings. Previously learned adjustment patterns are no longer adequate as these shifts occur. Adolescence presents new and often conflicting pressures. Heterosexual interests involve marked changes in interpersonal relationships, and marriage entails setting up a new household, accepting new responsibilities and adapting to a new kind of living. Changes also occur constantly within the individual. The relative calm of the preadolescent "latency" period is followed by a time of general upheaval in which even the process of physical growth is uneven. The sexual maturity that is attained is rarely accompanied by mature judgment, competence or the overall requirements for independent living. Apart from such dramatic periods, life includes broad and somewhat overlapping stages in which changes take place as growth begins, proceeds rapidly, then tapers off and declines. In addition, the individual's ability to adapt is further complicated by the special demands of his particular life situation.

The earlier developmental stages are marked by differentiation of functions and increase in dexterity, strength, emotional control and personality integration. At maturity, psychological and emotional organization tends to stabilize and then to become more rigid, a process which tends to make change increasingly stressful. The greater plasticity of the young makes adaptive changes easier, although independence and change may be sought for their own sake rather than for realistic values. Older generations, on the other hand, tend to think of change as a threat and may react with intolerance, opposition and overt resentment. These differences are highlighted currently by the open attack on former behavioral norms and values, giving impetus to the "under thirty" and "over thirty" dichotomy commonly called the "generation gap."

Further complicating the developmental picture is the fact that an individual's abilities are acquired, reach a plateau and decline at different rates and stages of life. Reaction times, for example, start to drop in early adulthood, while overall efficiency may increase throughout maturity and even into old age. These gains are made chiefly by increased psychological organization, a process which induces stability in attitudes, values and behavior. Greater tolerance for frustration, well-established habit patterns, ability to work consistently for long-range goals, economic pressures and concerns about later security can often offset some of the disadvantages of biological aging for a considerable period of time.

While a combination of emotional stability and physical health is favorable, successful adaptation to life changes also depends on factors such as the ability of the individual to adjust his goals appropriately as he ages. The dependence and lack of responsibility of the child are inappropriate in an older person, and the special language and sartorial tastes of the adolescent do not become the more mature. When such anachronisms occur, they frequently imply that the person is attempting to retain an inappropriate picture of himself—he is reacting like the child who borrows his parents' clothes and plays at being grown up.

Aging

The time at which aging is experienced as a handicap varies. Culturally determined attitudes toward the elderly are highly relevant. In some European and Asian cultures, the elderly are treated with respect and deference. In the United States, however, the "youth cult" dominates our culture. Recent youth movements involve even younger age groups, who may regard the generation of their parents as virtually senile. The theater, advertising and most mass media appeal increasingly to the young, who have significant buying power. Adults, urged on by unrealistic advertisements and wishful thinking, attempt to retain the appearance of youth as long as possible. Age has become synonymous with uselessness and futility. Such attitudes make it difficult for the individual to face aging with serenity and confidence.

The aging process itself is usually gradual, but it may be accelerated by unexpected reversals which overtax the individual's adaptive capacities. Even apart from such precipitating events, the aging person usually faces numerous threats to his independence and self-respect. Intellectual and physical abilities tend to decrease in accuracy as well as speed. Memory functions decline, with recent recall showing impairment earlier than memory for remote events. An elderly person will often have difficulty in remembering the events of the previous day, although he can recall occurrences in his childhood. In senility the individual may actually disregard current happenings and become increasingly preoccupied with the past. Although physical deterioration is closely related to such changes, studies have also shown that environmental and psychological factors influence the extent of impairment in the elderly. The social climate in which a person lives has much to do with the extent of the threat which he perceives. A society which places major value on independence, competitiveness, physical prowess and sexual potency tends to induce special stress in the aging. Employment is hard for the elderly to find, and mandatory retirement is often regarded as the end of usefulness. Deaths among contemporaries increase feelings of depression and loneliness. Forced abandonment of earlier interests, especially those involving physical activity and mental acuity, add to feelings of inadequacy and uselessness.

The aging have a number of additional problems, including anxieties related to increasing dependency and fear of dying. As the need for supervision increases, the prospect of living with the children in our society often arouses pronounced ambivalence on both sides, while the idea of going to an institution promotes feelings of rejection in the elderly and guilt in the children. Aging tends to be a period in which stress tolerance lowers and the perception of threat increases. While cultural, emotional and health factors affect the aging process to a large extent, biological deterioration induces increasingly apparent behavioral changes during old age, and some aspects of aging are often accompanied by the disorganization of senility.

LOSS AND ADAPTATION

Loss implies that the individual has been deprived of something desirable and must now adjust to a condition that is more or less unacceptable to him. The loss of something undesirable, such as a persistent headache, is unlikely to induce a stress reaction. Yet if illness has been utilized to elicit sympathy and attention from others, it may be an essential part of the individual's adaptation. In that event, the loss of pain may be regarded at some levels as threatening. Unless a person is very flexible, he is likely to experience disruption when he is forced to give up his usual adjustment patterns. The perceived threat lessens as he sees acceptable alternatives. The loss of a job, for example, may be catastrophic and even incapacitating unless the individual can find a suitable substitute. His previously learned adaptive patterns are major factors in determining how he will respond to subsequent loss.

Grief is a normal reaction to serious loss of any kind.[12] Much as mourning follows the loss of a loved one, a mourning period following the loss of a valued bodily function or body part is to be expected. In previously well-functioning individuals, the duration of this period is usually brief. Signs of recovery and constructive adaptation sometimes appear within days or weeks. However, recovery may be retarded when a sense of threat persists over a long period of time. A chronic depressive state may result, inhibiting and even preventing the "working through" of the initial shock reaction. At best a person confronted with a serious loss goes through a period of mourning and preoccupation as part of the transition to a realistic adjustment.

Body Image and Disability

Body image is one aspect of the larger concept of self-image. It may be regarded as the perception of a physical self which develops as the individual experiences his body in different situations, perceives the reactions of other people to it and associates it with values, attitudes and emotional responses of his own. Kolb[13] uses the term body image to include both a postural model of the body and also the person's related perceptions, attitudes, emotions and personality reactions. The term "body image disturbances" involves a conflict or disagreement between the body image an individual actually holds and the one he would prefer. If this discrepancy is extreme, the affected person may fail to accept or even refuse to recognize bodily changes which have taken place, maintaining his premorbid body image and attempting to adjust on that basis. The phantom limb is one of the most dramatic examples of the persistence of an earlier body image in spite of subsequent bodily changes.

The continuing improvement in the person-environment relationship which a healthy adjustment demands requires a realistic acceptance of the bodily changes incurred by disabilities and the gradual setting up of a realistic new body image. This process may require considerable time. Body image disturbance may thus be acute after a sudden disability, since the disabled person must alter his premorbid body image in order to attain a reasonably healthy adaptation. Until he is able to make these necessary shifts his recovery is seriously hampered, and he may be unable to cope with the reality of the situation.

Disability and Adaptation

An individual is most likely to react to a new disability in the same way that he had reacted to previous deprivation and loss. Loss is one of the more important meanings of disability, be it loss of a body part, a sensory capacity, an ability or competency, an established place in society or a cherished person. A distinction is also made between "disability" and "handicap"[17] that agrees with the ecological viewpoint and the individual perception which it stresses. A disability is regarded as an objective condition that can be physical, mental or emotional. A handicap is the degree to which a person is at a disadvantage in relation to a desired life objective. A similar distinction may be made between an "impairment," which refers to the loss itself, and a "disability" which in this context involves the total effect on the person sustaining the loss. Whether a disability represents a handicap to the affected person depends partly on his perception of himself and partly on how society regards him. It is important in rehabilitation to help a disabled individual evaluate his loss realistically so that a healthy long-range adaptation is facilitated.

While a person's self-perception, his evaluation of the loss, and the structure of his premorbid personality will affect his perception of his disability, there are also a number of other factors to which he must adjust. Physical functions may be curtailed, activities previously accomplished with ease may now demand considerable effort and pain and discomfort may be experienced. Threats to personal independence and to economic security may weaken the individual's sense of worth, and the need to adapt to new family, social and occupational roles may severely tax his stress tolerance as areas of conflict and frustration increase. The ability to minimize the sense of handicap is a major factor in enabling a disabled person to achieve his maximum potential. The self-image of a disabled person is not necessarily related to the actual severity of his loss. The loss of a foot or even of a toe may incapacitate one individual, while another may function well after losing one or even both legs.

Human ecology sees a disabled individual as a whole person interacting with his environment. Both the individual and the environment must adapt to the disability if a constructive person-environment relationship is to be maintained. In the case of a recent, severe disability, changes will be required at many levels simultaneously. Interpersonal involvements often alter both qualitatively and quantitatively, and shifts in the individual's physical environment are often necessary. He may have to accept reduced levels of aspiration and altered goals, adjusting to role changes in his family, his society and his work. Adjustments must also be made by those around him, since they too are affected by his disability. His family and his society must accept him as he is, as he must accept himself. Both must learn to recognize and focus on present and potential assets. Only then can the potentially disruptive effects of disability be minimized and a harmonious person-environment interaction be achieved.

SUMMARY

In this chapter we have discussed some of the salient aspects of human motivation and adaptive capacities from the viewpoint of human ecology, a theoretical approach in which man is studied in his natural setting and his behavior is regarded in the light of person-environment interaction. Human development, maturation and learning are discussed from this point of view, as are the individual's general adaptive patterns and his motivational system. Conflict, frustration and stress are also considered, with primary emphasis on how they influence man's adaptive potential. The human ecological interpretation of health and disease is discussed, followed by a brief account of the effects of change on the adaptive state of the individual throughout the life cycle. The chapter concludes with sections on shifts in adaptive patterns induced by loss. Alterations in body image and other special problems in adaptation which disabilities may entail are included.

REFERENCES

1. Berelson, B. and Steiner, G. A.: *Human Behavior: an Inventory of Scientific Findings.* New York, Harcourt, Brace & World, Inc., 1964.
2. Cammer, L.: *Outline of Psychiatry.* New York, McGraw-Hill Book Company, 1962.
3. Cannon, W. B.: *The Wisdom of the Body.* New York, W. W. Norton and Company, Inc., 1932.
4. Chapman, L. F., Thetford, W. N., Berlin, L., Guthrie, T. C. and Wolff, H. G.: Studies in human cerebral function: Impairment of cerebral hemisphere functions following prolonged life stress in man. *In:* First International Congress of Neurological Sciences, Brussels, 1957 (Proceedings). New York, Pergamon Press, 1959. Vol. 1: Sixth International Congress of Neurology, pp. 203–218.
5. Chapman, L. F., Thetford, N. W., Berlin, L., Guthrie, T. C., and Wolff, H. G.: Highest integrative functions in man during stress. Res. Publ. Assoc. Nerv. Ment. Dis., *36*:491–534, 1958.
6. Coleman, J. C.: *Abnormal Psychology and Modern Life,* 3rd ed. Chicago, Scott, Foresman & Company, 1964.
7. Friedman, A. P. and Merritt, H. H. (eds.): *Headache: Diagnosis and Treatment.* Philadelphia, F. A. Davis Company, 1959

8. Fromm, E.: *The Sane Society.* New York, Holt, Rinehart & Winston, Inc., 1955.
9. Goldstein, K.: Functional disturbances in brain damage. *In:* Arieti, S. (ed.): *American Handbook of Psychiatry.* New York, Basic Books, 1959, vol. 1, pp. 770–796.
10. Hinkle, L. E., Jr., Christenson, W. N., Kane, F. D., Ostfeld, A., Thetford, W. N., and Wolff, H. G.: An investigation of the relation between life experience, personality characteristics, and general susceptibility to illness. Psychosomat. Med. *20*:278–295, 1958.
11. Hinkle, L. E., Jr., Plummer, N., Metraux, R., Richter, P. et al.: Studies in human ecology. *In:* Rabkin, L. Y. and Carr, J. E. (eds.): *Sourcebook in Abnormal Psychology.* Boston, Houghton Mifflin & Co., 1967, pp. 342–350.
12. Janis, I. L., and Leventhal, H.: Psychological aspects of physical illness and hospital care. *In:* Wolman, B. B. (ed.): *Handbook of Clinical Psychology.* New York, McGraw-Hill Book Company, 1965, pp. 1360–1377.
13. Kolb, L. C.: Disturbances of the body-image. *In:* Arieti, S. (ed.): *American Handbook of Psychiatry.* New York, Basic Books, 1959, pp. 749–769.
14. Kolb, L. C.: Psychiatric and psychogenic factors in headache. *In:* Friedman, A. P. and Merritt, H. H. (eds.): *Headache: Diagnosis and Treatment.* Philadelphia, F. A. Davis Company, 1959.
15. Krech, D., Crutchfield, R. S. and Livson, N.: *Elements of Psychology,* 2nd ed. New York, Alfred A. Knopf, Inc., 1969.
16. Michaels, J. and Schucman, H.: Observations on the psychodynamics of parents of retarded children. Am. J. Ment. Defic., *66*:568–573, 1962.
17. Neff, W. S. and Weiss, S. A.: Psychological aspects of disability. *In:* Wolman, B. B. (ed.): *Handbook of Clinical Psychology.* New York, McGraw-Hill Book Company, 1965, pp. 785–825.
18. Selye, H.: *The Stress of Life.* New York, McGraw-Hill Book Company, 1956.
19. Simmons, L. W. and Wolff, H. G.: *Social Science in Medicine.* New York, Russell Sage, 1954.
20. Schucman, H.: Further observations on the psychodynamics of parents of retarded children. Train. Sch. Bull., *60*:70–74, 1963.
21. Schucman, H. and Thetford, W. N.: Expressed symptoms and personality traits in conversion hysteria. Psychol. Rep., *23*:231–243, 1968.
22. Schucman, H. and Thetford, W. N.: A comparison of personality traits in ulcerative colitis and migraine patients. J. Abnorm. Psychol., *76*:443–452, 1970.
23. Thetford, W. N.: An organismic approach to frustration. *Personality, 1*:1–19, 1951.
24. Thetford, W. N.: An objective measurement of frustration tolerance in evaluating psychotherapy. *In:* Wolff, W. and Precker, J. A. (eds.): *Success in Psychotherapy.* New York, Grune & Stratton, Inc., 1952, pp. 26–62.
25. Thetford, W. N., Goldberger, L., Hinkle, L. E., Jr. and Wolff, H. G.: Personality features and their cultural interrelationships in a group of Chinese. *In: Fifteenth International Congress of Psychology,* Brussels, 1957, (proceedings). Acta Psychol., *15*:541–542, 1959.
26. Thetford, W. N. (Chairman): Human ecology: studies in social and personality adaptation. American Psychological Association, 72nd Annual Convention symposium, Los Angeles, September, 1964 (unpublished).
27. Thetford, W. N., Schucman, H. and Farmer, C.: Psychological testing of children afflicted with headaches. *In:* Friedman, A. P. and Harms, E. (eds.): *Headaches in Children.* Springfield, Ill., Charles C Thomas, 1967, pp. 82–114.
28. Thetford, W. N. and Schucman, H.: Personality patterns in migraine and ulcerative colitis patients. Psychol. Rep., *23*:1206, 1968.
29. Thetford, W. N. and Schucman, H.: Self-choices, preferences, and personality traits. Psychol. Rep., *25*:659–667, 1969.
30. Wolff, H. G.: *Stress and Disease,* 2nd ed. Revised and edited by S. Wolf and H. Goodell. Springfield, Ill., Charles C Thomas, 1968.

Chapter 19

PAIN

by W. Crawford Clark, Ph.D., and Howard F. Hunt, Ph.D.

Pain is an unpleasant subjective experience familiar to all of us. Most of the time it signals that something is wrong: some tissue has been injured or has become inflamed, or our body is being assaulted by extremes of heat, cold or some other noxious stimulus. Though we cannot know precisely how another person or organism feels and cannot share his urgent experience of pain, we can infer its presence by changes in his behavior. When an injured or inflamed part is touched, he winces or writhes and attempts to minimize or terminate the stimulation. He may show autonomic symptoms such as pallor, flushing or perspiration, and his general pattern of activity may be altered so he becomes restless or, alternatively, relatively immobile. Most important, he generally complains of pain or vocalizes in a characteristic way; his behavior appears to have become focused around his reported pain as if the experience had pre-empted his consciousness and altered his motivation.

The initial assessment of pain by the practitioner is based upon observable behavior (as described above) and the signs and symptoms of the patient. The subjective report of the patient may be very useful to the examiner because a wide variety of pains exist which are differentially associated with various disorders. For example, a report of burning, searing pain could support a diagnosis of causalgia; a paroxysmal facial pain touched off by pressure on the gum could support a diagnosis of trigeminal neuralgia. Pain varies in intensity, locus and constancy. It may be dull and diffuse or sharply localized, deep or superficial. Vascular headaches of the "migraine" type throb, while "tension" headaches, from muscular tension, do not. Pain arising from the body surface

373

tends to be sharp and well-localized, while internal pain arising from muscles and viscera tends to be diffuse, aching and often poorly localized. The patient's report can aid diagnosis by indicating what circumstances initiate, ease or exacerbate pain, or change its quality. As with other symptoms, detailed observation and inquiry are essential aspects of the diagnostic work-up. Even greater care than usual must be exercised, however, to avoid suggesting symptoms because of the major contribution of psychic factors to symptomatic pain, as discussed later in this chapter.

Because we can observe in ourselves the painful subjective consequences of stimulation by excessive heat or cold, injury, electric shocks or inflammation, and observe that such stimulation changes the behavior of others just as it changes our behavior, we can derive the functional class of noxious (painful) stimuli or conditions. We observe that others behave as we do under comparable circumstances, and infer that they feel as we think we would. At this level of analysis, the methods and assumptions are similar to those used in the identification of adequate stimuli for visual, auditory and other senses.

PROBLEMS IN THE DEFINITION OF PAIN

Most discussions of pain begin with a definition, which quickly reveals its inadequacy, followed by a quasi-philosophical discussion of the mind-body problem, with the author finally opting for dualism, psychophysical parallelism or some kind of monism in which the pain experience is epiphenomenal to the "real" events taking place in the tissues and nervous system. Commonly, pain is defined as "an unpleasant experience which we primarily associate with tissue damage or describe in terms of tissue damage or both" (Mersky and Spear, 1967, p. 21). This definition implies (1) an experience correlated with (2) actual (or conceived by the subject) tissue damage. Usually the total complex of events defining pain also specifies typical overt behaviors: verbalization and complaint, motoric responses (e.g., withdrawal, tension), and often signs of autonomic arousal (e.g., perspiration, circulatory changes).

This approach, however straightforward, has its difficulties. Not only can damage occur without pain (as in some malignancies, sunburn, or tooth decay), but pain also can occur without apparent damage (as in electrical stimulation of tooth pulp, brief applications of radiant heat to the skin, or trigeminal neuralgia). Further, the same amount of tissue damage, insofar as this can be determined, may produce quite different intensities of pain in different individuals or in the same individual at different times. Objective and detectable tissue damage, although it usually produces pain, may represent only a part of the total complex of conditions producing the experience of pain and determining its intensity, and in some cases a vanishingly small part of that complex.

As one of the senses, then, pain is paradoxical in the extent of dissociation between the presumed intensity of the noxious stimulus (amount of apparent damage) and the subjective or behavioral reactions to it. That is to say, the report of pain, particularly in the case of clinical pain, is less veridical than the reports of other senses. The situation is very different from hearing or vision, in which the reaction can be predicted quite exactly in most instances once the intensity and frequency of the adequate stimulus are known. For example, photons at a wavelength of 700 nanometers arriving at the retina will be perceived as a red light by just about everyone (except for a small, colorblind minority). In contrast, the urgency of our subjective discomfort under given noxious conditions can be influenced substantially by distraction and redirection of attention, by expectations of relief or exacerbation, by a physician or dentist convincing us that nothing is wrong or predicting catastrophic illness, or, in little children, by a mother's kiss to "make it stop hurting."

The reasons for these special characteristics, and the limiting conditions, of pain, are far from clear. Probably, these reasons relate largely to the power of noxious stimulation to serve not only as a signal (as any other stimulus) to which responses can be conditioned, but also as a reinforcing (in conditioning) and motivating stimulus that evokes behavior in its own right. Noxious stimuli are biologically important for the organism, as indicated by the ease with which they interrupt fundamentally important appetitive behavior (such as eating) and produce emotional disturbances. Noxious stimuli peremptorily motivate the organism to act to minimize their impact or to terminate them altogether (escape); introduction of noxious stimuli can serve to punish other behavior, and their termination can serve as a reward. In a sense pain as an experience (and a noxious stimulus as it produces subjective pain) carries with it meaning and implications for action to a degree not commonly found in simple stimulation of the other sensory modalities (except for those involved in nausea, sexual excitation, vertigo and, perhaps, olfaction). The complaint of pain, and such external manifestations of it as winces and grimaces or changes in motility, thus may be mediated by several kinds of control: one in which the complaint is evoked by acute subjective discomfort and one or more in which the complaint is at least partially controlled by its consequences (e.g., what other people and the person himself do about the complaint) to acquire special significance in the individual's adaptive economy.

In a pioneering paper, Kolb (1962) spelled out a number of ways in which the experience of pain, and the complaint, become organized into an individual's total pattern of personality adaptation. He pointed out that the experience of pain has multiple functions. It implies to the patient that he has tissue damage or some functional derangement. When communicated to the physician (or friends and relatives) as a complaint, the implication is that there is something wrong with the patient's body—that there is something that must be done to relieve the discomfort. While the experience of pain appears to be an innate response to injury to the organism, the associated verbal complaint may be modified by learning processes established in the family and the culture. Thus the complaint may not only signal that some tissue damage has occurred but also convey a message of social importance—a bid for help or attention, an attempt to gain emotional support from another person or to dominate him, and so on. Psychic factors participate in determining the intensity of the complaint, independently of the severity of the organic injury, to produce intense complaints in persons with little or no discernible injury or to attenuate complaints in those badly damaged. Kolb, then, saw pain as a complex percept: a combination of sensation, action or responses and affect, and not as a simple sensory phenomenon mediated through peripheral pathways alone.

In other pioneering work, Beecher (1959, 1966) has commented on these special problems in pain and has suggested that clinical pain includes not only a basic sensory component, but also a substantial "reaction component" based largely on anxiety aroused by the circumstances and the significance of the pain to the subject (including the implied tissue damage). As an anesthesiologist, Beecher worked primarily with clinical pain and generally emphasized one class of pain indicators: verbal responses in which subjects request relief by analgesic medication or report relief as a result. He found not only large individual differences in pain sensitivity, but also wide variations in sensitivity within single cases over time. He has proposed that in clinical cases the major effect of analgesics is on the reaction component. This is usually weak or absent in most experimental procedures for studying pain, explaining their relative uselessness for evaluating clinical analgesics. Similarly, he has argued that placebos primarily influence the reaction component—placebos give relief to as high as 35 per cent of clinical cases but to only about 3 per cent of subjects in the usual experimental pain studies. It is important to note, however, that he did not employ other indicators of pain, such as physiological indicators and overt bodily responses (Sternbach, 1968), and that he has more recently adopted experimental pain procedures that reliably reflect the effects of analgesic drugs (Beecher, 1968).

Generally workers concerned with pain as a clinical problem recognize that the severity of the reported pain (and perhaps of the phenomenally experienced pain as well) is based not only on sensory input but also on one or more kinds of "central processing," reflecting more complex nervous system function. The details of such processing are still obscure, but anxiety and motivation related to the perceived significance of the pain and learning related to personal adaptation as influenced by the individual history and by family and cultural practices probably contribute significantly. Feedback mechanisms, both physiological and psychophysiological, also complicate the picture. For example, a pain-induced muscle spasm may augment the original pain; or attention to a headache may cause fear, which increases blood pressure which, in turn, increases the headache.

Goals, purposes and general activity levels also appear to modulate the pain experience. In some circumstances the reaction of individuals to ordinarily painful tissue damage may be surprisingly slight, as in "painless childbirth" or in primitive puberty rites (e.g., penile incision among the Polynesians of Mangaia). A football player who cracks an ankle bone in an active scrimmage may not feel a great deal of pain until later when the excitement has subsided and he is physically inactive. Here sensory inputs that might ordinarily be perceived as painful signify the achievement of valued goals; activity and excitement are at a high pitch. The general, intense sensory input can distract the subject, and the coding of this input lends cognitive significance to the situation to modify "central processing," and thus the experience.

Finally, it may be, as Petrie (1967) suggests, that some people have low "perceptual reactance" and tend to reduce subjectively what is perceived, while others tend to augment it. Petrie reported such a general dimension or perceptual typology for many aspects of perception other than suffering, but it is of interest to note that contact athletes, as compared with nonathletes, tend to be "reducers" and to have high pain tolerances (Ryan and Kovacic, 1966).

The clinician dealing with the complaint of pain must skillfully unravel this complex skein if he is to initiate the proper treatment, particularly in paradoxical "problem" cases in which the patient's physical condition and symptomatic complaints seem at odds. And it is important in such cases to remember that there is no evidence that so-called "psychogenic pain" (without observable physical cause) is any less distressing than pain which appears to arise from demonstrable physical damage. "Psychogenic pain" simply requires different treatment, even though the patient refers it to some sort of bodily injury (Mersky and Spear, 1967). Finally, it is important to note that the interaction between the basic sensory input and "central processing" is probably multiplicative rather than additive. We think, on balance, that only a multiplicative interaction could explain the dramatic discrepancies that often occur between perceived pain and observable physical trauma.

Thus, our discussion will be oriented around three aspects of pain: (1) pain as a sensation, discriminated from touch and other modalities, (2) pain as a producer of or an aspect of affect, and (3) the total pain response (including subjective experience) as a product of higher nervous system processing of the primary sensory input.

EXPERIMENTAL APPROACHES TO PAIN

Space limitations preclude anything more than a cursory glance at this extensive field of study. Any real understanding of pain mechanisms, however, requires attention to a few major findings.

Most experimental approaches to sense modalities emphasize the application of controlled and graded intensities of the adequate stimulus, and utilize procedures that require the subject (the observer) to make some judgment as to the presence or absence of the stimulus, as indexed by his subjective experiences, with the major interest being in thresholds. Procedural and statistical controls, to minimize the intrusion of error in these reports, usually are elaborate and include special training of subjects, placebo controls, single or double blind controls and, more recently, analyses that separate sensory sensitivity from the observer's expectations and bias. Careful control of the stimuli and the conditions of testing give the findings the kind of stability required for reproducibility and for analysis of the functions of the sensory systems involved.

Though pain studies could employ many different techniques to produce tissue damage and pain, practical and ethical considerations usually have dictated the use of just a few that have only short-term and reversible effects (e.g., electrical stimulation of tooth pulp or skin, immersion of the hand in ice water, stimulation of the skin with radiant heat short of burning of the tissue and tourniquet procedures that produce ischemic pain by obstructing circulation).

Hardy, Wolff and Goodell (1952) have investigated most extensively the algesic properties of radiant heat. They approached the problem of pain with the procedures of classic psychophysics and emphasized the determination of thresholds. Their studies revealed a great deal about the psychophysics of pain, distribution of pain sensitivity over the body surface and other matters of interest in sensory psychology. Beecher (1959) and others, however, found the radiant heat technique of very limited value in studies of analgesic drugs and the relief of clinical pain, presumably because the "reaction component" (anxiety) was absent in experimental pain from radiant heat. In support of the importance of anxiety in pain, Hill et al. (1952) have reported that subjects tested under anxiety-provoking conditions tended to overestimate the intensity of electric shocks (feel them as more painful) and that this overestimation was eliminated by morphine, while subjects run under relaxed conditions were more accurate in their estimations, with morphine having little or no effect.

While subjects ordinarily would be expected to see an experimental situation as generally benign, the possibility of some slip-up in procedure could loom large to individuals liable to anxious apprehension. Clark (1969), in his review of experimental studies in which anxiety was manipulated as a variable, has concluded that anxiety-prone subjects and those deliberately made apprehensive by the procedure appear to have lower thresholds for experimental pain than control subjects, as thresholds are usually determined. The matter is still unsettled, however (Sternbach, 1968).

Some investigators have sought more objective pain indicators than verbal report, which is easily influenced by nonsensory variables such as attitude, expectation and the social demand character of the situation (Orne, 1962). (Here social demand simply refers to the compelling influence on the subject of what is expected of him by an audience or, implicitly, by the social norms for the situation; for example, males are supposed to be "strong" and "not to cry" in mixed company, while females may shriek, cry or express emotion with more impunity.) A variety of physiological responses not ordinarily considered to be under voluntary control have been employed: increased pulse rate and blood pressure, shift of blood flow from viscera to striated muscles, inhibition of salivary and gastric secretion, dilatation of pupils and bronchioles, changes in blood glucose levels, increased secretion of adrenalin, palmar skin potential, altered electroencephalogram and increased corticosteroid levels, along with reflexive wincing and withdrawal. Unfortunately none of these is truly specific to pain (as opposed to fear, for example), and some may be produced by a wide range of variables (e.g., hunger, surprise or expectation). People not only differ considerably in their patterns of physiological responses to painful stimulation, but also can produce some of these responses upon simply being instructed to imagine a painful stimulus. Furthermore, evidence is now accumulating to indicate that many supposedly involuntary visceral responses can be placed under the same kind of conditioned control as so-called voluntary behavior (Miller, 1969). Thus, physiological responses may be useful adjuncts to verbal report, but they clearly are not infallible in determining what a subject is experiencing.

Recent developments in psychophysical measurement, particularly signal detection or sensory decision procedures, offer great promise in the measurement of pain (Green and Swets, 1966). These procedures separate the sensory component of the threshold from its psychological or attitudinal component (response bias or psychological criterion for calling a sensation painful). The method is complex, but with proper adaptations it can be used with untrained subjects and applied not only to verbal report but also to physiological and motor indicators of pain. In essence it (1) determines response bias by noting the tendency of the subject to call a known nonpainful or blank stimulus painful and his tendency to call known painful stimulus intensities nonpainful, and (2) it assesses sensory sensitivity by noting the accuracy with which the subject distinguishes between high and low stimulus intensities independently of his response bias. In a recent study in which he used these methods, Clark (1960) was able to show that all of the elevation in pain threshold produced by a placebo was produced by changes in response bias or the criterion for pain, while sensory sensitivity remained unchanged. Conventional psychophysical methods in this experiment simply showed a higher pain threshold for the placebo subjects. Again using the same approach, Clark and Mehl (1971) demonstrated that the elevated pain threshold of older subjects reflected their higher criterion for pain, not a decrease in sensory sensitivity to stimulation by radiant heat. Possibly the older subjects, who may have suffered to some extent from chronic aches and pains, had become partially adapted to pain and found the brief, mild radiant heat stimuli rather innocuous. These new procedures are now being applied to the study of analgesic drugs, hypnotic analgesia, effects of central nervous system lesions and the effect of chronic and severe suffering among clinical cases upon sensory sensitivity and response bias or criterion for pain. Hopefully these studies will help to disentangle the relation between experimental and clinical pain.

Probably one of the main difficulties in relating experimental to clinical pain is that in clinical pain one is dealing more with tolerance to severe pain than with the threshold for detection of mild stimulation that can be called painful, but which is limited in extent and duration. Methods for study of experimental pain, for the most part, produce superficial, brief, localized sensations rather than continued, diffuse and deep pain. Interestingly enough, the experimental procedure that shows the most promise of relating closely to clinical pain is the ischemic or tourniquet method. In Beecher's modification the subject, after an inflated cuff has occluded the circulation in his arm, squeezes a spring-loaded hand-grip exerciser 20 times, squeezing for 2 seconds and resting for 2 seconds in each cycle. With the tourniquet remaining inflated, the subject reports on his pain according to a 1 to 4 scale at intervals of a few minutes over the next hour. The cuff is removed at the end of the hour, or sooner if the subject reports severe pain "4"; the time taken to reach each rated level of pain is the indicator. Presumably, local metabolites sensitize the relevant receptors. Both aspirin and morphine offset this ischemic pain in a reasonably good dose-effect relationship, as shown by increased time to report a given level of pain as a function of dosage (Lim and Guzman, 1968; Beecher, 1968). Workers in Hilgard's laboratory (Voevodsky et al., 1967) have developed a comparable modification of the cold-pressor test (immersion of the hand in water at approximately 0° C), with ratings of pain from 1 to 10 and time to removal of the hand from the water as indicators. This procedure, however, is complicated by the effect of temperature reduction on sensory receptors themselves, as well as upon the blood vessels and circulation.

As people who have experienced various forms of pain, both experimental and clinical, we intuitively feel that ischemic and cold-pressor pain seem closer in quality and urgency to clinical pain than do brief shocks and pin-points of pricking heat that quickly go away (particularly when the tolerance or withdrawal threshold is determined). One feels that "something serious could go wrong," and experiences a desire to escape; and as action is postponed, affect begins to develop. Though space limitations preclude much comment on animal testing methods, it is interesting to note that those animal procedures of greatest sensitivity to analgesics (e.g., titration or "flinch-jump" test) also call for action on the part of the animal and produce strong emotional behavior if the action is blocked (Weiss and Laties, 1959; Weitzman and Ross, 1962; Evans, 1962). In contrast to pain-detection thresholds, which are well below the shock intensity required to get the animal to *do* something about the shock, these escape thresholds, being similar to tolerance thresholds, are the indicators showing the greater sensitivity to analgesics.

If these experimental procedures fulfill their promise, and if the variables influencing sensitivity to them are further clarified, we should be approaching a better understanding of the variables affecting clinical pain.

THE PAIN SYSTEM AS A SENSORY SYSTEM

Abundant experimental and clinical evidence indicates that, up to a point, the pain system is organized and responds in much the same way as other sensory systems. Under controlled conditions, given moderate levels of stimulation and minimal involvement of central processing mechanisms, good psychophysical functions can be obtained relating subjects' judgments of pain to intensity of physical stimulation as in vision or audition. To this degree, and it is a limited one, a "specificity theory" of pain can be entertained (i.e., that an invariant relation exists between stimulus intensity and magnitude of sensation, and that there is a relatively fixed, direct input from the periphery to "higher" pain centers in the brain.) This view encounters difficulties, as we have seen, and they intrude even at the simplest level. For example, a specificity model implies a system which transmits pain information and nothing else; yet very few fibers have been found that respond only to noxious stimulation, and pain input appears to share neural pathways with other senses such as touch, heat and cold. Even so, the basic pain transmission system should be understood if more adequate and complex models are to be accurate and meaningful.

The neuroanatomical aspects of pain have been treated in detail by White and Sweet (1955), Cassinari and Pagni (1969) and in three recent symposia (Knighton and Dumke, 1966; Way, 1967; and Soulairac, Cahn and Charpentier, 1968). Many details remain to be elucidated, and substantial disagreement exists; but there appears to be reasonably general agreement on the following major points.

There are two major systems concerned with transmission of pain. The spinothalamocortical system, which is phylogenetically recent, involves few neurons and mediates short-latency, accurately localized brief pain that is precisely discriminated with respect to intensity and duration. This classic "sensory-discriminative" pain system resembles the other sensory systems and is probably the one largely involved in experimental pain and the pain of minor trauma; it may project to the sensory cortex. The spinoreticulothalamic system, a phylogenetically older system, has complex multisynaptic connections and is believed to mediate diffuse, poorly localized pain that has a long latency and persists after the noxious stimulus has been removed. It projects to the limbic system of the brain and is implicated in emotional responses to pain and reflexive withdrawal or attack. It is probably responsible for the physiological responses of the adrenosympathetic system to pain and for the response of the pituitary-adrenal axis in hormonal stress reactions to prolonged pain as classically described by Selye (1956).

The stimulus for pain may be thermal, mechanical, chemical or electrical. The adequate stimuli for pathological pain are less clear, but presumably these include mechanical deformation or chemical changes such as are produced in anoxia. The receptor for pain appears to be fine unmyelinated nerve endings. It is possible to elicit pain from the cornea which contains only fine endings. Such endings appear in a variety of tissues which are pain sensitive: skin, serous membrane, tendon, periosteum and adventitia of blood vessels, particularly the arteries. While it has been implied that these fine nerve endings subserve only pain, and that specialized endings such as the end bulb of Krause mediate the other sensations, this view has recently been discarded. Membranes containing only free nerve endings have also been shown to be sensitive to touch, warmth and cold, as well as to pain stimuli.

Stimulation of the skin with a fine needle produces tissue damage and a sensation of touch, but often no pain, suggesting that some minimum number of free nerve endings must be stimulated to produce pain. As touch is even more ubiquitous than pain, it appears likely that these fine nerve endings subserve this sense as well. Whether the same or different free nerve endings subserve both pain and touch (and perhaps other modalities) by responding with different rates or patterns of neural activity remains unknown at present. Sensitivity of different parts of the body to various types of stimulation varies widely: cornea, teeth and arteries, viscera and striated muscle give rise to almost no sensation other than pain; differences in sensitivity reflect differences in the density of fibers, and probably their type.

Nerve fibers in the peripheral nerve trunks serving the terminal neural fields in the skin have been classified into A fibers (myelinated, large diameter, fast conduction) and C fibers (unmyelinated, small diameter, slow conduction); strenuous efforts have been made to correlate fiber type with different sensations, but this has not been resolved. In general, though, the large A fibers are thought to mediate epicritic sensation (i.e., nonpainful stimuli of heat, touch, and others), while smaller A fibers (the delta epsilon group) have been associated with sharp pain, which begins immediately upon trauma. C fibers have been associated with dull, throbbing, diffusely localized pain, which appears after a delay. Kenshalo's book (1968), however, reports a number of studies that emphasize the limitations of introspective neurophysiology. Kenshalo stresses the complexity of the relationship between fiber type and function. For example, studies in which nerve trunks were experimentally asphyxiated indicated that pain may be transmitted by A fibers larger than the delta group and that A-delta fibers may carry sensations of temperature and touch as well as pain.

The distribution of sensibility on the body surface appears to be somewhat "spotty," rather than even and continuous, with each spot innervated by several different nerve fibers. This insures multiple projections to the neuraxis. Each of these sensory areas, which may be less than 1 cm in diameter, transmits a unique pattern of excitation to higher centers, permitting localization and two-point discrimination. Because of the multiple overlap, a section of one sensory nerve generally fails to eliminate completely sensibility in any area, though thresholds are raised by the decrease in the number of receptive units. The various fibers, serving temperature, touch and pain in a given region, come together as a peripheral nerve on their way to the spinal cord. The sensory territory of any peripheral nerve is widely overlapped by that of adjoining nerves, and each spinal nerve branches into at least three segments. Thus, a number of peripheral nerve trunks or dorsal roots usually must be cut to eliminate pain in a particular area. The amount of overlap varies widely in different regions of the body, but every locus on the skin appears to be supplied by at least two dorsal roots. Individual variations in sensory loss following the section of a posterior root are extremely large, however.

The distribution of pain sensibility in deeper tissues is less well understood, but it is known that a deep branch of a spinal nerve may supply areas in fascia, skeletal muscle and periostium that are remote from the superficial areas supplied by other branches of the same nerve. Finally, the referred locus of deep pain (e.g., muscle or periostium) resulting from stimulation of a spinal root during a root section operation may be quite different from the subsequent area of cutaneous sensory loss. Thus, there may be a poor correlation between a patient's sensitivity to cutaneous stimulation and his report of clinical pain. Peripheral nerve and dorsal root section are often unsatisfactory procedures for the relief of pain.

It is now clear that viscera do have pain sensibility, particularly when the whole organ is involved and a sufficient number of the sparsely distributed receptors are stimulated. Adequate stimuli include rapid distension or contraction of hollow organs, distension of the capsule of solid organs such as the liver, damage to blood vessels and muscle ischemia. Visceral pain fibers are more sparsely distributed than the somatic fibers that carry pain from deep somatic tissues such as muscles and periostium. These visceral afferents run in mixed trunks along with sympathetic efferent fibers to smooth muscles and glands, but they are no different from the other somatic afferents and are not part of the sympathetic system. However, intense pain from deep somatic structures and viscera often produces such autonomic symptoms as nausea, decreased blood pressure and syncope, though these effects are mediated through the neuraxis.

Pain from a deep source may be referred to the corresponding cutaneous dermatome served by other branches of the same nerve, but the sensation is poorly localized and is usually experienced as a dull ache, as it probably is transmitted over slow C fibers (e.g., left arm pain in coronary thrombosis). At one time, it was considered that the sensation was referred to the superficial area because that area was more richly supplied with sensory endings, under more vigorous and varying stimulation and, consequently, more prominently represented at higher levels of the nervous system and in awareness. Now, however, it is increasingly recognized that nonpainful impulses from the referent area may play a significant role in triggering or potentiating central processes that lead to the experience of referred pain. This revised view is more consonant with the phenomena of referred pain inasmuch as viscera are not unique in producing it; referred pain is commonly experienced with toothache, for example, and teeth are well supplied with sensory innervation and well represented in awareness.

The peripheral nerves carry the axons (A and C fibers) of the primary sensory neurons, at the distal end terminating in free nerve endings for pain or other reception; at the proximal end, these axons enter the cord through the dorsal root, bifurcate into ascending and descending branches and send collaterals into the substantia gelatinosa. Their cell bodies make up the dorsal root ganglia (or the equivalent ganglia of the sensory cranial nerves). In the phylogenetically younger spinothalamocortical system the branches of the A fibers synapse on the cells of "second order neurons" lying in the posterior horn, whose axons, for the most part, cross to the contralateral side of the cord (some remain ipsilateral) through the anterior commissure to ascend as the lateral spinothalamic tract and terminate in the specific relay nuclei of the thalamus with good somatotopic organization (nucleus posterolateralis, nucleus ventralis posteromedialis or arcuate nucleus). The "third neurons" in this classic pain system, the spinothalamocortical system, project to the parietal cortex. This is the sensory-discriminative fast system; its main course is mainly contralateral and as it is quite direct, interruption of the pain signals it carries is relatively simple. Thus the major effect of hemisection of the spinal cord in man should be contralateral analgesia. This classic system also appears to send collaterals to the more diffuse spinoreticulothalamic system at all levels.

The older and more primitive spinoreticulothalamic system receives the proximal axons of the C fibers that have cell bodies in the dorsal root ganglia. The axons bifurcate, enter the tract of Lissauer and synapse in the multisynaptic net of the substantia gelatinosa instead of on the second order neurons of the classic system. The substantia gelatinosa is a long column of small cells extending the length of the spinal cord. The spinoreticulothalamic system then ascends both contralaterally and ipsilaterally through (1) the polysynaptic systems of the cord and brain stem and (2) the long fibers of the spinoreticular and spinotectal tracts to the reticular system of the medulla, pons and midbrain before ending on the nonspecific nuclei of the thalamus. The spinoreticulothalamic system and its thalamic terminus and projections are not somatotopically organized to give discrete spatial and temporal information, but represent a diffuse conduction system. It is open to considerable interaction with other sensory systems, via its connections with the reticular formation, and projects into the limbic system (including the hippocampus, amygdala and other rhinencephalic structures). The limbic system also has connections with the hypothalamus, and is implicated in avoidance, emotions, and defensive reactions.

Thalamotomies for intractable pain have yielded information on the role of thalamic nuclei with respect to touch, temperature and pain. In reviewing the work of Mark and his colleagues (1960), Sternbach (1968) has identified three syndromes resulting from destruction of different thalamic nuclei: (1) A loss of sensitivity to touch, temperature and pin-prick, without relief of chronic pain, from lesions in nucleus ventralis posteromedialis (one of the specific relay nuclei); (2) complete pain relief without other sensory loss from lesions in the nonspecific parafascicular and intralaminar nuclei; and (3) slight diminution of pain, with great increase in euphoria, from destruction of dorsal, medial and anterior thalamic nuclei. The last syndrome causes the patient to ignore external stimuli. These findings indicate that pain can be manipulated independently of touch and temperature and that pain does not always arise from excessive stimulation of touch and temperature systems. The "double pain" theory also receives support: in the first syndrome, patients became insensitive to pin-prick but continued to feel clinically significant pain. Fast, pricking pain, originating in the skin, is believed to be mediated by the classic spinothalamocortical pain system, while persistent deep pain involves the nonspecific parafascicular and intralaminar nuclei of the spinoreticulothalamic system.

Little is known about cortical representation of pain in man, even though the classic spinothalamocortical system projects directly and with good somatotopical organization to the sensory cortex from the specific relay nuclei in the thalamus. Electrical stimulation of this parietal cortex has occasionally produced pain, but usually produces only nonpainful tactile sensations. Localized extirpation of parietal cortex produces little, if any, reduction in peripheral sensitivity to pain. Unlike the other senses which, in humans, require intact cortex for proper functioning, sensitivity to significant pathological pain requires neural integrity only to the thalamus, even though the spinoreticulothalamic system does project diffusely to the cortex. Some patients with parietal lesions show analgesia or hypoalgesia and occasionally atypical pain sensations of central origin. Removal of an entire cerebral hemisphere does produce bilateral sensory deficit in pain, but some contralateral pain perception may still be spared, in spite of almost complete degeneration of thalamic nuclei involved, suggesting bilateral representation of the diffuse pain system in the cortex, the thalamus, or both.

Removal or isolation of the anterior and orbital parts of the frontal lobes (lobotomy, leucotomy), even though cortical areas not ordinarily regarded as sensory, produces a marked reduction in response to pain. Following the operation, which is done for patients with intractable neoplastic pain, subjects report that they feel the pain but that it does not hurt. Interestingly enough, their pain thresholds may be reduced (King, Clausen and Scarff, 1950). Presumably this means that they detect a high level of sensory input but that it does not have the quality of pain. Because nonspecific thalamic nuclei project to this area, and receive fibers from it and also to and from the limbic system, the operation should produce changes in the functioning of the diffuse spinoreticulothalamic system and thus in the affective component of pain.

Although the details are probably complex and certainly obscure, the neocortex and other cephalic structures (including thalamus, hypothalamus and limbic system) obviously participate in the modification of pain experience in central processing. Further, corticofugal fibers reach thalamic nuclei and subthalamic relay stations right down to the level of the first synapse in the afferent pathways and, as newer theories of pain suggest, may actually modify the afferent input to the system. The involvement of higher centers suggests ways in which experience, attention, input from other senses and, perhaps, hypnotic suggestion could modify the pain experience through central processing mechanisms.

The structural and functional details of the pain transmission system bring out three points of importance in the management of pain: (1) Overlapping innervation and multiple pathways that are widely distributed, both unilaterally and bilaterally, appear at every level of the nervous system from the receptor to the brain. (2) There are substantial individual differences in the details of anatomical distribution of pain pathways. The same operative procedure may not yield similar results in all cases. (3) Recovery of pain sensation following destruction of primary, classic pain pathways (e.g., in the spinothalamocortical system) can and does occur. Lesions which permanently destroy the original pain pathway do not always insure lasting relief. Even two or more years after surgery, secondary pathways can develop (presumably involving the diffuse spinoreticulothalamic system) and begin to transmit pain and other sensations. In view of these complexities, a patient with intractable pain that has not been relieved by operative treatment may have a legitimate basis for his complaint. Certainly the complaint should not be considered psychogenic without careful investigation.

MODULATION OF PAIN BY SENSORY INPUT AND AROUSAL

A full appreciation of new developments in the theory of pain perception (e.g., the "gate" theory of Melzack and Wall, 1965, 1968) requires prior discussion of the modulation of pain by sensory input and arousal and of the phenomena of paradoxical pain (e.g., causalgia, phantom limb).

It is common knowledge, as indicated earlier, that injuries sustained during strenuous physical activity may go unnoticed at the time or be perceived as not especially painful. The power of counter-irritant or masking stimuli to relieve pain seems firmly implanted in folk medicine; it appears, for example, in the human tendency to grasp firmly an area adjacent to a limb injury and has received some validation in laboratory studies. Apparently, however, the mechanisms by which pain attenuation is produced can be quite varied. For example, direct application of heat sometimes raises thresholds for pain as a consequence of vasodilatation, but vasodilatation also sometimes lowers these thresholds. Similarly, different degrees of cooling may alter thresholds by changing blood supply and by altering the activity of receptors. Furthermore, continuous stimulation can produce adaptation. Such effects could be largely local.

Wall and Sweet (1967) found that electrical stimulation of large diameter sensory (A) fibers relieved chronic pain resulting from peripheral nerve damage. The relief persisted for a long period after termination of the stimulating current. Distraction and suggestion were ruled out because stimulation of neighboring nerves and dorsal roots had no effect on the pain. Blitz and Dinnerstein (1968a) found that contralateral cold stimulation raised pain threshold. Wall and Sweet interpreted these findings as indicating that activity of the large fibers (which presumably mediated touch, temperature and other stimuli) inhibited activity of the pain pathways. These effects would appear to have involved segmental mechanisms in the spinal cord.

Gardner, Licklider and Weisz (1960) reported that high intensity sound (white noise) effectively reduced pain in routine dental operations, presumably because the noise input produced inhibition of pain pathways. Camp, Martin and Chapman (1962), however, were unable to replicate this finding experimentally, using electrical stimulation of tooth pulp. The modulation of pain by sound through direct inhibitory mechanisms thus would appear to be small, if it exists at all.

This is not to imply, however, that loud noise has no effect on the complaint or experience of pain. Green (1962), using a continuous (von Bekesy) procedure for determining threshold for cutaneous electrical pain, found that a multimodal sensory barrage increased pain threshold in a majority of his subjects. The barrage included white noise, flashing light and vibration of the subject's chair, and could be graded in composition and intensity. On balance, he interpreted his data as indicating that the effect on threshold represented distraction and redirection of attention rather than direct intermodular neural inhibition. Attention, its direction and redirection, involves neural interaction, of course, and selective, inhibitory and facilitory functions. This interpretation only suggests that crucial interactions in the nervous system took place at levels higher than those of the primary sensory inputs.

Here it should be stressed that the Gardner et al. (1960) procedure applies to a primarily clinical situation: real discomfort that had to be endured could be anticipated. This made it a better situation than a primarily experimental setting for demonstrating analgesic effects. In the clinical situation, loud noise or music can mask the sound of the drill which, to many people, is unpleasant itself and a harbinger of pain (a conditioned stimulus for pain responses). Also, commercial models of the apparatus give the subject control of the volume so it can be increased in moments of expected crisis. In addition to powerful expectancy or placebo effects introduced by the very reliance on a sound apparatus by a practicing dentist, such anticipatory control over the situation, however illusory, has been shown to raise pain thresholds (Jones, Bentler and Petry, 1966). (It is interesting to note in this connection that some dentists have found that patients derive comfort from having control of an over-ride switch that turns off the drill, even though they do not use it often.) Psychic factors, which are difficult to localize neurophysiologically, are almost impossible to eliminate completely in pain perception.

Arousal and stress can influence central processing of pain in other ways. A number of physiological changes in arousal prepare and sustain an individual during great physical exertion. Increases in secretion of epinephrine and changes in the blood supply to viscera and superficial tissues can play a role in the reduction of pain. More prolonged arousal, producing a stress reaction, mobilizes a defense system that involves the pituitary-adrenal axis, with release of ACTH stimulating production of hydrocortisone. Henkin (1971) showed that excess adrenal cortical secretion dulls taste, hearing and proprioception. Such neurohumoral changes in aroused and stressed individuals may similarly influence pain perception, though they have received far less attention than neural processes.

PARADOXICAL PAIN AND CENTRAL PAIN

The amount of pain experienced in certain syndromes, such as causalgia, phantom limb or central pain, is paradoxical in that it is out of all proportion to the apparent quantity or quality of sensory input. This disproportion poses problems for any approach that views pain as a simple sensory modality. It also poses problems for those who suffer from the disabilities as well as those who attempt to treat them.

Causalgia is characterized by intense and continuous pain that the patient may describe as burning. It is an occasional sequel to peripheral nerve injury. In an attack there may be vasomotor changes, profuse sweating and the skin of the affected limb may become smooth and glossy. An attack may arise spontaneously, or in response to weak peripheral touch stimulation or even as a result of emotional stress. The symptom of dysthesia—a lowered threshold to pain accompanied by an elevated threshold to touch—is of particular interest. Dysthesias in causalgia led Noordenbos (1959) to suggest that the disorder was caused by damage to the relatively faster conducting myelinated A fibers, leading to an imbalance in the ratio between fast A and slow C fiber inputs. The finding that electrical stimulation through the intact skin (which stimulated peripheral nerves) stops causalgic pain for a while supports this hypothesis. Also, cool, moist wrappings of the affected limb relieve causalgia, presumably by increasing the amount of A fiber input.

Postherpetic neuralgia may occur subsequent to herpes zoster, an infectious disease characterized by inflammation of dorsal root or cranial nerve ganglia and the distal portion of the nerves. The spontaneously occurring pain is intense and may be accompanied by unbearable itching. Though the affected area shows decreased sensitivity to non-noxious touch and temperature stimulation, repeated mild stimulation of the area (a trigger zone) can evoke an excruciating attack after a brief delay. The condition may last for years and resist all forms of therapy, including procaine block, nerve, dorsal root or ganglion resection or excision of sensory cortex. As in causalgia, the increased threshold for weak stimuli suggests that reduction in the fast A fiber population plays an important part in producing a predilection to spontaneous or easily evoked paroxysmal pain. In this connection Kerr and Miller (1966) have demonstrated degeneration in the largest myelinated fibers in the trigeminal ganglia of patients with trigeminal neuralgia.

Most recent amputees have a complex of sensations patterned in a way that makes them feel as if they still had a limb of normal size, shape and movement. Usually this phantom limb eventually disappears, but in some 4 or 5 per cent of cases, persistent and severe pain is reported in the phantom. Neuromas frequently develop at the end of the severed nerves at the amputation site, and these can be stimulated accidentally. Neurosurgery or local anesthetic injected at the site can eliminate this peripheral source of pain, though often only temporarily. Campbell (1966), however, has successfully treated phantom limb pain by encasing, in a special way, the stumps of nerves that have developed neuromas.

The patients who are not improved by surgery pose a problem, however. What is the source of the spontaneously recurring pain? Even dorsal root resections that remove all pain sensibility from the stump itself may not eliminate the phantom limb pain. Kolb (1954), discussing the problem from the point of view of central and peripheral mechanisms, demonstrated that psychotherapy was of value for certain patients. On the other hand, Noordenbos (1959) believes that the phantom limb sensations result from faulty or distorted information from the periphery: there is a lack of fast A fiber input from the stump, as the fibers that do regenerate tend to be the small, slow C fibers. If this interpretation is correct, mild exercise of the stump, which would increase afferent input of the fast fiber type, should reduce phantom limb pain. Melzack (1970) has reported precisely this result.

Central pain, which is recurring and excruciating, may be caused by vascular, traumatic or degenerative lesions at any level of the neuraxis, but it occurs more frequently with thalamic and mesencephalic lesions than with lesions at lower levels. Cassinari and Pagni (1969) concluded that isolated lesions of the spinoreticulothalamic system, the multisynaptic, phylogenetically old system organized for diffuse transmission, do not seem sufficient to produce true central pain. Rather, it appears to arise from lesions of the spinothalamocortical fibers, the "paucisynaptic" sensory-discriminative pain system which is phylogenetically new and somatotopically organized. Pure lesions of the lemniscal fibers of the epicritic system (subserving localizing non-noxious touch and temperature sensibility), however, produce only paresthesias, not pain. This suggests that a "paucisynaptic" pain system, but not the epicritic system (possibly large A fibers), modulates the activity of the old, diffuse multisynaptic pain system, a view that seems partly at variance with the views of Noordenbos and of Melzack.

Thus, paradoxical pain is characterized not only by pain that is out of all proportion to the discernible stimulus, but also by the following: (1) Gentle touch may produce extreme pain, yet additional stimulation sometimes will relieve it. (2) The pain response may be delayed and may persist long after stimulation has ceased. (3) Touch stimulation at superficial sites far removed from the pathologic tissue may trigger an attack (hence, "trigger zones"). (4) Surgical lesions of the pain pathways frequently fail to produce lasting relief, and sometimes offer little or no relief.

THE GATE CONTROL THEORY OF PAIN

Melzack and Wall (1965, 1968; see also Casey and Melzack, 1967) have proposed a conceptual model that organizes diverse clinical and experimental observations on pain and tactile sensibility into a comprehensive theory.

As in the general view of transmission systems presented earlier, Melzack and Wall also see two afferent transmission systems: the classic neospinalthalamic (i.e., spinothalamocortical) system, somatotopically organized for fast transmission of localizing information, and a phylogenetically older, diffuse paramedial ascending (i.e., spinoreticulothalamic) system having access to the limbic system in the forebrain and implicated in the affective and motivational aspects of pain. The higher centers, not to be confused with "central pain centers" of the old specificity theories, analyze input in terms of information (epicritic, spatial and temporal summation, and intensity), and through efferent connections generate motor and other responses and influence each other. More important, efferents from higher centers (the central control) descend to modulate the activity of lower levels of the neuraxis and, particularly, modulate the transmission characteristics of the spinal receptive fields in the substantia gelatinosa and dorsal horn of the cord at the level of primary sensory input as a part of the "gate control" system in the spinal cord. Here, the gate modulates the amount of input transmitted from peripheral afferent fibers through the dorsal horn transmission (or T) cells to the ascending fibers in the cord, and thus to higher levels of the neuraxis. The number of impulses transmitted per unit of time by the T cells is determined by the ratio of large and small fiber inputs, by their intensity and by efferent impulses descending from higher central control activities in the brain. The output of the T cells is monitored centrally and integrated over time; when it reaches or exceeds a critical intensity, it triggers an action system consisting of those neural mechanisms responsible for the complex motoric and experiential affective reactions characteristic of pain.

According to the gate control theory, cells and fibers in the substantia gelatinosa modulate the synaptic transmission of afferent nerve impulses from the periphery before these signals affect the first transmission, or T cells, in the dorsal horn. The control is probably presynaptic on the afferent fiber terminals and determines the excitation transmitted to the thalamus. Inputs to the cells of the substantia gelatinosa and T cells arrive from the periphery over large and small fibers. The relative balance between these inputs is considered to be critical for pain perception. In the absence of stimulation, the large myelinated fibers are quiet, while the small myelinated and unmyelinated fibers are spontaneously active, constantly bombarding cells in the substantia gelatinosa and causing the gate to be held in a relatively open position. Mild sensory stimulation activates the epicritic system, the large myelinated sensory fibers subserving nonpainful tactile stimuli. This activation alters the ratio of large to small fiber activity, causing the gate to close partially, and decreasing the activity of the T cells. As these large fibers tend to adapt quickly, their input to the gate soon decreases. The proportional or relative contribution to input by the small fibers increases, opening the gate, and in the event of noxious stimulation, the output of T cells rises and pain may be perceived. If, however, the subject rubs his skin or otherwise increases large fiber activity at that spinal level, the gate closes and pain diminishes, as T cell activity decreases as a result of the closing of the gate.

The central control mechanism, as indicated above, influences the gate control system through efferent fibers descending to spinal levels and entering the substantia gelatinosa where they join in the modulation of sensory input. This central control is postulated to explain alterations of pain through attention, learning, expectancy and other complex psychological processes. The activation of descending efferent fibers by stimulation of the brain experimentally suggests that such a mechanism is possible; and from the work of Henkin, cited earlier, it seems that a general hormonal action on the gate is a distinct, though as yet unexplored, possibility.

According to the gate theory, then, the perception of pain depends upon (1) the balance between large and small fiber inputs and (2) upon the modulating functions of the central control mechanism. In relation to the pain paradoxes discussed earlier, a decrease in large-fiber input, with small-fiber input maintained, would open the gate, creating hyperalgesia but higher thresholds for touch and temperature. Because normal presynaptic inhibition by the gate control system would be reduced, even non-noxious stimuli could trigger central T cells transmitting pain (as in causalgia, neuralgia, and phantom limb pain). As the smaller fibers show a relatively higher spontaneous level of activity in the absence of external stimulation, the loss of A fibers and the operation of the gate could explain spontaneous pain attacks. On the other hand, if the A fiber system is relatively intact, non-noxious epicritic sensory input could serve to close the gate and relieve pain. Thus, gentle tapping of the stump sometimes relieves phantom limb pain, and mild electrical stimulation, to which larger fibers have a lower threshold, may reduce causalgic pain.

The central control mechanism, as it influences the gate by a tonic input from higher levels, could produce centrally controlled inhibitions or closings of the gate that could account for the poor correlation often found between amount of tissue damage and severity of reported pain. Thus, central processing variables such as past experience, selective attention, level of arousal and activity, and emotion could act to alter the openness of the gate, and thus the pain experience. Nevertheless, the effectiveness of these psychological factors depends in part upon the sensory input, particularly the fast, discriminatory inputs carried up through the dorsal and dorsolateral fasciculi of the cord. If these epicritic systems are damaged, or if the pain rises very rapidly (as in colic or cardiac pain), central inhibition of the gate (closing it) might not occur rapidly enough to block the pain experience. Probably then, the more gradually rising pain inputs are easier to manage by conscious, psychological maneuvers.

Also, the central control mechanisms can be highly specific. For example, Beecher (1959) has described how men wounded at the Anzio beach head complained of little pain from the wounds but complained bitterly about inept venous punctures. Thus, the general excitement of the situation and the relief of escaping from battle with a "good" wound did not make them generally anesthetic; rather the perception of pain was highly selective. Similarly, dogs that repeatedly receive food (as an unconditioned stimulus) immediately after shock or burn (as a conditioned stimulus) soon stop reacting in the usual way to these noxious stimuli and begin salivating when they occur. Very small changes in the locus and character of the noxious stimulation, however, produce the usual vocalizations, arousal and attempts to escape, replacing the previously conditioned salivation (Pavlov, 1927). In this connection, it is important to note that the theory specifically suggests that the organized perceptual response of the whole organism can be actually blocked or attenuated (the subject does not experience pain) by the central control mechanism as it "reaches down to close the gate." This is somewhat different from other approaches that involve a psychological loop, in which the pain sensation may be initially perceived, only to be offset in some way subsequently by higher mental processes and reactions (e.g., Beecher's reaction component).

The Melzack-Wall theory has important therapeutic implications, related to the control of pain (1) by increasing input from large A fibers, (2) favoring this increase and also mobilizing central control mechanisms through specific training. Thus, hydrotherapy, massage and manipulation should decrease pain, provided the proper level of sensory input is achieved. Similarly, exercise, if persistent, in the face of pain should eventually dampen the pain experience itself. Two somewhat different possibilities emerge here. In the first, the patient may have to be effectively encouraged to attempt and maintain initially painful exercises that are therapeutically important. Operant conditioning techniques will be helpful here (Reynolds, 1968; Schaefer and Martin, 1969) largely because they provide for control of behavior through manipulation of its consequences. Specific tasks and goals can be set, and the patient deliberately rewarded by concrete information concerning his progress and by other social reinforcers such as praise, appreciation and attention. (Often in busy rehabilitation centers, patient motivation is poor, and such behavior—maintaining feedback and attention is left to chance, with reliance placed largely on occasional exhortation.) Also, visual and auditory displays should be available to provide the feedback necessary to allow the patient to control his behavior and, thus, his experienced pain.

To produce the largest and most durable behavioral changes, reinforcements should be carefully scheduled: at first, they should be given for each effort, but later on an intermittent schedule based on the satisfaction of specified work or output requirements. Such "ratio schedules" generate high work outputs in animals and man (as in piecework in a factory); they are most effective if the amount of work required for each reward varies randomly or irregularly around some suitable average value. These "random ratio schedules" resemble the pay-off schedules gamblers encounter in slot machines or in the casino; they effectively maintain stable, high outputs of behavior in the face of irregular and infrequent reward. Also, they create behavior that is resistant to extinction through nonreward.

Once the patient begins effective exercise, other conditioning may take place very much as with the dogs Pavlov shocked and then fed. Some pain and discomfort will become an indicator that the performance has been adequate and qualifies as "good" or "sufficient." By association of the discomfort with the reward, central control mechanisms may develop (if Melzack and Wall are correct), and the subjective distress will be progressively and ultimately reduced as it comes to signify that an endpoint has been achieved. Long distance runners learn to exert themselves "until it hurts" as an indicator that they have done enough for the day's training. As training progresses, not only the amount they can do increases, but the discomfort of the "hurt," as endpoint, decreases, even though the runners retain the ability to discriminate what amounts to a proper amount of training.

Just as psychiatric patients have been returned to their homes after being taught to modify their psychotic behavior, there is no reason that beneficial behaviors such as dieting and exercise cannot be induced by behavioral methods in rehabilitation medicine (see Wilson, 1950).

Additional Psychosocial Determinants of Pain

The efferent central control mechanism of Melzack and Wall suggests how the activity of higher centers can bear upon the pain process at the level of primary sensory input. It is helpful to know that such a mechanism could exist and that all psychic modulation of pain need not be confined exclusively to intracortical or even intracerebral neurophysiological transactions. We derive little understanding from that schema, however, as to the extent and manner in which psychic or behavioral factors influence pain experience and report. At the present time, that can be handled best within the metaphor of the psycho-social sciences. In this section we will discuss those additional aspects of psychic and experiential contributions to pain perception not covered in the introduction, the section on definition or elsewhere.

Adequate pain perception and response ordinarily develop under normal rearing conditions in animals (and probably man) without any specially directed training. Normal life experience, however, appears to be necessary for the development of normal responsivity to pain. Dogs raised from infancy under isolation conditions that deprived them of normal sensory experience showed atypical responses to noxious stimulation at maturity (Melzack and Scott, 1957). These dogs failed to respond appropriately when stepped on. They repeatedly poked their noses into a flame, showing curiosity rather than pain. They also endured pin-pricks with little evidence of pain other than reflex movements, but electric shock and complex audiovisual inputs evoked violent excitement. These findings suggested that sensory input was not blocked, at least not completely, at the periphery as it might have been had deprivation prevented development of receptors; but they also suggest that perceptual learning is necessary for the development of adequate and normal response to pain.

Conditioned and cognitive factors strongly influence pain tolerance. Kanfer and Goldfoot (1966) found that instructions and direction of attention modified the length of time subjects would endure a cold-pressor test. Members of a group forced to focus upon the pain sensation by being required to report on it were least tolerant, while those told to expect severe pain were more tolerant; a control group remained in between these levels of tolerance. The two most tolerant groups were (1) one that viewed and described projected slides during the test (distraction) and (2) one that watched a clock with the goal of setting high tolerance standards (control over pain).

Other experiments suggest that human subjects will seek information about intensity and timing of forthcoming unavoidable electric stimulation (Jones, Bentler and Petry, 1966). Here reduction of uncertainty about coming stimulation reduced anxiety, provided that a basis for cognitive control ("I can relax for another minute") was available, giving the subject time to elaborate some preparatory motor response (clenching the fist, for example) that could generate proprioceptive input to compete with the noxious stimulus.

There is evidence that warning signals and the opportunity to make preparatory responses for receiving shock reduce the noxiousness of that stimulus in both humans (Lykken, 1959) and rats (Lykken, 1962). The noxiousness or aversiveness of the warning signal, and the disturbance it produces, however, may be greater than the disturbance produced by the shock itself. Hare et al. (1966) have reported that human subjects tend to choose to take shock sooner rather than later, whether it is heavy or light, certain (given 100 per cent of the trials) or uncertain (50 per cent of the trials). And in rats, Gibbon (1967) has found that subjects will press a lever and take an immediate shock in order to get rid of a signal that warns that that very shock is coming eventually and unavoidably.

In a complex experiment, Nesbitt and Schachter (1966) gave subjects a pill (actually a placebo) that was supposed to be a new drug being tested for its effect on skin sensitivity. Half of the subjects were told that the pill would produce side-effects (resembling emotional arousal) such as tremor, palpitation, and so on; the other half were told to expect quite irrelevant side effects (not related to arousal). (Ostensibly the experiment was supposed to determine proper shock intensities for electroconvulsive shock therapy.) Then, all were tested for detection and pain thresholds for cutaneous shock and finally for tolerance to suprathreshold shocks ("The shock's too painful to endure." "Stop!"). Though both groups showed similar detection and pain thresholds, the group expecting arousal side effects showed much higher tolerance than the other group. Subjects believing themselves to be aroused by the pill not only failed to attribute their real arousal symptoms (produced by shock) to the shocks, but also found shock less painful and were willing to take stronger shocks. These findings indicate that cognitive labeling of experience can significantly influence its perceived noxiousness.

Ethnocultural factors influence not only experimental pain thresholds, but also the ways in which the subject labels, perceives and responds to his pain. This can be a serious complication in clinical work and is an important factor in assessing reported symptomatic discomfort in different ethnocultural groups (Kolb, 1962). Pain thresholds have been reported as higher among northern Europeans than among Mediterranean people and Negroes. "Irish Catholics" and "Yankee Protestants" have been reported to have higher thresholds than Italians and Jews. For almost every study that reports a difference due to ethnocultural factors, however, another disagrees. Wolff and Langley (1968) list a number of studies suggesting that attitudinal factors do influence response to pain among ethnocultural groups. For example, minority groups who were informed that they were unable to stand pain, as compared with some majority group, increased their tolerance to noxious stimulation significantly. Also, if the experimenter came from a different ethnic group than the subjects, they tended to withstand higher intensities of noxious stimulation before reporting pain.

Similarly, biological variables such as age and sex have been considered to affect pain perception, but again the literature is confusing. Some workers find that pain thresholds increase with age; others do not. Some find women more sensitive to experimental pain than men, in spite of folklore to the contrary with respect to pathological pain; others do not.

A large number of studies have explored the effect of anxiety produced by such things as threat of shock, an impersonal and rigid experimenter, unfamiliar apparatus, inability to control or anticipate intensity and time of occurrence of shock. Generally such anxiety (as well as the anxiety found among some types of psychiatric patients) tends to produce lower thresholds for experimental pain. And there is some evidence that persons tending to be extroverted and scoring high on a "psychopathic" personality index have higher thresholds to experimental pain.

The comparatively small differences in threshold found with personality type and anxiety, ethnocultural and religious differences and biological variables of age and sex suggest that these factors influence a subject's criterion or response bias rather than his sensory sensitivity to pain. Most of the experimental studies covered in this chapter employed traditional psychophysical methods rather than signal detection methods that distinguish between these two aspects of threshold determination. The work of Clark and Mehl (1971), mentioned earlier, showed that the increase in threshold among older people reflected differences in criterion for pain or report bias but no difference in sensory sensitivity. In this connection, the strongest verbal, autonomic and skeletal response of pain ever emitted by one of the writers occurred when the radiant heat stimulus was misdirected at the wall instead of his arm; instead of the expected pain, there was a bright flash of light. The result was an extreme "pain" response, after which he was forced to admit that absolutely no pain had been experienced. Until much of the work on pain thresholds among various groups and under various conditions is repeated using signal detection – sensory decision theory techniques – we cannot even hope to expect unambiguous results or clarification of the present confusing situation.

Even then, there remain problems in method that can lead to error. For example, Hall and Stride (1954) found that subjects who were not told they were in a pain experiment had radiant heat pain thresholds averaging 89 mcal per sec per cm^2 higher than informed subjects. Blitz and Dinnerstein (1968b) raised both threshold and tolerance to pain by appropriate instructions. In Clark's own work, using the new methods, he has produced a 40 mcal per sec per cm^2 rise in threshold merely by elevating the range of stimulus intensities used. Apparently when subjects know that they are involved in a pain experiment, they assume they must emit some "pain" responses. If the experimenter uses only a range of low intensities, the subject will deliver his pain responses to some of those low intensities rather than withhold them altogether. Some sort of psychophysical anchor effect, determined by the spectrum of intensities that the trials sample in a session, may be involved with the subject's standards. If the experimenter uses a range of high intensities, the subject tends to reserve pain responses for the highest intensities in this higher range, thus raising the threshold. Such factors influence subject expectation and illustrate the operation of the effects of demand variables implicit in the situation (i.e., "It is a pain experiment, so some but not all stimuli should be painful.").

Effects of Placebo and Hypnosis

Suggestion, particularly if supported by a placebo or a procedure that operates as one (e.g., an ineffective but established and respectable medication or treatment), exerts powerful effects on the patient's behavior. Placebos, in the form of inert substances properly packaged, often have startling effects, many of which are described by Hass, Fink and Härtfelder (1959). This review indicates that, besides apparently relieving symptoms of clearly organic disorders such as infections, placebos have been reported to produce side effects including observable physiological responses (e.g., rashes and changes in corticosteroid levels). Placebo effects introduce serious bias into clinical drug trials

(Wilson, 1962); and their elimination requires special care if correct primary analgesic potency is to be determined for a particular substance. Beecher (1955, 1959) reviewed studies of patients suffering severe pathological pain and found that approximately 70 per cent of the patients obtained relief with 10 mg of morphine. Thirty-five per cent however, received satisfactory relief from placebos!

Placebo responses apparently involve a wide variety of psychological factors—the personality of the physician and the patient, their motivations, expectations and anxieties—yet no clear, fixed personality type appears to characterize the placebo reactor who shows these effects. Religious, ethnocultural and socioeconomic factors appear to play significant roles, along with prior experience with other physicians. As with hypnosis, the mechanism of the placebo response is unclear, but shift of attention, reduction of anxiety and the necessity of coping with difficult personal situations can play significant parts; response or reporting bias no doubt plays a role, as in Clark's study (1969) of placebo effects on pain threshold. In addition, the patient has been conditioned by previous experience with medication and physicians to expect relief; treatment in some ways could act as a conditioned stimulus that might even evoke a physiological response. Assuming the validity of Melzack and Wall's central control mechanism, the quality of sensory input entering the transmission systems of the spinal cord and brain might even be altered as a basis for the reported subjective relief that is found in the placebo response. Finally, because placebo responses tend to be found much more often in clinical than in experimental pain situations, the motivational and affective aspects of the total situation almost certainly are vital components.

A reaction this powerful deserves more careful study than it has received. Much effort has been devoted to controlling it as an artifact which interferes with more important determinations. Perhaps the trend should be reversed and a greater effort made to learn more about its mode of action. A skeptic viewing contemporary research in hypnosis might argue that this is precisely what is going on in that area. Such a view, however, really does not do full justice to either topic.

Hypnosis and suggestion, with or without administration of formal placebos, clearly alters pain-related behavior in a significant proportion of patients: reports of pain decrease, autonomic indicators change and requests for analgesics decline. Such phenomena pose serious problems for those who view pain as a simple function of amount and kind of sensory input, in accordance with specificity theory. Indeed, they pose problems for those who view pain thoughtfully in any way at all! Hypnosis is less an answer to how pain perception works than a series of unanswered questions about a way of investigating the problem.

Reports of psychological relief of pain go back to antiquity, but careful, clinical accounts were not really widely available before the middle of the nineteenth century when Esdaile reported on the use of mesmerism as an anesthetic in his surgical practice in India. No one who reads his account can doubt his sincerity, care in observation and the startling (for the time) nature of the phenomena he reported, however dated his explanations. He assumed, however, as do a substantial number of contemporary workers, that the behavioral effects produced by hypnotic analgesia (in his case anesthesia) reflected decreases in subjectively experienced pain. Conclusive evidence on this point is difficult to obtain, perhaps, impossible by its very nature. More likely, the question is really meaningless and reflects metaphorical traps the "modern" thinker easily falls into as he struggles with the old mind-body problem. A more scientific approach conducts a functional analysis of the problem, seeking to determine what procedures, hypnotic and other, produce what aspects of the phenomena—which are necessary, which are sufficient, which are irrelevant and which phenomena are important in producing effective analgesia. (For example, the characteristics of the "trance" itself have changed drastically from the dramatic productions presided over by Mesmer, through the rigid posture and motoric activity considered necessary in the days of Esdaile and Charcot, to the staid and undramatic behavioral situation characterizing experimental and medical hypnosis today. What part of the present spectrum of behavior we call the trance is really necessary?)

Investigators differ widely concerning the essential nature of hypnosis (see Shor and Orne, 1965). Sarbin and Anderson (1964) feel that the hypnotized person is unconsciously enacting the role expected of a hypnotized person. Barber and Hahn (1962) and Barber (1963) take the extreme view that all of the hypnotic phenomena can be found in the performance of unhypnotized subjects given similar, but forceful, task-motivating instructions. Barber suggests that the hypnotic trance may be extraneous and unnecessary in ameliorating pain in situations described as hypnotic; the important things are suggestions of pain relief given in a close interpersonal setting. Much of the relief, he feels, is superficial and consists largely of an unwillingness to admit that pain had been experienced. London and Fuhrer (1961) have also reported remarkable instructional effects among nonhypnotized subjects.

Orne (1959) takes a more moderate view. He has investigated in great detail the ways in which hypnotized subjects may be distinguished objectively from simulating unhypnotized subjects. (For his most explicit discussion of simulation controls, see O'Connell, Shor and Orne, 1970.) The hypnotized subject will tolerate perceptual inconsistencies; for example, he readily reports and is unconcerned when a person he has hallucinated in one part of the room simultaneously appears elsewhere in the flesh. The hypnotized subject will report both the image and the real person, but the simulator reports only one. Hypnotized subjects (in accordance with contemporary fashions in trance behavior) do differ from nonhypnotized subjects: they appear to lack internal, spontaneous motivation; are relatively immobile; and have a narrow focus of attention.

Much of the controversy, including failure of investigators to replicate each other's work in different laboratories, arises from the fact that subjects differ widely in susceptibility to hypnosis. Though there are standardized scales for depth of trance, which hopefully permit accurate control of this variable in replications and experimental comparison, these may measure only coarsely obscure aspects of the trance that are critical to producing certain kinds of effects (e.g., amount of fantasy as discussed by Spanos, 1971). Finally, laboratories and workers may differ in subtle but important ways with respect to expectations, implicit definitions of appropriate performance and care in considering and properly engineering the entire social context of the experiment to produce maximum effects. For example, Fisher (1954) has reported how the appearance or nonappearance of a posthypnotic suggestion in a subject's behavior could be determined by implicit and indirect social cues which indicate whether the experiment was finished or not. Hypnotic subjects are actually alert, literal and very sensitive to such subtleties. Also, they can reliably report and discriminate presence and depth of trance (Hilgard, 1965).

There are many well-documented studies of the efficacy of hypnotic analgesia in pathological pain in which verbal report, motoric activity and physiological indicators suggest reduction or relief of pain. Definitive studies of hypnotically induced reduction in experimental pain are much rarer. A recent study by McGlashan, Evans and Orne (1969) is worth examining in detail, particularly because it demonstrates the attention to experimental control and scientific objectivity now to be found in the best experiments in this area. Subjects who were highly susceptible to hypnosis (by clinical tests and objective ratings) and subjects who were extremely resistant performed a motor task that produced ischemic pain under three conditions: control, analgesic-hypnosis and a placebo condition. The pain threshold of nonsusceptible subjects increased during analgesic hypnosis, but this rise was no greater than under the placebo condition. On the other hand, the susceptible subjects, particularly those convinced of the "reality" of the analgesia, showed a much greater rise under the analgesic-hypnosis condition, a rise significantly greater than under the placebo condition. The authors concluded that hypnotic analgesia had two components. One is essentially a response to instructions of the experimenter, a response to demand characteristics of the situation and which is common to all experiments, whether hypnosis is involved or not. The other component may be regarded as a distortion of perception induced during deep hypnosis, a true analgesia.

Though verbal and motor reactions and perception of experimental pain may be altered by hypnotic analgesia, what about effects on objective physiological indicators of pain such as blood pressure? Hilgard et al. (1967) initiated a program of experiments on hypnotic analgesia, one study of which (Sachs, 1970) investigated that very problem. In this study cold-pressor ischemia served as the pain source; subjective ratings during the session (pain-state reports) and blood pressure recordings, both obtained every five seconds, indexed the subject's reaction. After special training in developing hypnotic analgesia, all subjects were hypnotized and exposed to the ischemia, some first under hypnotic analgesia and later under relaxation suggestions, and the remaining subjects in the reverse order. Under analgesia, pain-state reports all stayed at zero, indicating no subjective experience of pain under both the lowest and highest blood pressure conditions, but blood pressure showed some progressive elevation as a function of the time the subject's arm was in ice water. Although the analgesic condition produced far greater effect on pain report than on blood pressure, each subject's blood pressure scores were lower under analgesia than under relaxation. In relaxation, the pain-state reports and blood pressure readings showed a respectable correlation. Hypnotic analgesia effectively dissociated those two indicators.

One might wonder which indicator was the more valid. Hilgard (1969), however, has found that the pain-state report under waking conditions is capable of discriminating finer differences in stimulus conditions, is more reliable on repeated measurement under the same conditions and is more regularly and lawfully related to changes in stimulus conditions than any of the physiological indicators of pain. Thus, the credentials of the pain-state report are superior to those of the physiological indicators, by ordinary standards under ordinary circumstances. With this in mind, does it make better sense to ask "Did the pressor test 'really hurt' during analgesia?" or to ask "How does one alter each of the various aspects of the pain response most effectively, and which alterations are of greatest advantage to the subject?"

The mechanisms that produce hypnotic analgesia are unknown, although the attentional focus on the hypnotist instead of the subject's body and the tolerance for perceptual inconsistencies are probably important. Perhaps re-labeling of sensation (Nesbitt and Schacter, 1966) contributes. Changes in states of consciousness without formal hypnosis are frequently reported, particularly under conditions of strong emotional pressure. Effective autosuggestion and informal, partial autohypnosis may be much more frequent than we realize. Occasionally, sophisticated observers report dramatic instances of deliberately induced analgesia without hypnosis in any formal sense. For example, Reis (1966) reported her own experiences in undergoing major surgery with neither formally induced hypnosis nor chemical anesthesia. As an operating room nurse, she had observed both hypnotic and chemical anesthesia. When she required surgery herself, she decided that there was no reason why she could not manage the problem of operative pain by autosuggestion. She did so, required no physical restraints on the operating table and experienced only slight cutaneous sensations, but no pain or discomfort.

As a closing comment, we present an interesting case study by Kaplan (1960) which dramatizes the interpretive dilemma in hypnotic analgesia. A highly trained subject was placed in a very deep trance and given two sugges-tions: that his left arm was analgesic and insensitive, and that his right hand would perform automatic writing continuously throughout the experiment. The analgesic left arm was pricked four times with an hypodermic needle; during reception of this stimulus, the subject's right hand wrote, "Ouch, damn it, you're hurting me." A few minutes later, the subject turned to the experi-menter and asked when he was going to begin the experiment, apparently having "forgotten" that he had already received the painful stimuli. Kaplan interpreted these findings as indicating that hypnotic suggestions of analgesia produce artificial repression and denial of pain, but that pain is experienced at "some" level and experienced as discomfort.

Kaplan's interpretation may be entirely correct, although a behaviorist would see it as replacing one unknown with another. The behaviorist, however, has his troubles too. With the idea that overt behavior represents the only dependable scientific data in this field, he would paraphrase the old saying to the effect that: "As a man doeth, so is he." But what was Kaplan's subject "doing"?

REFERENCES

1. Barber, T. X., and Hahn, K. W.: Physiological and subjective responses to pain producing

stimulation under hypnotically suggested and waking-imagined "analgesia." J. Abn. Psychol., 65:411-418, 1962.

2. Barber, T. X.: The effects of hypnosis on pain: A critical review of experimental and clinical findings. Psychosomatic Med., 25:303-333, 1963.

3. Beecher, H. K.: The powerful placebo. J. Amer. Med. Assoc., 159:1602-1606, 1955.

4. Beecher, H. K.: *Measurement of Subjective Responses: Quantitative Effects of Drugs.* New York, Oxford University Press, 1959.

5. Beecher, H. K.: Pain: One mystery solved. Science, 151:840-841, 1966.

6. Beecher, H. K.: The measurement of pain in man: A reinspection of the work of the Harvard group. In: A. Soulairac, J. Cahn, and J. Charpentier (eds.): *Pain*, pp. 201-214. New York, Academic Press, 1968.

7. Blitz, B., and Dinnerstein, A. J.: Pain attenuation by contralateral cold stimulation. Psychonomic Science, 10:395-396, 1968a.

8. Blitz, B., and Dinnerstein, A. J.: Effects of different types of instructions on pain parameters. J. Abn. Psychol., 73:276-280, 1968b.

9. Camp, W., Martin, R., and Chapman, L.: Pain threshold and discrimination of pain intensity during brief exposure to intense noise. Science, 135:788-789, 1962.

10. Campbell, J. B.: Painful phantom limb: Relief through peripheral nerve surgery. In: R. S. Knighton and P. R. Dumke (eds.): *Pain*, pp. 255-271. Boston, Little, Brown, 1966.

11. Casey, K. L., and Melzack, R.: Neural mechanisms of pain: A conceptual model. In: E. L. Way, (ed.): *New Concepts in Pain and Its Clinical Management*, pp. 13-32. Philadelphia, F. A. Davis, 1967.

12. Cassinari, V., and Pagni, C. A.: *Central Pain: A Neurosurgical Survey.* Cambridge, Harvard University Press, 1969.

13. Clark, W. C.: Sensory-decision theory analysis of the placebo effect on the criterion pain and thermal sensitivity (d'). J. Abn. Psychol., 74:363-371, 1969.

14. Clark, W. C., and Mehl, L.: Thermal pain: A sensory decision theory analysis of the effect of age and sex on d', various response criteria, and 50% pain threshold. J. Abn. and Social Psychol., 1971. In press.

15. Esdaile, J.: *Mesmerism in India.* Silas Andrews and Son, Hartford, England, 1847. (Reprinted in part as: Esdaile, J.: *Hypnosis in Medicine and Surgery.* New York, Julian Press, 1957.)

16. Evans, W. O.: A comparison of the analgetic potency of some analgesics as measured by the "flinch-jump" test. Psychopharmacologia, 3:51-54, 1962.

17. Fisher, S.: The role of expectancy in the performance of post-hypnotic behavior. J. Abn. and Soc. Psychol., 49:503-507, 1954.

18. Gardner, W. J., Licklider, J. C. R., and Weisz, A. J.: Suppression of pain by sound. Science, 131:1583-1588, 1960.

19. Gibbon, J.: Discriminated punishment: Avoidable and unavoidable shock. J. Exper. Anal. Behav., 10:451-460, 1967.

20. Green, D. M., and Swets, J. A.: *Signal Detection Theory and Psychophysics.* John Wiley & Sons, New York, 1966.

21. Green, E. E.: A preliminary study of sensory barrage using pain threshold as an indicator. Unpublished Ph.D. dissertation, University of Chicago, 1962.

22. Hall, K. R. L., and Stride, E.: The varying response to pain in psychotic disorders: A study in abnormal psychology. Brit. J. Med. Psychol., 27:48-60, 1954.

23. Hardy, D. J., Wolff, H. G., and Goodell, H.: *Pain Sensations and Reactions.* Baltimore, Williams and Wilkins, 1952.

24. Hare, R. D., Krebs, D. L., Creighton, T. D., and Petrusic, W. M.: Latency of self-administered shock as a function of its intensity and probability. Psychon. Sci., 6:79-80, 1966.

25. Hass, H., Fink, H., and Härtfelder, G.: Das Placeboproblem. Fortschritte der Arzneimittelforschung, 1:279-454, 1959. (Translation of selected parts in Psychopharmacology Service Center Bulletin, 2:1-65, 1963.)

26. Henkin, R. I. The neuroendocrine control of perception. In: D. Hamburg (ed.): *Perception and Its Disorders.* Proceedings of the Association for Research in Nervous and Mental Diseases, pp. 54-107. Baltimore, Williams and Wilkins, 1970.

27. Hilgard, E. R.: *Hypnotic Susceptibility.* New York, Harcourt, Brace and World, 1965.

28. Hilgard, E. R., Cooper, L. M., Lenox, J., Morgan, A. H., and Voevodsky, J.: The use of pain-state reports in the study of hypnotic analgesia to the pain of ice water. J. Nerv. Ment. Dis., 144:506-513, 1967.

29. Hilgard, E. R.: Pain as a puzzle for psychology and physiology. Amer. Psychologist, 24:103-113, 1969.

30. Hill, H. E., Kornetsky, C. H., Flanary, H. G., and Wikler, A.: Effects of anxiety and morphine on discrimination of intensities of pain. J. Clin. Invest., 31:473-480, 1952.

31. Jones, A., Bentler, P. M., and Petry, G.: The reduction of uncertainty concerning future pain. J. Abn. Psychol., *71*:87–94, 1966.
32. Jones, M. H.: Second pain: Fact or artifact? Science, *124*:442–443, 1956.
33. Kanfer, F. H., and Goldfoot, D. A.: Self-control and tolerance of noxious stimulation. Psychological Reports, *18*:79–85, 1966.
34. Kaplan, E. A.: Hypnosis and pain. Arch. Gen. Psychiat., *2*:567–568, 1960.
35. Kenshalo, D. R. (ed.): *The Skin Senses*, pp. 223–260. Springfield, Ill., Charles C Thomas, 1968.
36. Kerr, F. W. L., and Miller, R. H.: The pathology of trigeminal neuralgia. Arch. Neurol., *15*:308–319, 1966.
37. King, H. E., Clausen, J., and Scarff, J. E.: Cutaneous threshold for pain before and after prefrontal lobotomy. J. Nerv. Ment. Dis., *112*:93–96, 1950.
38. Knighton, R. S., and Dumke, P. R.: *Pain*. Boston, Little, Brown, 1966.
39. Kolb, L. C.: *The Painful Phantom: Psychology, Physiology, and Treatment*. Springfield, Ill., Charles C Thomas, 1954.
40. Kolb, L. C.: Symbolic significance of the complaint of pain. In: W. H. Mosberg, (ed.): *Clinical Neurosurgery*, Vol. 8, Baltimore, Williams and Wilkins, 1962.
41. Lim, R. K. S., and Guzman, F.: Manifestations of pain in analgesic evaluations in animals and man. In: A. Soulairac, J. Cahn, and J. Charpentier (eds.): *Pain*. pp. 119–152. New York, Academic Press, 1968.
42. London, P., and Fuhrer, M.: Hypnosis, motivation, and performance. J. Personality, *29*:321–333, 1961.
43. Lykken, D. T.: Preliminary observations on the preception phenomenon. Psychophysiol. Measmt. Newsltr., *5*:2–4, 1959.
44. Lykken, D. T.: Preception in the rat: autonomic response to shock as a function of length of warning signal. Science, *137*:665–666, 1962.
45. Mark, V. H., Ervin, F. R., and Yakovlev, P. I.: The treatment of pain by stereotaxic methods. Confinia Neurologica, *22*:238–245, 1962.
46. McGlashan, T. H., Evans, F. J., and Orne, M. T.: The nature of hypnotic analgesia and placebo responses to experimental pain. Psychosomatic Med., *31*:227–246, 1969.
47. Melzack, R., and Scott, T. H.: The effects of early experience on the response to pain. J. Comp. and Physiol. Psych., *50*:155–161, 1957.
48. Melzack, R., and Wall, P. D.: Pain mechanisms: A new theory. Science, *150*:971–979, 1965.
49. Melzack, R., and Wall, P. D.: Gate control theory of pain. In: A. Soulairac, J. Cahn, and J. Charpentier (eds.): *Pain*, pp. 11–31. New York, Academic Press, 1968.
50. Melzack, R.: Phantom limbs. Psychol. Today, *4*:63–68, 1970.
51. Merskey, H., and Spear, F. G.: *Pain: Psychological and Psychiatric Aspects*. London, Bailliere, Tindall, and Cassell, 1967.
52. Miller, N. E.: Learning of visceral and glandular responses. Science, *163*:434–445, 1969.
53. Nesbitt, R. E., and Schachter, S.: Cognitive manipulation of pain. J. Exper. Social Psychol., *2*:227–236, 1966.
54. Noordenbos, W.: *Pain*. New York, Elsevier Pub. Co., 1959.
55. O'Connell, D. N., Shor, R. E., and Orne, M. T.: Hypnotic age regression: an empirical and methodological analysis. J. Abn. Psychol. Monogr., *76*, No. 3, Part 2:1–32, 1970.
56. Orne, M. T.: The nature of hypnosis: Artifact and essence. J. Abn. Psychol., *58*:277–299, 1959.
57. Orne, M. T.: On the social psychology of the psychological experiment. Amer. Psychologist, *17*:776–783, 1962.
58. Pavlov, I. P.: Conditioned Reflexes. Oxford, Milford, 1927.
59. Petrie, A.: *Individuality in Pain and Suffering*. Chicago, University of Chicago Press, 1967.
60. Reis, M.: Subjective reactions of a patient having surgery without chemical anesthesia. Amer. J. Clin. Hypnosis, *9*:122–124, 1966.
61. Reynolds, G. S.: *A Primer of Operant Conditioning*. Glenview, Ill., Scott Foresman, 1968.
62. Ryan, E. D., and Kovacic, C. R.: Pain tolerance and athletic participation. Perceptual and Motor Skills, *22*:383–390, 1966.
63. Sachs, L. B.: Comparison of hypnotic analgesia and hypnotic relaxation during stimulation by a continuous pain source. J. Abn. Psychol., *76*:206–210, 1970.
64. Larkin, T. R., and Anderson, M. L.: Role-theoretical analysis of hypnotic behavior. In: J. Gordon (ed.): *Handbook of Hypnosis*, New York, Macmillan, 1964.
65. Schaefer, H. H., and Martin, P. L.: *Behavioral Therapy*. New York, McGraw-Hill Book Co., Inc., 1969.
66. Selye, H.: *The Stress of Life*. New York, McGraw-Hill Book Co., Inc., 1956.
67. Shor, R. E., and Orne, M. T.: *The Nature of Hypnosis*. New York, Holt, Rinehart, and Winston, 1966.
68. Sternbach, R. A.: *Pain, a Psychophysiological Analysis*. New York, Academic Press, 1968.
69. Soulairac, A., Cahn, J., and Charpentier, J. (eds.): *Pain*. New York, Academic Press, 1968.

70. Spanos, N. P.: Goal directed fantasy and the performance of hypnotic test suggestions. Psychiatry, *34*:86-96, 1971.

71. Voevodsky, J., Cooper, L. M., Morgan, A. H., and Hilgard, E. R.: The measurement of supra-threshold pain. Amer. J. Psychol., *80*:124-128, 1967.

72. Wall, P. D., and Sweet, W. H.: Temporary abolition of pain in man. Science, *155*:108-109, 1967.

73. Way, E. L.: *New Concepts in Pain and Its Clinical Management.* Philadelphia, F. A. Davis Co., 1967.

74. Weiss, B., and Laties, V. C.: Titration behavior on various fractional escape programs. J. Exper. Anal. Behav., *2*:227-248, 1959.

75. Weitzman, E. D., and Ross, G. S.: A behavioral method for the study of pain perception in the monkey. Neurology, *12*:264-272, 1962.

76. White, J. C., and Sweet, W. H.: *Pain: Its Mechanisms and Neurosurgical Control.* Springfield, Ill., Charles C Thomas, 1955.

77. Wilson, A. J.: *The Emotional Life of the Ill and Injured.* New York, Social Sciences Publishers, 1950.

78. Wilson, C. W. M.: Suggestion and the placebo. In: C. A. Keele and R. Smith (eds.): *Assessment of Pain in Man and Animals,* pp. 213-228. Universities Federation for Animal Welfare, Potters Bars, Herts. (U.K.), 1962.

79. Wolff, B. B., and Langley, S.: Cultural factors and the response to pain: A review. Amer. Anthropologist, *70*:494-501, 1968.

Biomathematics

Chapter 20

MATHEMATICAL MODELS
IN PHYSIOLOGY

by Charles E. Huckaba, Ph.D.

Mathematics traditionally has been confined to a rather peripheral role in the medical field. Applications most frequently have involved problems in the preclinical sciences such as physiology and biochemistry. Increased cooperation between engineers and physicians during the past decade, however, has produced exciting new insights regarding the relevancy of mathematical analysis to clinical studies with respect to both improved diagnoses and patient care.

The purpose of this chapter is to provide a brief introduction to the philosophy and methodology of applied mathematics in the context of medical applications. It is not necessary that the physician gain complete manipulative facility in order to avail himself of the broadened insights frequently provided by considering problems from a mathematical point of view.

Systems engineering concepts implemented via computers appear to have particular revelancy to the study and management of the human body. Just as these methods have revolutionized the professional practice of engineering in recent years, there are strong indications of imminent breakthroughs in the dispensing of high quality health care on a broad scale as engineer-physician teams extend these techniques into the medical field. Thus it appears quite likely that within the next decade even those physicians in individual private practice or those affiliated with small clinics will find it necessary to utilize some of these procedures in such areas as diagnostic assistance and automated laboratory services. It behooves the physician, then, to acquire at least a limited acquaintance with the language and philosophy of this rapidly developing aspect of health care in order to insure that his practice remains viable and competitive.

Through the use of familiar clinical and laboratory examples, an attempt will be made to demonstrate the utility of several elementary mathematical concepts. Certainly it is just as important to recognize the limitations of mathematics as it is to appreciate its advantages.

MATHEMATICS — A SHORTHAND LANGUAGE

In the medical field communications are usually effected by means of words and pictorial representations involving either sketches, as in anatomy, or plots of data. Mathematics is merely a third means of communicating — *mathematics is simply a language!* When properly appreciated, it is recognized as an extremely concise and efficient language that greatly facilitates computations in many fields.

Since mathematics is a language, it is possible to translate from English to mathematics in a manner that is analogous to translating from English to another language such as French. For each equation in our books and journals, there is an equivalent English word expression. The English counterpart may be lengthy and awkward, but it can be made precise and exact. For example, consider the following simple algebraic equation and its word equivalent:

Mathematical Statement	*Word Equivalent*	
$(3x - 10) = 7(10 - x)$	There is a number less than ten. If this number is multiplied by three, the result is a product which is seven times as much more than ten as the number itself is less than ten.	(1)

The word equivalent is not only ten times longer than the equation and also difficult to comprehend, but it would be even more difficult to determine a value of the unknown quantity without reverting to some form of symbolic notation. Thus, the shorthand mathematical language of Equation (1) is not only extremely concise, but it also converts a potentially troublesome problem into one that can be manipulated with relative ease to obtain the number in question.

The whole point, then, is that mathematics, when properly understood, can become a valuable aid to the physician. In the next section some of the basic ideas relative to mathematical modeling will be introduced. Later we shall learn how a limited working knowledge of these principles can lend valuable assistance in tackling a variety of practical clinical and laboratory problems.

MATHEMATICAL MODELS

The term "mathematical model" is a currently fashionable expression used to refer to an equation or a set of equations that describe a physical system. Mathematical modeling involves nothing more than writing down an equation to represent something; thus, "equation writing" or "equation formulation" are equally good designations of this activity. The expression "mathematical model," however, does perhaps help us to realize that in many instances we can construct a mathematical model just as we can build a physical model of something such as a boat or an airplane. Furthermore, the mathematical model can go beyond the inherent bounds of a geometric model in that the behavior of a system, in addition to its geometric description, can be represented. Just as the operating characteristics of a steam heater, for example, can be expressed meticulously in words, in charts, or by a combination of both, in some cases a more concise and more readily comprehended description is obtained by writing the mathematical model (i.e., by translating from English into the language of mathematics).

Mathematical models are most conveniently classified in terms of the type of mathematical language involved in the equations comprising the model. Thus, a mathematical model in the form of an algebraic equation is designated as an "algebraic" model. Later we shall learn that a "differential" model involves a differential equation.

The type of model required to describe any physical phenomenon depends upon both the geometric configuration of the phenomenon and its mode of functioning. For instance, the model describing the steady heat loss from a resting patient will be different from one that describes a changing rate of heat loss when a subject moves from a hot to a cold environment. At first thought, it might appear that there would be a large variety of mathematical models. However, use of an appropriate scheme for characterizing both the system being studied and its mode of behavior can result in a very concise listing of models.

The Mathematical Model as a Guide to Effective Experimentation

Frequently in scientific work there is a distinction made between the "experimental approach" versus the "theoretical approach" to a problem, the implication being that the two are mutually exclusive. Rapid strides during recent years in the development of general mathematical modeling techniques, however, have led to a fresh viewpoint. In many areas it is now recognized that the optimum approach to an investigation involves concurrent mathematical analysis and laboratory observation. The guiding and coordinating influence of a mathematical model can lead to more effective and efficient experimentation.

As applied to clinical studies, whether for research or diagnostic purposes, the combined approach offers exciting possibilities. Clinical reports usually take the format of listing values obtained from a number of separate tests and measurements. When the patient must be subjected to repetitive testing over a period of time, these data can become quite voluminous and difficult to comprehend. On the other hand, a mathematical model can help to interrelate and condense these data into correlations of manageable proportions. Moreover, the model can be used to predict the future course of a patient, so that in many cases corrective therapy can be instituted before a crisis develops. For instance, a model representing the genesis and defervescence of fevers should help the clinician both to anticipate episodes of high fevers and to decide the optimum therapeutic regimen. An analogous situation has already been realized in the chemical industry in which mathematical models, no longer merely a research aid, are recognized as an essential tool for maintaining smooth plant operation.

The next decade will be marked by an upsurge of demands for increased medical care for the public with no significant increase in medical personnel. The only hope for coping with this situation is through increased automation of clinical procedures and the use of computers. The implementation of this approach requires the development of computer programs based on appropriate mathematical models. Although the practitioner need not have a detailed knowledge of these methods, he must gain at least a conceptual understanding in order to apply these new techniques effectively and to interpret the results with confidence.

CLASSIFICATION OF PHYSIOLOGICAL SYSTEMS

For purposes of mathematical analysis, physiological systems must be considered in terms of their behavior with respect to geometric and time variables. From the geometrical standpoint, these systems fall into one of two possible categories:

1. Well-stirred (i.e., uniformly mixed) systems such as a metabolic pool (e.g., glucose pool, urea pool). In this case it is assumed that the entire body content of glucose, for example, may be adequately approximated as residing in one well-mixed "pool" of uniform composition.

2. Non-uniformly distributed (or distributed-parameter) systems, such as the heat content of the body. We know the body is hottest in the interior and becomes progressively cooler as heat moves toward the skin surface for dissipation to the environment. In this case the level of heat content as reflected by temperature varies continuously with the geometric variable, distance, from interior to surface.

Because of the greater complexity of the distributed systems, they are frequently approximated as being uniform at some average value. With reference to heat content, for instance, an entire arm or a leg might be considered to be at a uniform temperature, the average of interior and skin surface values. When this approximation is employed, we say that we "lump" the distributed values into a single uniform value. The resulting system is frequently designated as a "lumped-parameter" system.

Likewise, we must be concerned with possible changes of the variables with time. Most body parameters under normal conditions are maintained constant within narrow limits, so that time variations are minimized by means of appropriate compensatory or control measures. There are only two possibilities:

1. Steady-state conditions—in which there is no variation of pertinent variables with time.

2. Unsteady-state conditions—in which time variations do occur.

It is essential, of course, not to confuse variations in geometry with variations in time. To avoid this, we merely ask ourselves, "At a fixed point in geometry, is there any variation with time?" For example, under steady-state conditions skin temperature along an arm will vary all along the length of the arm; however, if unsteady-state conditions prevail, the temperature at any fixed point on the arm will be changing with time.

Dependent versus Independent Variables

A little later we shall learn how to predict the types of mathematical models that apply to various physiological systems in terms of the number of *independent* variables involved. Therefore, it is essential that we be able to separate the independent variables from the dependent variables in a problem. Actually this is quite easy as long as we understand the basic distinction between the two categories.

Suppose that we wish to follow a patient's oxygen consumption (V_{O_2}) over a period of time (t) after the initiation of exercise. We might be interested in the values of V_{O_2} at the beginning of the study (time = 0) and at subsequent half-hour intervals. In setting up these stipulations, it is clear that we might have made free (i.e., *independent*) choices of the values of time of interest. Then the values of V_{O_2} that we record in the study will be *dependent* upon the values of t which we have selected. There are several alternative ways of stating this relationship:

a. "Word equation": Oxygen consumption is
a function of time. (2)

b. Mathematical notation: $V_{O_2} = f(t)$ (3)

c. Plot:

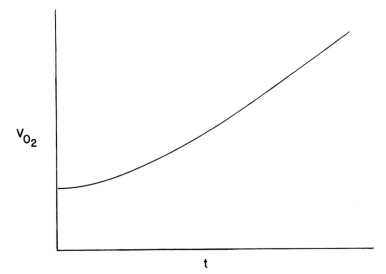

V_{O_2}

t

Figure 20–1

d. Representation of this curve in the form of a specific mathematical equation:

$$V_{o_2} = at^b + c \tag{4}$$

where a, b, and c are the constants required to make the general expression of Equation (3) apply specifically to the curve shown in Figure 20-1.

In all four methods of stating this relationship, however, t is the *independent* variable and V_{O_2} is the *dependent* variable.

In another instance we might be interested in the variation of skin temperature (T_s) along the length (L) of an arm from the shoulder to the tip of the finger. We would first select locations of interest and specify them in terms of distance from the shoulder. Then we would measure the temperature at each of these points. Mathematically we would be determining skin temperature as a function of distance:

$$T_s = f(L) \tag{5}$$

where L is the independent variable over which we have control and T_s is the dependent variable. Note that in Equation (3) time, t, is the independent variable, whereas in Equation (5) the geometric parameter, L, is independent.

We may summarize by stating that for any functional relationship,

$$y = f(x) \tag{6}$$

where x is the independent variable and y is the dependent variable. Furthermore, there are only four basic independent variables. Suppose that we have two uninsulated metal blocks as shown in Figure 20-2. Block A is hot and block B is cold. If we now move the blocks so that they are in contact, heat will move from A to B, and temperatures will vary in all three directions. Since this heat flow will continue until the temperatures in both blocks are equal, there will be

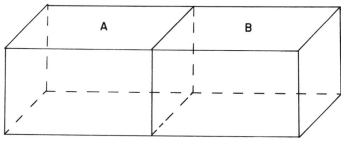

Figure 20–2

a continuous variation of temperature with time until a state of equilibration has been achieved. Thus, temperature in this example can vary only in three geometric directions and also with time. Since there is no other way in which variations can occur, we see that there is a *maximum* of four independent variables. In a later section we shall find that the type of mathematical equation required to describe a physical situation is determined by the number of independent variables involved. Usually only one or two of the possible four must be taken into account.

Calculus Made Easy

Without overemphasizing the details of manipulation, we shall review a few of the basic concepts of calculus as an appropriate introduction to mathematical models involving differential equations. What is a differential? How big is it? Why do we need it? How can anything seemingly so vague be of practical value? What is integration?

Returning to our concepts of mathematics as a shorthand notation, let us consider the two basic symbols of calculus, which are described in an informal manner by Thompson* as follows:

1. d, which merely means "a little bit of." Thus, dx means a little bit of x; or du means a little bit of u. Ordinary mathematicians think it more polite to say "an element of" instead of "a little bit of." Just as you please. But you will find that these little bits (or elements) may be considered to be indefinitely small.

2. $\int$, which is merely a long S, and may be called (if you like) "the sum of." Thus, $\int dx$ means the sum of all the little bits of x; or $\int dt$ means the sum of all the little bits of t. Ordinary mathematicians call this symbol "the integral of." Now any fool can see that if x is considered as made up of a lot of little bits, each of which is called dx, if you add them up together, you get the sum of all the dx's (which is the same thing as the whole of x). The word "integral" simply means "the whole."

Although it is helpful to have an appreciation of each of these basic concepts, it is not necessary for modeling purposes to be concerned with the manipulative details of differentiation and integration with which calculus courses are usually preoccupied.

TYPES OF MATHEMATICAL MODELS

For physiological systems we need to be concerned only with the following types of equations or models:

1. An *algebraic model* is simply one in which the mathematical description of the process takes the form of an algebraic equation.
2. A *differential model* is merely one which contains a derivative (or two differentials), which means that it applies to "a little bit of" the system.
   A. If the situation involves only one independent variable, the model takes the form of an *ordinary* differential equation, as signified by the notation "d"; e.g., dy, dx, or dV/dt.

---

*S. P. Thompson: Calculus Made Easy, Third Edition. New York, St. Martins Press (Papermac 132). 1965

B. If two or more independent variables are involved, a partial differential equation results with another symbol "∂" (a rounded "d") being used to distinguish a partial derivative, $\partial V/\partial t$, from the ordinary derivative, dy/dt.

Although partial differential models are beyond the scope of this introductory chapter, it is well to note in passing at least the type of situation requiring their use as well as the difference in notation employed. In the remainder of the chapter several situations giving rise to both algebraic and differential models are considered.

BASIC MODELING TECHNIQUES

The mathematical modeling of both physical and physiological systems proceeds by writing equations as suggested by the laws of science. Among the more useful of these principles are the laws of conservation of mass and energy, which aid in the solution of a wide variety of problems.

Fortunately, the application of these conservation principles follows an extremely simple format:

$$\text{Input} - \text{Output} = \text{Change in inventory} \tag{7}$$

The inherent logic of this equation can be readily visualized by consideration of an ordinary tank or pool, as shown in Figure 20-3. It is obvious that the change in inventory or volume, V, is dependent upon the relative rates of input feed, F, and output product, P. If F exceeds P, V will increase; conversely if P exceeds F, V will decrease; only when F equals P is change in V equal to zero.

The practical consequences of these situations can be seen by considering the container as a feed tank to a chemical reactor. In this instance if F should exceed P for a significant length of time, the feed tank would overflow; if P should sufficiently exceed F, the tank would tend to run dry. Obviously neither of these conditions would lead to stability of operation.

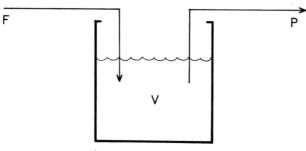

Figure 20-3 Storage tank.

The foregoing illustration provides us with the basis for stating a few simple rules that may be used as a helpful starting point in the solution of a wide range of problems:

1. State a basis of computation.
2. Draw a sketch, identifying the inputs, outputs and inventory of the system.
3. Substitute the absolute magnitudes of the quantities into Equation 7.

Before considering the application of these rules to a specific problem, I might offer a few general suggestions. In the usual case, there will be flows of material streams involved. The basis of computation is specified as a convenient period of time. With flow rate stated, for example, as 100 mg per min, using one minute as the basis is equivalent to choosing 100 mg of that material for the computation. Since each rate of flow is thus stated in terms of its corresponding mass, these quantities can be substituted directly into a mass balance in the form of Equation 7.

Occasionally we might be concerned about the proper signs to be affixed to the quantities in the generalized conservation equation. Perhaps a little faith will be required for the moment, but it is only necessary to use each quantity in terms of its absolute magnitude, i.e., $|P|$ or $|10|$. In other words, whether the quantity is an input or an output, the absolute magnitude is substituted as indicated in Equation 7, and the signs will *automatically* take care of themselves. The following examples should reassure you of this point. Although these problems are concerned only with simple flow situations, in the next section we shall consider metabolic and physiological pools that function in an analagous manner.

EXAMPLE 1.   CHANGE IN INVENTORY OF A STORAGE TANK

A distilled-water storage tank has a volume of 200 liters. The maximum capacity of the still producing this water is 3 liters per min. However, during periods of heavy demand the outflow rate from the tank will reach 5 liters per min. How long can this mode of imbalanced operation be maintained before the liquid in the tank will drop to the minimum operational level of 50 liters?

Solution.

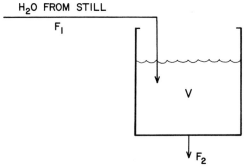

F = flow rate in liters per min.

V = tank inventory in liters

Preliminary Analysis:

a. Since the inventory in the tank is changing *continuously* with time, this is an unsteady-state situation for which the basis of computation must be a differential increment of time, dt.

b. Time is the only independent variable.

c. We anticipate, therefore, an ordinary differential model.

Basis: dt

We proceed by writing the material balance, following the format of Equation (7).

$$|\text{Input}| - |\text{Output}| = |\text{Inventory change}| \tag{7}$$

$$|F_1 dt| \quad - \quad |F_2 dt| \quad = \quad |dV| \tag{8}$$

Although F_1 is a finite rate, it acts only through a differential increment of time, dt. Thus, $|F_1 dt|$ is the differential amount of flow into the tank during this time.

Rearranging the equation,

$$|F_1| - |F_2| = \left|\frac{dV}{dt}\right| \tag{9}$$

and substituting flow rates

$$|3| - |5| = \left|\frac{dV}{dt}\right| \tag{10}$$

Since we are now finished setting up of the model, we drop away the "absolute magnitude" symbols.

$$\frac{dV}{dt} = -2 \tag{11}$$

$$-2dt = dV \tag{12}$$

This ordinary differential model must be integrated to obtain the desired finite answer. The limits for the integrals are readily stated from information given in the problem statement:

$$\text{at } t = 0 \text{ min, } V = 200 \text{ liters}$$
$$t = t \text{ min, } V = 50 \text{ liters}$$

Accordingly,

$$-2 \int_0^t dt = \int_{200}^{50} dV \tag{13}$$

$$t = 75 \text{ min.}$$

Note that the negative sign in Equation 11 automatically results when absolute values are substituted into the basic equation. Since the inventory in the tank is falling with time, we intuitively know in this simple case that the sign should be negative. However, in more complex situations, involving more than one input and output, it is not so easy to decide the direction of the inventory change. Adherence to the suggested procedure using absolute magnitudes to set up the model will always produce the correct result.

EXAMPLE 2.   CHANGE OF CONCENTRATION IN A MIXING TANK

A mixing tank contains 200 liters of a saline solution having a concentration of 0.63 gm per liter. At a given instant pure water starts flowing into the tank at a rate of 5 liters per min. An agitator provides uniform mixing at all times. In order to maintain a constant liquid level in the tank, saline is pumped out of the tank also at a rate of 5 liters per min. Changes in density of the saline solution with composition may be considered negligible.

A. Set up a mathematical model describing how the concentration in the tank varies with time.

B. Use the model to calculate the concentration of the solution in the tank one hour after pumping has begun.

Solution

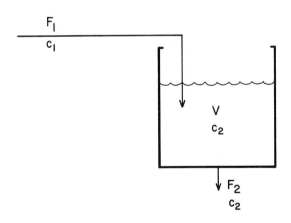

F = flow rate, liters per min
c = composition of salt in the solution, gm per liter
V = volume of tank contents, liters

Preliminary Analysis:
Input: no salt in incoming water.
Inventory of Tank: saline solution is diluted by incoming water; thus, well-mixed composition, c_2, is changing continuously with time.
Output: salt leaves with the outflowing stream with composition, c_2, equal at any instant to the uniform composition in the tank.

Conclusion: Since c_2 is a function of time, but there are no variations of c_2 with geometry (i.e. uniformly mixed), there is only one independent variable. Therefore, we anticipate that the model expressing $c_2 = f(t)$ will take the form of an ordinary differential equation.

Basis: dt (for same reasons as explained for Example 1)

In this instance the material balance principle leads to two equations: one based on the total contents (i.e., solute + solvent) and a second based on solute alone.

Total Balance:

$$| \text{Input} | - | \text{Output} | = | \text{Inventory change} | \tag{7}$$

$$| F_1 dt | - | F_2 dt | \quad = | dV | \tag{14}$$

$$F_1 - F_2 \quad = \frac{dV}{dt} \tag{15}$$

In this case $F_1 = F_2$; thus,

$$\frac{dV}{dt} = 0 \tag{16}$$

which means that the total contents of the tank do not change with time.

Solute (Salt) Balance:

$$| F_1 c_1 dt | - | F_2 c_2 dt | = | d(Vc_2) | \tag{17}$$

$$F_1 c_1 \quad - \quad F_2 c_2 \quad = \frac{d(Vc_2)}{dt} \tag{18}$$

Expanding the derivative,

$$F_1 c_1 - F_2 c_2 = V\frac{dc_2}{dt} + \frac{c_2 dV}{dt} \tag{19}$$

However, from Equation 16, $dV/dt = 0$,

$$F_1 c_1 - F_2 c_2 = V\frac{dc_2}{dt} \tag{20}$$

Also, $F_1 = F_2$, so we can drop the subscripts

$$F(c_1 - c_2) = V\frac{dc_2}{dt} \tag{21}$$

Solving the differential equation

$$c_1 = 0 \text{ for all values of time, } t$$

$$-Fc_2 = V \frac{dc_2}{dt} \tag{22}$$

$$dt = -\frac{V}{F} \frac{dc_2}{c_2} \tag{23}$$

This is the ordinary differential model relating concentration to time.

At $t = 0$ min, $c_2 = 0.63$ gm per liter
$t = t$ min, $c_2 = c_2$ gm per liter

$$\int_0^t dt = -\frac{V}{F} \int_{0.63}^{c_2} \frac{dc_2}{c_2} \tag{24}$$

$$t = -\frac{200}{5} \ln\left(\frac{c_2}{0.63}\right) \tag{25}$$

At the end of 1 hour:

$$t = 60 \text{ min}$$

$$60 = -40 \ln\left(\frac{c_2}{0.63}\right) \tag{26}$$

$$-1.5 = \ln \frac{c_2}{0.63}$$

$$e^{-1.5} = \frac{c_2}{0.63}$$

$$c_2 = 0.63\, e^{-1.5} \tag{27}$$

$$c_2 = 0.63\,(0.223) = 0.141 \text{ gm/liter}$$

Although these two examples represent simple physical situations, they nevertheless provide realistic applications of the basic modeling principles discussed at the beginning of this chapter. In the next section we shall consider the application of these methods to analogous physiological situations.

SIMPLE PHYSIOLOGICAL MODELS

In a previous section it was pointed out that most physiological situations can be described adequately in terms of either algebraic or differential models. The purpose of this section is to consider well-known examples which lead to both types of models.

Algebraic Models

A familiar example is the measurement of hepatic blood flow via indocyanine green clearance. One technique involves continuous infusion of this dye into

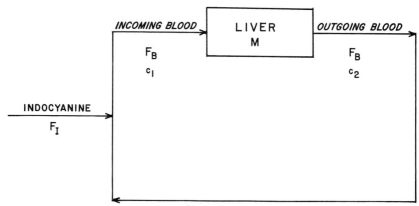

Figure 20–4 Hepatic blood flow. F_B = blood flow rate (ml/min); F_I = indocyanine infusion rate (ml/min); c_1 = indocyanine concentration in incoming blood (mg/ml); c_2 = indocyanine concentration in outgoing blood (mg/ml); M = rate of removal of indocyanine (mg/min).

the blood stream. The change in concentration of indocyanine in the plasma during passage through the liver is indicative of the rate of blood flow through this organ. Since the dye is not removed from the blood in any other part of the circulation, the inlet composition can be determined from blood samples obtained at any convenient upstream location. On the other hand, the samples for assessing outlet composition must be obtained directly from the hepatic vein.

Schematically the situation may be depicted as shown in Figure 20-4. No change in blood flow occurs across the liver, and the rate of infusion of indocyanine, F_I, is adjusted to achieve constant values of both c_1 and c_2. Since these concentrations are determined only after this steady-state condition has been achieved, the mathematical model takes the form of a simple algebraic equation.

EXAMPLE 3.   DETERMINATION OF HEPATIC BLOOD FLOW.

Develop the mathematical model required for calculating the liver blood flow using the technique just described and illustrated in Figure 20-4.

Solution

Material balance around the liver:
Basis: unit of time, e.g., one minute

$$\text{Input} - \text{Output} = \text{Inventory change} \tag{7}$$

$$F_B c_1 - \quad F_B c_2 = M \tag{28}$$

At steady-state condition the rate of removal, M, must be equal to the rate of infusion, F_I, of indocyanine. Making this substitution,

$$F_B(c_1 - c_2) = F_I \tag{29}$$

or
$$F_B = \frac{F_I}{c_1 - c_2} \tag{30}$$

Since the values of F_1, c_1 and c_2 are measured, this algebraic model can be used to calculate the hepatic blood flow, F_B.

Although not routinely administered because it requires catheterization of the hepatic vein, this test can be of considerable value in the clinical diagnosis of suspected liver malfunction.

Other familiar physiological examples which give rise to algebraic models occur in connection with renal clearance studies and the determination of cardiac output using the Fick principle. This type of model frequently can be developed by intuition, but, if in doubt, the format of Equation 7 as demonstrated in Example 3 can offer virtually a fool-proof method of approach.

Ordinary Differential Models

An ordinary differential model is one that takes the form of a first order, ordinary differential equation. In plain language, this means that the equation contains only ordinary differentials such as dx or dy; i.e., no higher derivatives, d^2y/dx^2 nor partial derivatives, $\partial y/\partial x$, are involved.

In the previous section we considered models of this type in connection with a simple storage tank. In that example there was variation of the pertinent variable with respect to only a *single* independent variable. Therefore, as a result of our earlier discussion, it came as no surprise that this situation was described by an ordinary differential equation. In this section we wish to consider several physiological situations that also lead to ordinary differential models and to demonstrate further the great versatility of the differential equation as a tool of the clinical investigator.

Much of the current work related to studies of rates of metabolism of carbohydrates, proteins and fats involve the concept of homogeneous "pools" of reactants, intermediate products and final products. Since these pools are inaccessible for direct study, a widely used approach is to obtain information indirectly through use of labeled components such as C^{14}-glucose and N^{15}-alanine. There is a need then for appropriate mathematical models for use in deducing from experimental data both the sizes of these pools and the overall rates of chemical and physical interactions among them.

The concept of a homogeneous "pool" bears a direct analogy to the "well-stirred tank" or "continuous stirred-tank reactor" (CSTR) used in the study of industrial chemical reaction systems. Accordingly, information developed by chemical engineers relative to the modeling of this type of equipment and to associated computation methods is of direct relevance to the corresponding metabolic studies.

The magnitude of the errors caused by the lumping of inherently distributed elements into "pools" or "tanks" must be assessed and considered acceptable before proceeding with the model development. The assumption of uniform composition may introduce errors of indeterminate magnitude.

Example 4. Glucose Metabolism

Figure 20–5 shows a glucose metabolic pool for which we must derive a mathematical model that represents the variation of labeled C^{14}-glucose with time. The following treatment follows closely that presented by Baker et al.,[1] but it is entirely analogous to the procedure used for the tanks in the previous examples.

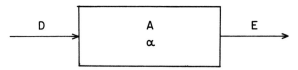

Figure 20–5 Glucose pool. D = dietary input (gm C/day); A = pool size (gm C); E = output (gm C/day); α = amount of labeled component (counts per minute C^{14}); α/A = concentration of C^{14}.

A typical study is initiated by injection of a measured amount of C^{14}-glucose, α_0, which is assumed to disperse rapidly throughout the glucose pool to produce a uniform concentration at time zero. As oxidation proceeds, the relative amount of labeled glucose falls, since the replacement glucose from the dietary input, D, is not labeled. The mathematical model representing change of C^{14}-glucose with time can be derived by writing a C^{14}-glucose balance around the glucose pool shown in Figure 20–5. Since α varies continuously with time, we must start by writing a material balance for a differential increment of time, dt.

Basis: dt
C^{14}-glucose balance (as explained, input of C^{14}-glucose after the initial injection is zero):

$$| \text{Input}| - |\text{Output}| \quad = |\text{Inventory change}| \tag{7}$$

$$\left| 0 \right| - \left| E\left(\frac{\alpha}{A}\right) dt \right| = |d\alpha| \tag{31}$$

As shown in Figure 20–5, since α is amount of labeled glucose, (α/A) is the concentration.

$$-E\frac{\alpha}{A} = \frac{d\alpha}{dt} \tag{32}$$

let $\lambda = E/A$

$$-\lambda \alpha = \frac{d\alpha}{dt} \tag{33}$$

Equation 33 is the ordinary differential model relating α to t. This result was fully expected since there is continuous variation of the dependent variable of interest, α, with a single independent variable, t.

The finite equation corresponding to this differential model is obtained by integrating the differential equation in the same fashion as demonstrated in Example 1.

$$\frac{d\alpha}{\alpha} = -\lambda dt \tag{34}$$

at $t = 0$, $\alpha = \alpha_0$

$$\int_{\alpha_0}^{\alpha} \frac{d\alpha}{\alpha} = -\lambda \int_{0}^{t} dt \qquad (35)$$

$$\ln \frac{\alpha}{\alpha_0} = -\lambda t \qquad (36)$$

In exponential form,

$$\alpha = \alpha_0 e^{-\lambda t} \qquad (37)$$

Because of the form of this equation, this phenomenon is sometimes referred to as the "exponential decay" of the labeled component (Figure 20–6).

Studies of this type not only are of value in developing basic physiological and biochemical data, but also have relevance to the clinical treatment of patients who have experienced severe trauma associated with surgery, injuries or burns. Long et al.[6] in a series of studies on a group of elective surgery patients, found that both glucose pool size and rate of oxidation were greater postoperatively than preoperatively. Increased sugar content in the blood, therefore, apparently results from a cause other than the frequently assumed explanation of a reduction in the rate of oxidation. Accordingly, a prescribed clinical regimen can be more closely attuned to the actual state of the patient when information supplied by the mathematical model is available for consideration.

Mathematical analysis of protein metabolism studies using a labeled amino acid such as N^{15}-alanine, as described by San Pietro and Rittenberg,[11] leads to the same type of ordinary differential model as Equation 33 and a finite exponential expression analagous to Equation 37. It is clear at this point, then, that the well-stirred tanks of the chemical engineer and the metabolic pools of the biochemist are described by the same form of mathematical model. The only difference lies in the nomenclature which has been developed independently for the two areas.

Another physiological situation which leads to an ordinary differential

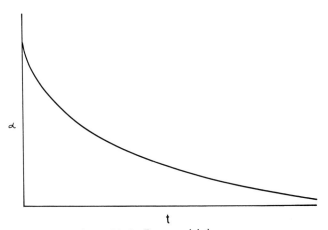

Figure 20–6 Exponential decay curve.

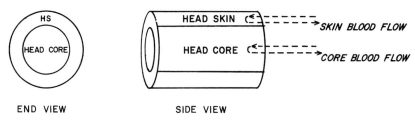

END VIEW   SIDE VIEW

Figure 20-7 Heat model of head.

model is the dissipation of heat from various portions of the body. Stolwijk and Hardy,[15] for instance, have approximated the head as two concentric cylinders, as shown in Figure 20–7. One area of interest involves the effect on heat flow in both the head core and the head skin when the body is subjected to a change in ambient temperature conditions. Since the dependent variable, temperature (T), is a function of only one independent variable, time (t), an ordinary differential model will describe this dynamic heat flow situation.

Head Core:

Heat Inputs:
    1. Heat given up by circulating blood $= w_{HC}\rho_B c_B(T_{CB} - T_{HC})$
where $w_{HC} =$ blood flow rate to head core, liters per min
    ρ_B = density of blood, gm per liter
    c_B = heat capacity of blood, $\dfrac{cal}{(gm)(°C)}$
    T_{CB} = temperature of blood from central blood source, °C
    T_{HC} = temperature of blood leaving head core, °C
    2. Heat generated by the fraction of total body metabolism that occurs in the head core $= M_{HC}$, cal per min.

Heat Outputs:
    1. Heat lost by conduction from head core to head skin $= kA(T_{HC} - T_{HS})$
where k = thermal conductance of head core,

$$\frac{cal}{(sq\ m)(min)(°C)}$$

    A = area at zone between head core and head skin
    T_{HC} = head core temperature, °C
    T_{HS} = head skin temperature, °C

    2. Heat losses by respiration are assumed to be negligible in this development.

Rate of change in heat inventory $= m_{HC}c_{HC}\,\dfrac{dt_{HC}}{dt}$

    where $m_{HC} =$ weight of head core, gm
        $c_{HC} =$ heat capacity of head core, $\dfrac{cal}{(gm)\ (°C)}$

$$\text{Input} - \text{Output} \qquad = \text{Inventory change} \qquad (7)$$

$$[w_{HC}\rho_B c_B(T_{CB} - T_{HC}) + M_{HC}] - kA(T_{HC} - T_{HS}) = m_{HC}c_{HC}\frac{dt_{HC}}{dt} \qquad (38)$$

This is the ordinary differential model with which one can calculate head core temperature as a function of time during periods of heat changes.

The same procedure could be used to develop a similar model for the head skin. In this case the heat leaving the head core by conduction constitutes an *input* to the head skin. The head skin, however, loses heat to the environment by both convection and radiation. In problems involving several inputs and outputs one merely needs to enter each quantity at the appropriate place in the generalized format of Equation 7. The paper by Stolwijk and Hardy illustrates the implementation of this technique for seven body compartments. The resulting model can be used to assess the effects of clinical procedures involving heating or cooling of the body. The physiological response to therapeutic heating as a physical medicine modality or to the use of a surgical cooling blanket for control of fevers can be anticipated more accurately when viewed in the light of the mathematical description.

The physiological models developed in this chapter are typical of many found throughout the life sciences literature. More complex situations usually can be viewed as consisting of two or more subsections, each of which can be handled by the standard format.

THE ROLE OF COMPUTERS

In the medical field electronic computers serve two principal functions: (1) as an information, recording, processing and retrieval system and (2) for making scientific computations. A hospital information system can include such items as patient data, laboratory results, monitored clinical data, pharmacy orders, billing and so forth. A medical information system can function as a massive repository of diagnostic data to which symptoms may be transmitted for comparison with accumulated knowledge of previous cases. A familiar example involves the use of such a system for assisting the physician in the interpretation of electrocardiograms from patients showing symptoms of coronary disease. In the second area of application, computers are employed to advantage in making computations which are either excessively tedious or numerous, especially when many repetitive steps are involved.

There are three types of electronic computers: (1) digital, (2) analog and (3) hybrid. A *digital computer* basically is an expanded high-speed desk calculator to which has been added a greatly enlarged memory storage. This type of computer derives its name from the fact that it processes data in the form of discrete increments or "digits." Although capable of performing only the elementary arithmetic operations of addition, subtraction, multiplication and division, its phenomenal speed and virtually unlimited memory capacity make it possible to execute any type of mathematical computation, such as differentiation and integration, of almost any degree of complexity or size. This is accomplished through the use of a custom-made, step-by-step detailed program of instructions which expresses every step of, the computation in terms of the four basic arithmetic processes in an orderly sequence. The preparation of this set of directions is carried out by a computer programmer. The resulting program is usually introduced to the computer by means of cards or tape.

An *analog computer* operates on the principle of continuous signal processing, in contrast to the incremental signals of the digital computer. This computer is so named because physical quantities are represented by analogous electrical circuits. In this case the program consists of instructions for wiring ("patching") a panel board to correspond to the desired computation. Although capable of performing directly the differentiation and integration operations of calculus, the analog computer is severely limited in scope because its mode of functioning as a continuously operating electrical circuit precludes an easily implemented memory system.

The *hybrid computer* represents an attempt to combine the computational advantages of the analog computer with the memory capabilities of the digital computer. This requires the use of an interface, an analog-digital converter, to translate continuous signals to incremental signals and vice-versa.

Except for certain computational or control applications in which an analog or hybrid computer is dedicated to a specific application, digital computers are used almost exclusively in the medical field. Recent advances in miniaturization make it possible to obtain a digital computer adequate for many clinical applications for a relatively small cost. Alternatively, a data terminal, providing the user with access to a large central computer on a time-sharing basis, can be purchased or rented at relatively low cost.

The mathematical models derived in this chapter are simple enough to permit solution by hand computation. However, more realistic representations of metabolism and body heat flow as well as most physiological situations of practical interest require the use of a computer for obtaining desired results. Moreover, the hospital and medical information systems described above require the formulation and solution of many mathematical models. Although the physician will usually rely on specialists to implement these procedures, he needs to acquire a sufficient appreciation of the basic concepts in order to participate effectively in both the planning and application of these systems.

CONTROL CONCEPTS

In the foregoing sections we have considered the mathematical modeling of individual transport processes. The normal functioning of the human body, however, involves many interactions and balances among the separate organs and vital functions. An assessment of the condition of well-being or illness of the body, in the final analysis, must consider the total system. For instance, the effects of poor circulation are not confined to the arterial-venous system alone, but permeate the entire body.

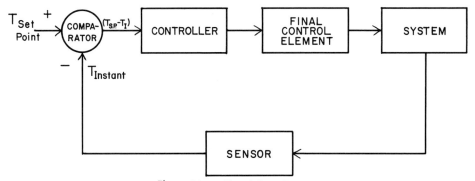

Figure 20–8 Signal flow diagram.

In order to achieve the delicate balance among its many separate functions, the body is equipped with a number of effective control systems. Illness or even death may occur because of the lack of maintenance of an acceptable value of a controlled variable, although no major organ has suffered physical failure per se. An understanding of the control mechanisms of the body utilizing systems concepts, therefore, can play an important role in both diagnosis and therapeutic prescription.

A control system is conveniently viewed as being composed of several basic elements, as shown in the engineering signal flow diagram in Figure 20-8. The operation of a simple laboratory constant temperature bath may be used to explain the role of each component represented by the diagram.

The *system* being controlled is the water contents of the bath. Temperature as an indication of the heat content of the bath is the *controlled variable*. The thermostat is adjusted to a preselected, desired temperature called the "*set point*." The thermal state of the bath must be monitored by means of a *sensor*, in this case an appropriate temperature indicator. The current condition of the system must be compared in an appropriate manner with the set point. When deviation of the controlled variable is greater than allowable, corrective action must be initiated by the *controller*, which implements its action through a *final control element* such as a valve or switch. In the simple case of a constant temperature bath a simple on-off control action is accomplished by means of an electric switch.

The "comparator," which is shown in the diagram, is merely a representation of the comparison of an instantaneous value of the controlled variable with the set point value. Deviations from the latter (i.e., $T_{set} - T_{instant}$) provide the motivating potential or "forcing function" required to activate the controller and, in turn, the final control element.

A large variety of industrial control systems, even though they may differ greatly in physical details, can be depicted functionally by the same type of signal flow diagram. The control action illustrated by the above example is termed "feedback" since observed information regarding the condition of the system is fed back to the source from which corrective measures can be taken. In the case of the water bath, this source of compensation is an electrical power supply that can be used in varying amounts as required to supply the heating element.

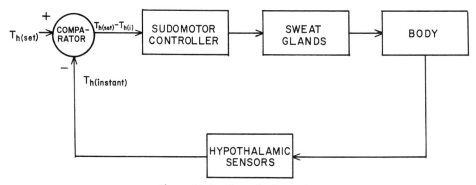

Figure 20–9   Control of sweating.

A portion of the human thermoregulatory system may be used to illustrate the functioning of a physiological feedback control loop. All that one must do to make Figure 20-8 apply to this case is to substitute appropriate physiological labels, as shown in Figure 20-9.

Central sensors located in the hypothalamus continuously monitor the temperature of the brain tissues. Instantaneous values of this hypothalamic temperature, T_h, are compared to the set point value of 37°C. As the temperature of the body increases above this value under heat stress, the comparator generates an error signal, $T_{h(set)} - T_{h(instant)}$, which activates the sudomotor controller. The response of the controller as transmitted to the sweat glands is in proportion to the magnitude of the deviation from the set point. As the sweat glands respond and evaporative cooling occurs, the body temperature moves back toward 37°C. This information is continuously fed back around the loop with the result that the sudomotor controller output is attenuated appropriately. Vasomotor action and metabolic response as induced by shivering can be explained in terms of additional feedback loops, which along with the sudomotor loop comprise the total thermoregulatory system.

Huckaba, Downey and Darling[3] have postulated a comprehensive multi-loop mechanism for the human thermal control system. Fever is viewed as an increase in set point (i.e., the body thermostat has been adjusted to a higher value). If this be so, then the use of body cooling to control fever can impose an added stress upon the patient, unless an antipyretic pharmacological agent, such as aspirin, is also administered to lower the set point back to the normal value.

Since heat flows freely throughout the whole body, an adequate representation of the thermoregulatory mechanism cannot be viewed accurately in terms of anything less than the complete system. Likewise, control of other physiological and biochemical functions appears to follow analogous feedback mechanisms encompassing the entire body. Therefore, systems concepts and viewpoints, as developed in the engineering field, appear to be equally well suited for extending our knowledge of and improving our methods for managing the human body both in sickness and in health.

REFERENCES

1. Baker, N., Shreeve, W. W., Shipley, R. A., Incefy, G. E., and Miller, M.: C^{14} studies in carbohydrate metabolism. I. The oxidation of glucose in normal human subjects. J. Biol. Chem. *211*:575–592, 1954.
2. Beaumont, J. O.: On-line patient monitoring system. Datamation *15*(5):50–55, 1969.
3. Huckaba, C. E., Downey, J. A., and Darling, R. C.: A feedforward-feedback mechanism for human thermoregulation. CEP Symposium Series Volume: *Advances in Bioengineering.* New York, Amer. Inst. of Chem. Engrs. In press (1971).
4. Huckaba, C. E. and Hahn, A. W.: A generalized approach to the modeling of arterial blood flow. Bull. Math. Biophys., *30*:645–662, 1968.
5. Kleppner, D. and Ramsey, N.: Quick Calculus: A Short Manual of Self Instruction. New York, John Wiley & Sons, Inc., 1965.
6. Long, C. L., Spencer, J. L., Kinney, J. M., and Geiger, J. W.: Carbohydrate metabolism in man: Effect of elective operations and major injury. J. Appl. Physiol. In press (1971).
7. Milhorn, H. T., Jr.: *The Application of Control Theory to Physiological Systems.* Philadelphia, W. B. Saunders Company, 1966.
8. Milsum, J. H.: *Biological Control System Analysis.* New York, McGraw-Hill Book Company, 1966.
9. Reilly, N. B.: Computers in medicine. Datamation, *15*(5):46–49, 1969.
10. Riggs, D. S.: *The Mathematical Approach to Physiological Problems.* Baltimore, Williams and Wilkins Company, 1963.
11. San Pietro, A. and Rittenberg, D.: A study of the rate of protein synthesis in humans. II. Measurement of the metabolic pool and the rate of protein synthesis. J. Biol. Chem., *201*:457–473, 1953.
12. Singer, J. P.: Computer-based hospital information systems. Datamation, *15*(5):38–45,1969.
13. Spencer, J. L., Kinney, J. M. and Long, C. L.: Material and energy balances on postoperative patients. Chem. Eng. Progr., Symp. Ser., *62*(66):124–130, 1966.
14. Stibitz, G. R.: *Mathematics in Medicine and the Life Sciences.* Chicago, Year Book Medical Publishers, Inc. 1966.
15. Stolwijk, J. A. J. and Hardy, J. D.: Temperature regulation in man: a theoretical study. Arch. Ges. Physiol., *291*:129–162, 1965.
16. Thompson, S. P.: *Calculus Made Easy,* 3rd ed. New York, St. Martins Press, Inc. 1966.
17. Yamomoto, W. S. and Brobeck, J. R. (eds.): *Physiological Controls and Regulations.* Philadelphia, W. B. Saunders Company, 1965.

INDEX